Essential Emergency Procedures

WITHDRAWN

Second Edition

Kaushal H. Shah, MD

Residency Director
Mt. Sinai Emergency Medicine Residency Program
Icahn School of Medicine at Mt. Sinai Medical Center
New York, New York

Chilembwe Mason, MD

Attending
Department of Emergency Medicine
Bronx-Lebanon Hospital Center
Bronx, New York

Reuben J. Strayer, MD, FRCPC, FAAEM

Safety/Quality Editor
Department of Emergency Medicine
Icahn School of Medicine at Mount Sinai/Elmhurst Hospital
NYU School of Medicine
New York, New York

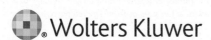 Wolters Kluwer

Philadelphia · Baltimore · New York · London
Buenos Aires · Hong Kong · Sydney · Tokyo

Acquisitions Editor: Jamie M. Elfrank
Product Development Editor: Ashley Fischer
Editorial Assistant: Brian Convery
Senior Production Project Manager: Alicia Jackson
Design Coordinator: Holly McLaughlin
Art Director: Jennifer Clements
Senior Manufacturing Coordinator: Beth Welsh
Marketing Manager: Stephanie Kindlick
Prepress Vendor: S4Carlisle Publishing Services (P) Ltd.

2nd edition

Library of Congress Cataloging-in-Publication Data
Essential emergency procedures / editor, Kaushal Shah; associate editor, Chilembwe Mason. — 2nd edition.
    p.; cm.
  Includes bibliographical references and index.
  ISBN 978-1-4698-9190-3 (alk. paper) — ISBN 1-4698-9190-5 (alk. paper)
  I. Shah, Kaushal, editor.   II. Mason, Chilembwe, editor.
  [DNLM: 1. Emergencies—Handbooks.   2. Emergency Medicine—methods—Handbooks.   3. Emergency Treatment--methods--Handbooks. WB 39]
  RC86.8
  616.02'5—dc23

                                                                                    2014044114

DEDICATION (KAUSHAL H. SHAH)

I'd like to dedicate this book to my two beautiful girls, Naya and Mila, who I hope never stop doing the "Daddy is home!" dance.

DEDICATION (CHILEMBWE MASON)

This book is dedicated to all the wonderful teachers I've had throughout my career: *nanos gigantum humeris insidentes (standing on the shoulders of giants)*.

CONTRIBUTORS

Gallane Dabela Abraham, MD
Assistant Professor
Department of Emergency Medicine
Icahn School of Medicine at Mount Sinai
New York, New York

Olabiyi Akala, MD
Emergency Physician
The Ronald O. Perelman Department
    of Emergency Medicine
NYU Langone Medical Center
New York, New York

Nissa J. Ali, MD, MEd
Department of Emergency Medicine
Beth Israel Deaconess Medical Center
Harvard Medical School Teaching Hospital
Boston, Massachusetts

Mara S. Aloi, MD
Associate Professor (Adjunct)
Department of Emergency Medicine
Temple University
Philadelphia, Pennsylvania
Program Director, Residency
Department of Emergency Medicine
Allegheny General Hospital
Pittsburgh, Pennsylvania

Matthew R. Babineau, MD
Resident
Department of Emergency Medicine
Beth Israel Deaconess Medical Center
Boston, Massachusetts

Naomi Jean Baptiste, MD
Resident
Department of Emergency Medicine
New York-Presbyterian Hospital
New York, New York

David Barlas, MD
Assistant Professor
Department of Emergency Medicine
NYU School of Medicine
New York, New York
Chief of Service
Cobble Hill Emergency Department
NYU Langone Medical Center
Brooklyn, New York

Joshua M. Beiner, MD
Fellow
Department of Pediatric Emergency Medicine
NYU/Bellevue Medical Center
New York, New York

Anthony Berger, MD, MS
Staff Physician
Department of Emergency Medicine
Kaiser South Sacramento Medical Center
Volunteer Assistant Clinical Professor
Department of Emergency Medicine
UC Davis Medical Center
Sacramento, California

Alicia Blazejewski, MD
Per Diem Attending
Department of Emergency Medicine
Baystate Medical Center
Attending
Steward Medical Group
Springfield, Massachusetts

Rebecca T. Brafman, MD, MA
Resident
Department of Emergency Medicine
Icahn School of Medicine at Mount Sinai
New York, New York

Calvin A. Brown III, MD
Assistant Professor
Department of Emergency Medicine
Harvard Medical School
Attending Physician
Department of Emergency Medicine
Brigham and Women's Hospital
Boston, Massachusetts

Simran Buttar, MD
Resident
Department of Emergency Medicine
Mount Sinai St. Luke's-Roosevelt Hospital
New York, New York

Amy B. Caggiula, MD
Assistant Professor
Department of Emergency Medicine
Icahn School of Medicine
Attending Physician
Department of Emergency Medicine
Mount Sinai St. Luke's-Roosevelt Hospital Center
New York, New York

David W. Callaway, MD
Associate Professor
Department of Emergency Medicine
Director
Division of Operational and Disaster Medicine
Carolinas Medical Center
Charlotte, North Carolina

Nicholas D. Caputo, MD, MSc, FAAEM
Assistant Professor of Emergency Medicine
Department of Emergency Medicine
Weil Medical College of Cornell University
New York, New York
Associate Chief
Department of Emergency Medicine
Lincoln Medical and Mental Health Center
Bronx, New York

Brian Chung, MD
Resident
Emergency Medicine Residency
New York Hospital Queens
Flushing, New York

Wendy Coates
Attending
Department of Emergency Medicine
Harbor-UCLA Medical Center
Torrance, California

Clinton J. Coil, MD, MPH
Associate Clinical Professor of Medicine
Division of Emergency Medicine
David Geffen School of Medicine at UCLA
Los Angeles, California
Chief Quality Officer
Department of Clinical Quality and Safety
Harbor-UCLA Medical Center
Torrance, California

Robert Dalton Cox, MD
Resident
Department of Emergency Medicine
Icahn School of Medicine at Mount Sinai
The Mount Sinai Hospital
New York, New York

Jason D'Amore MD, FACEP
Associate Professor Emergency Medicine
Hofstra-NSLIJ School of Medicine
Research Director
Department of Emergency Medicine
North Shore University Hospital
Manhasset, New York

David Diller, MD
Instructor
Department of Emergency Medicine
Oregon Health and Science University
Education Fellow
Department of Emergency Medicine
Oregon Health and Science University
Portland, Oregon

Nicole M. Dubosh, MD
Instructor
Department of Emergency Medicine
Harvard Medical School
Beth Israel Deaconess Medical Center
Boston, Massachusetts

Peter C. England, MD
Resident
Department of Emergency Medicine
Icahn School of Medicine
Mount Sinai St. Luke's-Roosevelt Hospital Center
New York, New York

Andrew J. Eyre, MD
Clinical Fellow
Department of Emergency Medicine
Harvard Medical School
Resident Physician
Department of Emergency Medicine
Brigham and Women's Hospital
Boston, Massachusetts

Robert P. Favelukes, MD, FACEP
Assistant Professor
Department of Emergency Medicine
Albert Einstein College of Medicine
Assistant Director
Department of Emergency Medicine
Bronx-Lebanon Hospital Center
Bronx, New York

Denise Fernández, MD
Medical Toxicology Fellow
Department of Emergency Medicine
NYU/Bellevue Hospital Center
New York, New York

Tsion Firew, MD
Resident
Department of Emergency Medicine
New York University
Bellevue Hospital
New York, New York

Elizabeth M. Foley, MD
Clinical Fellow
Department of Emergency Medicine
Harvard Medical School
Chief Resident
Department of Emergency Medicine
Beth Israel Deaconess Medical Center
Boston, Massachusetts

Ryan P. Friedberg, MD
Clinical Instructor
Departments of Medicine and Orthopedics
Harvard Medical School
Director
Musculoskeletal Education
Department of Emergency Medicine
Beth Israel Deaconess Medical Center
Boston, Massachusetts

Maureen Gang, MD
Associate Professor
Associate Residency Director
Department of Emergency Medicine
New York University School of Medicine
New York, New York

Jeffrey P. Green
Attending Physician
New York Hospital Queens
Flushing, New York

Hamza Guend, MD
General Surgeon
New York, New York

J. Michael Guthrie, MD
Resident
Department of Emergency Medicine
Icahn School of Medicine at Mount Sinai
New York, New York

Aldo Gutierrez, MD
Senior Resident
Department of Emergency Medicine
Mount Sinai Medical Center
New York, New York

Christopher K. Hansen, MD, MPH
Physician
Department of Emergency Medicine
Icahn School of Medicine at Mount Sinai
New York, New York

Raquel F. Harrison, MD
Chief Resident
Department of Emergency Medicine
Weill Cornell Medical College
Chief Resident
Department of Emergency Medicine
New York-Presbyterian Hospital
New York, New York

Timothy Horeczko, MD, MSCR
Assistant Professor
Department of Emergency Medicine
David Geffen School of Medicine at UCLA
Los Angeles, California
Faculty
Department of Emergency Medicine
Harbor-UCLA Medical Center
Torrance, California

Catherine H. Horwitz, MD, MPH
Attending Physician
Department of Emergency Medicine
Metrowest Medical Center
Framingham, Massachusetts

Jennifer V. Huang, DO
Assistant Professor
Department of Emergency Medicine
Icahn School of Medicine at Mount Sinai
Director of Ultrasound Education
Department of Emergency Medicine
Mount Sinai Hospital
New York, New York

Heather Huffman-Dracht
Department of Emergency Medicine
Harbor-UCLA Medical Center
Torrance, California

Jason Imperato, MD, MBA
Assistant Professor
Department of Emergency Medicine
Harvard Medical School
Boston, Massachusetts
Associate Chair
Department of Emergency Medicine
Mount Auburn Hospital
Cambridge, Massachusetts

Eric Ingulsrud, MD
Chief Resident
Department of Emergency Medicine
Mount Sinai Beth Israel
Icahn School of Medicine at Mount Sinai
New York, New York

Kimberly Kahne
Fellow
Department of Pediatrics Emergency
    Medicine
Mount Sinai School of Medicine
New York, New York

Amy H. Kaji, MD, PhD
Associate Professor
Department of Emergency Medicine
David Geffen School of Medicine
    at UCLA
Harbor-UCLA Medical Center
Torrance, California

Julie K. A. Kasarjian, MD, PhD
Resident
Department of Emergency Medicine
Harbor-UCLA Medical Center
Torrance, California

Raashee Sood Kedia, MD
Resident
Department of Emergency Medicine
Icahn School of Medicine at Mount Sinai
New York, New York

Raashee Sood Kedia, MD
Resident
Department of Emergency Medicine
Icahn School of Medicine at Mount Sinai
New York, New York

Amie M. Kim, MD
Resident
Department of Emergency Medicine
Bellevue Hospital Center
NYU Langone Medical Center
New York, New York

Andreana Kwon, MD
Assistant Clinical Professor
Department of Emergency Medicine
Weill Cornell Medical College
Attending Physician
Department of Emergency Medicine
New York-Presbyterian Lower Manhattan Hospital
New York, New York

Heidi E. Ladner, MD
Clinical Instructor Pending
Weill Medical College of Cornell University
Director of Emergency Ultrasound
Department of Emergency Medicine
New York Hospital Queens
Flushing, New York

Daniel Lakoff, MD
Assistant Professor
Department of Emergency Medicine
Icahn School of Medicine at Mount Sinai
New York, New York

Alden M. Landry, MD, MPH
Instructor
Department of Emergency Medicine
Harvard Medical School
Attending Physician
Department of Emergency Medicine
Beth Israel Deaconess Medical Center
Boston, Massachusetts

Lindsey Lawrence, MD, MPH
Resident, PGY-IV
Department of Emergency Medicine
Icahn School of Medicine at Mount Sinai
New York, New York

Jessica H. Leifer, MD
Resident Physician
Department of Emergency Medicine
Icahn School of Medicine at Mount Sinai
Resident Physician
Department of Emergency Medicine
Sinai St. Luke's-Roosevelt Hospital
New York, New York

Penelope Chun Lema, MD
Assistant Professor
Department of Emergency Medicine
SUNY University at Buffalo School
    of Medicine and Biomedical Sciences
Director of Emergency Ultrasound
    Fellowship
Department of Emergency Medicine
Buffalo General Hospital
Buffalo, New York

Meagan Lewis, MD
Emergency Medicine Physician
Pittsburgh, Pennsylvania

Resa E. Lewiss, MD
Associate Professor
Department of Emergency Medicine
    and Radiology
University of Colorado
Director of Point-of-Care Ultrasound
Department of Emergency Medicine and
    Radiology
University of Colorado
Aurora, Colorado

Carey C. Li, MD
Resident
Department of Emergency Medicine
Icahn School of Medicine
    at Mount Sinai
Mount Sinai Beth Israel
New York, New York

George Lim, MD
Resident
Department of Emergency Medicine
Mount Sinai Hospital
New York, New York

Allegra Georgian Long, MD
Resident Physician
Department of Emergency Medicine
Mount Sinai St. Luke's-Roosevelt Hospital
    Center
New York, New York

Jessica Hetherington Lopez, MD
Resident
The Ronald O. Perelman Department
    of Emergency Medicine
NYU Langone Medical Center
New York, New York

Chilembwe Mason, MD
Attending
Department of Emergency Medicine
Bronx-Lebanon Hospital Center
Bronx, New York

Todd A. Mastrovitch, MD
Director, Pediatric Education
Emergency Medicine Residency
New York Hospital Queens
Flushing, New York

Danielle K. Matilsky, MD
Department of Emergency Medicine
Mount Sinai St. Luke's and Mount Sinai
    Roosevelt Hospital
New York, New York

Alexander S. Maybury, MD
Resident Physician
Department of Emergency Medicine
New York University
New York, New York

Daniel C. McGillicuddy, MD
Adjunct Faculty
Department of Emergency Medicine
University of Michigan
Associate Chair
Department of Emergency Medicine
St. Joseph Mercy Hospital-Ann Arbor
Ann Arbor, Michigan

Maxwell Morrison, MD
Resident Physician
Department of Emergency Medicine
Mount Sinai St. Luke's-Roosevelt
New York, New York

Neil Patel, MD
Assistant Clinical Professor of Medicine
Department of Emergency Medicine
David Geffen School of Medicine
    at UCLA
Acting Chief
Division of Emergency Medicine
West Los Angeles VA Medical Center
Los Angeles, California

Jayson R. Pereira, MD
Chief Resident
Department of Emergency Medicine
Harvard University
Beth Israel Deaconess Medical Center
Boston, Massachusetts

Kenneth J. Perry, MD
Resident
Department of Emergency Medicine
New York-Presbyterian Hospital
New York, New York

Joseph R. Pinero, MD
Resident
Department of Emergency Medicine
Icahn School of Medicine at Mount Sinai
New York, New York

Armin Perham Poordabbagh
Resident
Department of Emergency Medicine
North Shore University Hospital
Manhasset, New York

Jennifer V. Pope, MD, FACEP
Assistant Professor
Department of Emergency Medicine
Harvard Medical School
Boston, Massachusetts
Chair
Department of Emergency Medicine
St. Luke's Hospital
New Bedford, Massachusetts

Brent T. Rau, MD
Emergency Medicine Physician
Pittsburgh, Pennsylvania

Kathleen G. Reichard, DO
Senior Attending Physician
Department of Pediatric Emergency Medicine
St. Luke's-Roosevelt Hospital Center
New York, New York

**David Riley, MD, MSc, RDMS, RDCS,
RVT, RMSK**
Assistant Professor of Medicine
Department of Emergency Medicine
Columbia University
Director of Emergency Ultrasonography
Department of Emergency Medicine
Columbia University Medical Center
New York, New York

Czarina E. Sánchez, MD
Clinical Fellow in Emergency Medicine
Department of Emergency Medicine
Beth Israel Deaconess Medical Center
Boston, Massachusetts

Jennifer E. Sanders, MD
Clinical Fellow
Department of Emergency Medicine
Icahn School of Medicine at Mount Sinai
New York, New York

Amy Sanghvi, MD
Department of Emergency Medicine
SUNY Downstate Medical Center
Brooklyn, New York

Fereshteh Sani, MD
Resident Physician
Department of Emergency Medicine
New York University
Resident Physician
Department of Emergency Medicine
Bellevue Hospital Center
New York, New York

Joseph Scofi, MD
Resident
Department of Emergency Medicine
Icahn School of Medicine at Mount Sinai
New York, New York

Jennifer Sedor, MD
Physician
Department of Emergency Medicine
Icahn School of Medicine at Mount Sinai
Physician
Department of Emergency Medicine
Mount Sinai Beth Israel
New York, New York

Tara S. Sexton, MD
Resident
The Ronald O. Perelman Department
    of Emergency Medicine
NYU Langone Medical Center
New York, New York

Anar D. Shah, MD, MBA
Chief Resident
Department of Emergency Medicine
Icahn School of Medicine
The Mount Sinai Hospital
New York, New York

Hiral H. Shah, MD, JD
Department of Emergency Medicine
North Shore University Hospital
Manhasset, New York

Kaushal H. Shah, MD
Residency Director
Mt. Sinai Emergency Medicine Residency
    Program
Icahn School of Medicine at Mt. Sinai
    Medical Center
New York, New York

Ashley Shreves, MD
Assistant Professor
Department of Emergency Medicine and
    Brookdale Department of Geriatrics
    and Palliative Medicine
Icahn School of Medicine at Mt. Sinai
New York, New York

Benjamin H. Slovis, MD
Chief Resident
Department of Emergency Medicine
Icahn School of Medicine at Mount Sinai
New York, New York
Chief Resident
Department of Emergency Medicine
Mount Sinai Hospital
New York, New York

Peter B. Smulowitz, MD
Instructor in Medicine
Department of Emergency Medicine
Beth Israel Deaconess Medical Center
Boston, Massachusetts

Jennifer B. Stratton, MD
Attending Physician
Department of Emergency Medicine
Mount Sinai
Attending Physician
Department of Emergency Medicine
Mount Sinai St. Luke's-Roosevelt Hospital
New York, New York

Alison E. Suarez, MD
Clinical Instructor of Emergency Medicine
Department of Emergency Medicine
Weill Cornell Medical College
New York, New York
Assistant Program Director
Department of Emergency Medicine
New York Hospital Queens
Flushing, New York

Anand K. Swaminathan, MD, MPH
Assistant Residency Director
The Ronald O. Perelman Department
    of Emergency Medicine
NYU School of Medicine
Assistant Clinical Professor
Department of Emergency Medicine
New York University-Bellevue
New York, New York

Felipe Teran, MD
Resident Physician
Department of Emergency Medicine
Icahn School of Medicine
New York, New York

Sarah W. Tochman, MD
Resident Physician
Department of Emergency Medicine
University of Michigan/St. Joseph
    Mercy Hospital Emergency Medicine
    Residency
Ann Arbor, Michigan

Jason A. Tracy, MD
Chief
Department of Emergency Medicine
South Shore Hospital
South Weymouth, Massachusetts

Lara Zucconi Vanyo, MSc, MD
Resident Physician
Department of Emergency Medicine
Mount Sinai Hospital
New York, New York

Michelle N. Vazquez, MD
Pediatric Emergency Medicine Fellow
Department of Emergency Medicine
Icahn School of Medicine at Mount Sinai
Pediatric Emergency Medicine Fellow
Department of Emergency Medicine
Mount Sinai Hospital
New York, New York

Kathryn A. Volz, MD
Assistant Medical Director
Department of Emergency Medicine
St Joseph Mercy Hospital
Ann Arbor, Michigan

Gina Waight, MD
Instructor
Department of Emergency Medicine
Albert Einstein College of Medicine
    of Yeshiva University
Attending Physician
Department of Emergency Medicine
Jacobi Medical Center
Bronx, New York

Jonathan Wassermann, MD
Assistant Professor
Department of Emergency Medicine
Icahn School of Medicine at Mount Sinai
Director of ED Trauma Services
Department of Emergency Medicine
St. Luke's-Roosevelt Hospital Center
New York, New York

Scott D. Weingart, MD, FCCM
Chief
Division of ED Critical Care
Stony Brook Medicine
New York, New York

Nelson Wong, MD
Instructor
Department of Emergency Medicine
Harvard Medical School
Assistant
Department of Emergency Medicine
Massachusetts General Hospital
Boston, Massachusetts

Joel Wussow, MD
Resident
Department of Emergency Medicine
New York-Presbyterian Hospital
New York, New York

Kris E. C. Zaporteza, MD, MBA
Attending Physician
Department of Emergency Medicine
United States Naval Hospital
Yokosuka, Japan

Julie A. Zeller, MD
Attending Physician
Department of Emergency Medicine
Emerson Hospital
Concord, Massachusetts

Section Editors

Wallace A. Carter, MD
Associate Professor
Department of Emergency Medicine
Weill Cornell Medical College
Columbia University College of Physicians &
    Surgeons
Program Director
Emergency Medicine Residency
New York-Presbyterian Hospital
New York, New York

Moira Davenport, MD
Associate Professor
Department of Emergency Medicine
Temple University
Associate Residency Director
Department of Emergency Medicine
Allegheny General Hospital
Pittsburgh, Pennsylvania

Natasha Desai, MD
Sports Medicine Fellow
University of Pennsylvania
Philadelphia, Pennsylvania

Jonathan A. Edlow, MD
Professor
Department of Medicine
Harvard Medical School
Vice-Chair
Department of Emergency Medicine
Beth Israel Deaconess Medical Center
Boston, Massachusetts

Sanjey Gupta, MD
Assistant Professor
Department of Emergency Medicine
Hofstra University School of Medicine
Hempstead, New York
Chairman
Department of Emergency Medicine
NSLIJ Franklin Hospital
Valley Stream, New York

Joseph Habboushe, MD, MBA
Assistant Professor
Department of Emergency Medicine
New York University
Associate Chief of Service
Emergency Department
Bellevue Hospital
New York, New York

Dara A. Kass, MD
Assistant Professor
Department of Emergency Medicine
NYU Langone Medical Center
Director Undergraduate Medical Education
Department of Emergency Medicine
NYU Langone Medical Center
New York, New York

Diana Kim, MD
Attending
Department of Emergency Medicine
Bronx-Lebanon Hospital
Bronx, New York

Elan S. Levy, MD, RDMS
Attending Physician
Department of Emergency Medicine
Lenox Hill HealthPlex
Greenwich Village, New York

Ari M. Lipsky, MD, PhD, FACEP
Research Director
Department of Emergency Medicine
Rambam Health Care Campus
Haifa, Israel

Bret P. Nelson, MD, RDMS, FACEP
Associate Professor
Department of Emergency Medicine
Icahn School of Medicine at Mount Sinai
Director of Emergency Ultrasound
Department of Emergency Medicine
Mount Sinai Hospital
New York, New York

Ram A. Parekh, MD
Clinical Assistant Professor
Emergency Department
Icahn School of Medicine at Mount Sinai
New York, New York
Attending
Emergency Department
Elmhurst Hospital Center
Elmhurst, New York

Joshua Quaas, MD
Assistant Professor of Emergency
  Medicine
Department of Emergency Medicine
Mount Sinai St. Luke's-Roosevelt
  Hospital
New York, New York

Leon D. Sanchez, MD, MPH
Associate Professor
Department of Emergency Medicine
Harvard Medical School
Vice-Chair for Operations
Department of Emergency Medicine
Beth Israel Deaconess Medical
  Center
Boston, Massachusetts

Louis A. Spina, MD
Assistant Professor, Fellowship
  Director
Pediatric Emergency Medicine
Department of Emergency Medicine
Icahn School of Medicine
  at Mount Sinai
Assistant Professor
Department of Emergency Medicine
Mount Sinai Medical Center
New York, New York

Scott G. Weiner, MD, MPH
Assistant Professor
Department of Emergency Medicine
Harvard Medical School
Attending Physician
Department of Emergency Medicine
Brigham and Women's Hospital
Boston, Massachusetts

PREFACE

Procedures in the emergency department (and the hospital in general) are frequent and varied. They range from simple suturing to complicated thoracotomies. Procedures that are performed for the first few times or infrequently are the ones that cause the most anxiety. The ability to review the procedure quickly from a reliable source is clearly invaluable to a physician (and the patient).

This procedure handbook is designed primarily for any physician, resident, or medical student who will be doing emergency procedures. The aim of the book is to have a bedside refresher of the key components of a procedure. This creates accuracy, confidence, and, likely, fewer complications. There will be times when you want to read an entire chapter to fully grasp every detail, and there will be times when you want just the critical information. This book was designed to meet both needs.

In keeping with the times, the highlights of this second edition include an interactive e-book, more critical care procedures, and a dedicated section on safety/quality that focuses on both procedural and cognitive pearls in every chapter. The readers will find wonderful pearls that will not only change practice but improve patient care.

Key chapters that are worth reviewing and very unlikely to be found in other procedure books are Delayed Sequence Intubation, No DESAT, Induction of Therapeutic Hypothermia, Occipital Nerve Block, and Open Joint Evaluation/Methylene Blue Injection.

There is no doubt that increased comfort with medical procedures translates to increased comfort as a physician. Enjoy the read.

ACKNOWLEDGMENTS

We are extremely grateful to all the original authors of the various chapters who made the first edition of this book a success.

CONTENTS

1

Intubation: Tracheal and Nasotracheal

Elizabeth M. Foley and Leon D. Sanchez

GENERAL

Rapid sequence intubation (RSI) is the preferred method of emergency airway management. It involves the near simultaneous administration of fast-acting induction and neuromuscular blocking agents to achieve optimal intubating conditions without the need for bag-mask ventilation. The following discussion of orotracheal intubation refers to RSI. Techniques for gum-elastic bougie insertion and nasotracheal intubation are also discussed.

INDICATIONS

- Failure to protect the airway
- Failure to maintain the airway
- Failure of ventilation
- Failure of oxygenation
- Predicted deterioration or anticipated clinical course requiring intubation

CONTRAINDICATIONS

- **Orotracheal and Nasotracheal Intubation**
  + Total upper airway obstruction
  + Total loss of facial landmarks
- **Nasotracheal Intubation**
  + Apnea
  + Basilar skull or facial fracture
  + Neck trauma or cervical spine injury
  + Head injury with suspected increased intracranial pressure (ICP)
  + Nasal or nasopharyngeal obstruction
  + Combative patients or patients *in extremis*
  + Coagulopathy
  + Pediatric patients

LANDMARKS

- Viewing the oropharynx from above, the tongue is the most anterior structure
- The pouchlike vallecula separates the tongue from the epiglottis, which sits above the larynx **(FIGURE 1.1)**
- The vocal cords sit as an inverted "V" within the larynx
- The larynx is anterior to the esophagus

TECHNIQUE FOR OROTRACHEAL INTUBATION

- **General Basic Steps**
  + **Preparation**
  + **Preoxygenation**
  + **Pretreatment**
  + **Paralysis and induction**
  + **Positioning**
  + **Placement of tube**
  + **Proof of placement**
  + **Postintubation management**

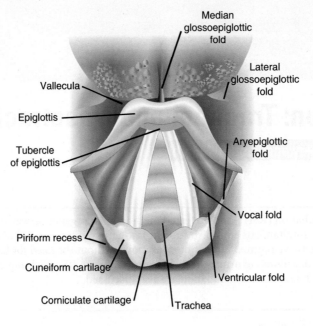

R.W.Williams

FIGURE 1.1 Larynx visualized from the oropharynx. Note the median glossoepiglottic fold. It is pressure on this structure by the tip of a curved blade that flips the epiglottis forward, exposing the glottis during laryngoscopy. Note that the valleculae and the pyriform recesses are different structures, a fact often confused in the anesthesia literature. The cuneiform and corniculate cartilages are called the arytenoid cartilages. The ridge between them posteriorly is called the posterior commissure. (Reused with permission from Redden RJ. Anatomic considerations in anesthesia. In: Hagberg CA, ed. *Handbook of Difficult Airway Management*. Philadelphia, PA: Churchill Livingstone; 2000:9.)

❏ Preparation
  + **Assess airway:** Use LEMON mnemonic to predict difficulty of airway
    + **Look externally:** If you sense that an airway appears difficult, it likely is
    + **Evaluate anatomy:** The "3-3-2 rule" (**FIGURE 1.2**)
      ▬ **Thyromental distance:** Should be approximately 3 finger widths. Significantly more or less suggests a difficult airway.
      ▬ **Mouth opening:** Less than 3 finger widths predicts poor visualization on laryngoscopy and a difficult airway
      ▬ **Hyomental distance:** More or less than 2 finger widths predicts a difficult airway
    + **Mallampati score:** Roughly correlates the view of internal oropharyngeal structures with intubation success. Graded as class I to IV (**FIGURE 1.3**).
    + **Obstruction/Obesity:** Any evidence of upper airway obstruction heralds a difficult airway. Obesity is also associated with difficult laryngoscopy.
    + **Neck mobility:** Crucial to obtaining the optimum view of the larynx. Hindrance to neck extension, including cervical spine immobilization, predicts difficulty in intubation.
  + **Equipment**
    + Endotracheal tube (ETT) and smaller backup (often 7.5 or 8.0 and 7.0)
    + 10-cc syringe
    + Laryngoscope blade
    + Laryngoscope handle
    + Suction
    + Rescue airway devices, including oral airway, gum-elastic bougie, and laryngeal mask airway
    + RSI pharmacologic agents

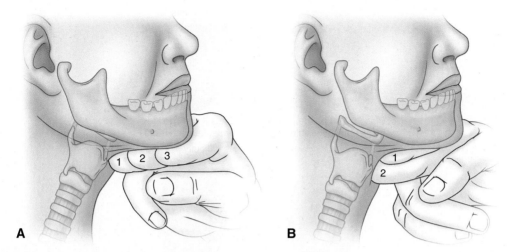

FIGURE 1.2 A: The second 3 of the 3-3-2 rule. **B:** The 2 of the 3-3-2 rule. (From Walls RM, Murphy MF. *Manual of Emergency Airway Management.* The 4th edition, 2012 version of the Walls Emergency Manual as well. Philadelphia, PA: Lippincott Williams & Wilkins; 2012:77, with permission.)

+ Check integrity of ETT cuff
+ Ensure that laryngoscope light source is working properly
+ Make sure IV is functioning
+ Ensure patient is appropriately monitored
+ Position patient and adjust bed height
+ Assign team roles
+ Prepare for possible surgical airway

▢ **Preoxygenation**
+ Theoretically, deliver 100% oxygen for 3 minutes via nonrebreather mask. (In reality, it delivers approximately 70% oxygen.)
  + This fills the functional residual capacity with oxygen, replacing nitrogen and allowing for a longer apneic period before desaturation
+ When time is critical, preoxygenation can be achieved in eight vital capacity breaths
+ Nasal cannula should be placed to augment preoxygenation and facilitate apneic oxygenation

▢ **Pretreatment**
This refers to the administration of medications to attenuate the potential adverse side effects of intubation. Medications are given 3 minutes prior to intubation. While evidence supporting pretreatment is not conclusive, it should be considered in the following groups of patients:
+ Elevated ICP: To mitigate ICP increase with laryngoscopy and intubation
  + **Lidocaine** 1.5 mg/kg
  + **Fentanyl** 3 μg/kg
+ Cardiovascular disease: To decrease sympathetic response
  + **Fentanyl** 3 μg/kg
+ Reactive airway disease: To reduce bronchospasm
  + **Lidocaine** 1.5 mg/kg
  + **Albuterol** 2.5 mg nebulized

▢ **Paralysis and Induction**
+ Give the induction agent, as a bolus, in sufficient dose to produce immediate loss of consciousness. Common agents are propofol (1.5–3 mg/kg) and etomidate (0.3 mg/kg).
+ Push the paralytic agent immediately following the induction agent. Succinylcholine (1.5–2 mg/kg) is the common first choice in RSI because of its rapid onset.
  + Fasciculations will occur 20 to 30 seconds after the administration of succinylcholine
  + Apnea and paralysis will occur almost uniformly by 1 minute

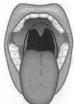
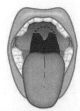

Class I: Soft palate, uvula,
fauces, pillars visible

No difficulty

Class II: Soft palate,
uvula, fauces visible

No difficulty

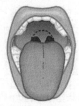
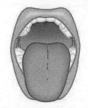

Class III: Soft palate, base,
of uvula visible

Moderate difficulty

Class IV: Hard palate,
only visible

Severe difficulty

FIGURE 1.3 The Mallampati Scale. (From Walls RM, Murphy MF. *Manual of Emergency Airway Management.* 4th edition, 2012 version of the Walls Emergency Manual as well. Philadelphia, PA: Lippincott Williams & Wilkins; 2012:78, with permission.)

Positioning
+ Place patient in "sniffing" position: Place a towel underneath the head to create slight flexion of lower cervical spine and then extend the head (**FIGURE 1.4**). This optimally aligns the pharyngeal and laryngeal airways.

Placement of the Tube
+ Open the mouth
+ Holding the handle in the left hand, insert the blade into the right side of the mouth and sweep the tongue fully to the left
+ Apply gentle upward and forward pressure (approximately 45 degrees) to lift the epiglottis and visualize the airway. Avoid the temptation to use the laryngoscope as a lever.
+ If cords are not immediately visible, try withdrawing the laryngoscope slowly to allow the cords to drop into view
+ If the view of the cords is limited, the gum-elastic bougie can be used to facilitate ETT placement (see discussion later)
+ If cords are adequately visualized, maintain direct visualization and ask someone to hand you the ETT
+ Pass the tube through the vocal cords and stop when the cuff is just past the cords
+ Remove the stylet and inflate the balloon

Proof of Tube Placement
+ Auscultate over the stomach and over the lungs
+ Confirm with qualitative (colorimetric) or quantitative (waveform) end-tidal carbon dioxide detection
+ Obtain postintubation chest x-ray

Postintubation Management
+ Maintain proper ventilator settings
+ Administer appropriate analgesia and sedation to keep the patient comfortable
+ Insert a nasogastric or orogastric tube to decompress the stomach
+ Obtain an arterial blood gas to assess for adequate oxygenation and ventilation

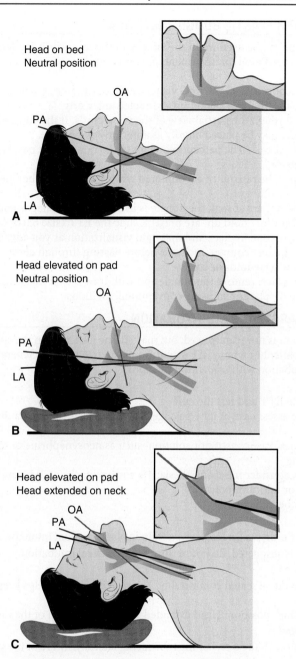

FIGURE 1.4 A: Anatomic neutral position. The oral axis (*OA*), pharyngeal axis (*PA*), and laryngeal axis (*LA*) are at greater angles to one another. **B:** Head, still in neutral position, has been lifted by a pillow flexing the lower cervical spine and aligning the *PA* and *LA* axes. **C:** The head has been extended on the cervical spine, aligning the *OA* with the *PA* and *LA* axes, creating the optimum sniffing position for intubation. (From Walls RM, Murphy MF. *Manual of Emergency Airway Management*. 4th ed. Philadelphia, PA: Lippincott Williams & Wilkins; 2012:56, with permission.)

TECHNIQUE FOR GUM-ELASTIC BOUGIE INSERTION

The gum-elastic bougie can be used when the view of the vocal cords is inadequate for confident ETT placement. Preoxygenation, pretreatment, paralysis, and positioning are executed as described earlier.

- Via direct laryngoscopy, obtain maximal visualization of the airway structures
- Orient the bougie such that the angled tip is directed anteriorly
- Carefully advance through the partial view of the vocal cords. If the cords are completely obscured, the bougie may be placed blindly as anteriorly as possible.
- Check for "palpable clicks": The perceptible snaps of the bougie as it passes over the rings of cartilage in the trachea
- Check for "hold up": The resistance encountered when the tip of the bougie reaches the carina or small bronchi
- If "clicks" and "hold up" are absent, the bougie is likely in the esophagus and should be removed
- If "palpable clicks" and/or "hold up" are present, slide the ETT (size 6.0 or larger) over the bougie. Keep the laryngoscope in place and maintain visualization as you advance.
- Rotate the ETT 90 degrees counterclockwise before passing through cords, to prevent the bevel tip from catching on arytenoids or cords
- Once the ETT is in place, remove the bougie and withdraw the laryngoscope
- Confirm tracheal ETT placement using conventional methods

TECHNIQUE FOR NASOTRACHEAL INTUBATION

Nasotracheal intubation is now rarely used, but may still be indicated in the spontaneously breathing and cooperative patient in whom RSI is contraindicated (FIGURE 1.5). General basic steps are similar to orotracheal intubation with some modifications.

- **Preparation**
  - Obtain 6.0 to 7.5 ETT and test the cuff
  - Inspect nares to assess ease of tube passage. The right naris is the default if there is no clear preference.
  - Administer topical vasoconstrictor solution, such as neosynephrine or oxymetazoline, to help prevent bleeding
  - If time permits, consider nasal anesthesia: 4% cocaine pack, 2% lidocaine jelly, or 4% nebulized lidocaine or lidocaine spray
  - Lubricate the tube and nostril
- **Preoxygenate**
- **Pretreatment and Paralysis Do Not Have a Role in Nasotracheal Intubation**
  - If elevated ICP is suspected, do not perform nasotracheal intubation
- **Positioning**
  - The patient should be seated comfortably. The seated position helps keep the tongue anterior in the airway.
  - Maintain "sniffing" position: Head extended with slight flexion of the lower cervical spine
- **Placement and Proof**
  - Enter the nostril with the bevel of the tube facing laterally, aware of the vascular supply along the anterior septum
  - Follow the floor of the nasal cavity directly back; the major nasal airway is located beneath the inferior nasal turbinate
  - Once the turbinate is reached, direct the tube slightly caudad
  - Slight resistance will occur in the posterior pharynx; rotate the tube such that the bevel is facing up to facilitate passage into the oropharynx
  - Once the oropharynx is entered, return the bevel to the lateral position and advance until breath sounds are best heard through the tube; the tube will be just above the vocal cords
  - Place pressure against the larynx with the nondominant hand and ask the patient to take a deep breath. As the patient is inspiring and the cords are abducting, gently advance the tube 3 to 4 cm.
  - Confirm tube placement as with orotracheal intubation

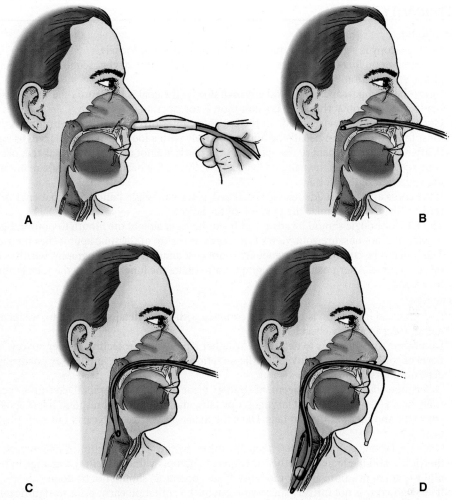

FIGURE 1.5 Nasotracheal intubation. (From Reichman EF, Simon RR. *Emergency Medicine Procedures*. New York, NY: McGraw-Hill; 2004, with permission.)

COMPLICATIONS

- Incorrect tube placement
  - Esophageal intubation: Remove ETT and ventilate via bag-valve mask (BVM) if oxygen saturation is less than 90%
  - Mainstem intubation: Pull back ETT to ventilate both lungs
- Hypoxia
- Aspiration
- Direct mechanical complications: Broken teeth, lip lacerations, pharyngeal injury, bleeding secondary to mucosal damage
- Pneumothorax and pneumomediastinum
- Cardiac dysrhythmia
- Complications or side effects from pharmacologic therapy, including hypotension

SAFETY/QUALITY TIPS

▣ **Procedural**

+ Laryngoscopy is a gentle procedure. Hold the laryngoscope loosely.
+ An assistant pulling the right corner of the mouth facilitates laryngoscope insertion and glottis visualization
+ Insert the laryngoscope gently and advance slowly; the goal is to identify the epiglottis
+ Inadequate suction at this stage is a common error; suction aggressively
+ Once the epiglottis is visualized, lift the epiglottis anteriorly. This maneuver requires the most force, but still can usually be done effectively with a loose grip on the laryngoscope.
+ If, after best displacement of the epiglottis, the cords are not adequately visualized, place your right hand under the patient's head and optimize the head position while maintaining your view of the glottis
+ If the cords are still not adequately visualized, place your right hand on the patient's thyroid cartilage and optimize the position of the larynx
+ The ETT or bougie should be advanced from the right side of the mouth to optimize geometry and not obscure your view of the cords as the tip of the tube approaches the glottis
+ The initial tube confirmation maneuver is not auscultation but capnography, which is far more accurate. After positive capnography, auscultate the lungs to verify the tube is above the carina.

▣ **Cognitive**

+ Endotracheal intubation is cognitively complex with many details to attend to; we recommend using an airway checklist
+ Do not use the gag reflex to determine whether a patient is protecting his/her airway. Level of consciousness, ability to handle secretions, voice, stridor, and airway posturing determine airway protection.
+ Determine your airway management strategy prior to the first attempt. Determine specifically how you will respond if laryngoscopy fails, and how you will respond if laryngoscopy fails and then ventilation fails. Have the materials you need to carry out your plan at bedside.
+ Once the laryngoscopic view has been optimized by the above-mentioned maneuvers, if the view is still inadequate, further or repeated attempts without making a change in technique (patient position, airway modality, blade, operator) should not be done
+ If laryngoscopy is not initially successful, establish ventilation early, prior to significant desaturation
+ The time immediately after intubation is high risk. Do not overventilate, mindfully attend to postintubation care (e.g. adequate analgesia/sedation, chest radiograph, blood gas), and monitor cardiorespiratory status carefully.

▣ **Acknowledgment**

Thank you to prior author Todd A. Seigel and Leon D. Sanchez.

Suggested Readings

Brown CA, Walls RM. Airway. In: Marx JA, ed. *Rosen's Emergency Medicine Concepts and Clinical Practice.* Philadelphia, PA: Saunders Elsevier; 2013.

Reichman EF, Freeman CJ. Airway procedures. In: Wolfson AB, ed. *Harwood-Nuss' Clinical Practice of Emergency Medicine.* 6th ed. Philadelphia, PA: Lippincott Williams & Wilkins; 2014.

Vissers RJ. Advanced airway support. *Emergency Medicine Manual.* New York, NY: McGraw-Hill; 2012.

Walls RM, Murphy MF. *Manual of Emergency Airway Management.* 4th ed. Philadelphia, PA: Lippincott Williams & Wilkins; 2012.

2

Video Laryngoscopy

Andrew J. Eyre and Calvin A. Brown III

INDICATIONS

- Routine intubation
- Rescue for failed direct laryngoscopy
- Anticipated difficult intubation (abnormal anatomy, reduced mouth opening, history of difficult intubations, cervical spine precautions, obesity)
- Intubation with desire for teaching or supervision of physician trainees

RELATIVE CONTRAINDICATIONS

- Brisk bleeding or copious secretions
- No oral access (angioedema)
- Provider discomfort or lack of training with indirect laryngoscopy and intubation

DEVICES

- Multiple devices are available
- Devices are broadly grouped into acutely curved blades (GlideScope, King Vision, C-MAC D-blade, Pentax airway scope) or traditionally shaped blades (C-MAC, GlideScope teaching blade)
- Traditionally shaped blades can be used as a direct and video laryngoscope to facilitate mechanical memory for direct laryngoscopy
- Some devices require free-hand placement of the endotracheal tube (ETT) (GlideScope, C-MAC, McGrath Series 5), while others have integrated ETT channels that require the device and ETT to be inserted together (King Vision, Pentax airway scope)

SUPPLIES

- Video laryngoscope system
- ETT
- ETT stylet (malleable or rigid)
- ETT lubricant
- 10-cc syringe for cuffed ETTs
- End-tidal carbon dioxide detector
- Tube securing device
- Bag-valve mask
- Oral and/or nasal airways
- Equipment for preoxygenation (facemask oxygen with reservoir)

TECHNIQUE—RAPID SEQUENCE INTUBATION

- **Preparation**
  - Vascular access
  - Monitoring: Cardiac monitor, blood pressure monitoring, and pulse oximetry
  - Suction device
  - Assemble necessary equipment (see above)
  - Obtain rapid sequence intubation (RSI) medications
  - Perform an airway assessment for difficulty
- **Preoxygenation**
  - Preoxygenate with nonrebreathing mask or bag-valve mask
  - Nasal cannula for passive oxygenation during intubation, especially for rapid desaturators

◻ **Positioning**
  ✚ Cervical spine extension and head elevation if no contraindication
  ✚ In-line cervical spine neutrality for patients with cervical spine precautions
◻ **Perform "Time Out"**
  ✚ Ensure that the team agrees on medications and dosing, devices to be used, and plan for
    a failed intubation
◻ **Administer Induction and Paralytic Agents**
◻ **Perform Intubation**
Traditionally shaped video system blades (C-MAC, GlideScope teaching blade)

  ✚ Open mouth with a finger/scissor or similar technique
  ✚ Insert the blade in the right paralingual gutter of the mouth, sweeping the tongue to the left
  ✚ Advance the blade in traditional technique with the goal of identifying epiglottis first (epi-
    glottoscopy), followed by placement of the tip of the blade in the base of the vallecula
  ✚ Using an upward motion, lift up on the handle and blade to obtain a view of the vocal cords
    by manipulating the hyoepiglottic ligament
  ✚ If an optimal direct view is not seen under direct vision, the operator may attempt optimiza-
    tion maneuvers such as backward upward rightward pressure, or "BURP," to improve view
  ✚ Alternatively, the intubator can opt for early recourse to the video screen to assess glottic
    view and intubate using the video screen
  ✚ Stylet should be shaped with a gentle curve to approximate the trajectory the blade has taken
    to the airway

Curved "indirect" video systems (standard GlideScope, C-MAC D-blade, McGrath video
laryngoscope, Pentax airway scope, King Vision video laryngoscope)

  ✚ Open mouth with a finger/scissor or similar technique
  ✚ Insert the device in the midline, staying opposed to the dorsal surface of the tongue
  ✚ Advance and rotate the blade around the tongue, staying in the midline, while watching on
    the video screen to identify key midline airway landmarks (uvula and tip of epiglottis)
  ✚ Advance until the blade rests in the vallecula
  ✚ Gently tilt the blade and cranially bring the vocal cords into view on the screen. Do not place
    the device too close to the glottic inlet as this impedes tube passage.
  ✚ If the device has a channel to hold and launch the ETT, gently push the tube through the
    channel and past the vocal cords after first ensuring the vocal cords are in the center of the
    video screen
  ✚ If the device requires the use of a stylet, preference should be made for a rigid preshaped
    stylet as these do not deform during intubation. Malleable stylets should be shaped with a
    more aggressive curve to mimic the shape of and trajectory taken by the blade.
  ✚ Place the stylet-loaded tube in the right corner of the mouth with the length of the tube par-
    allel to the ground (3 o'clock position). Advance the tube while rotating the tube in a counter-
    clockwise position until the tube aligns with the curvature of the blade (12 o'clock position).
    Advance the tube through the vocal cords. If unable to fully pass the tube, withdraw the stylet
    slightly to allow for more mobility. Withdraw the stylet.
  ✚ Inflate the cuff (for cuffed tubes)
◻ **Proof of Intubation**
  ✚ Confirm tube placement with breath sounds, chest rise, and colorimetric or quantitative end-
    tidal carbon dioxide
◻ **Postintubation Care**
  ✚ Secure the ETT
  ✚ Order portable chest x-ray
  ✚ Connect to a mechanical ventilator, if appropriate
  ✚ Strategy for ongoing sedation

COMPLICATIONS

- Failed intubation with hypoxic insult
- Need for surgical cricothyrotomy
- Esophageal intubation
- Airway bleeding and swelling
- Damage to vocal cords
- Damage to teeth, lips, or tongue
- Hemodynamic decompensation following RSI medications

SAFETY/QUALITY TIPS

- **Procedural**
  - Your eyes should start out looking in the mouth for blade placement, then shift to the screen for optimal blade advancement, then back to the mouth to place the tube near the tip of the blade, then back to the screen to deliver the tube through the cords.
  - When using video laryngoscopy, do not place the blade too close to the vocal cords as this limits the ability to easily pass the ETT. In practice, this means not trying to get the "best view of the cords" on the screen, rather, keeping a slightly suboptimal view of the cords on the bottom of the screen, which makes tube delivery much easier.
  - If you are having difficulty passing the tube through the vocal cords, withdraw the stylet and advance the tube
  - When able, use the proprietary stylet and adjunctive equipment. The proprietary stylets are designed to exactly match the curvature of the blade.
- **Cognitive**
  - Standard geometry video laryngoscopes will provide an excellent view of the glottis in most cases, can function using direct or indirect technique, and offer comparatively easy tube delivery. Hyperangulated geometry blades provide an excellent view of the cords in almost every case, including cases where standard geometry view is inadequate, but can only be used by the indirect/video approach, and tube delivery can be more challenging.
  - If the ETT needs to be adjusted, consider doing so under video guidance
  - Practice with the video laryngoscopy system before using it clinically, especially if the device features a hyperangulated geometry blade
  - Select the right device for the right patient. Standard geometry video laryngoscopy allows for direct visualization if secretions or blood obscure the screen. Hyperangulated geometry requires less lifting force and may be easier in patients requiring cervical spine immobilization.

Suggested Readings

Walls RM, Murphy MF. *Manual of Emergency Airway Management.* 4th Ed. Philadelphia, PA: Lippincott Williams & Wilkins; 2012.

3

Delayed Sequence Intubation

Nelson Wong and Scott D. Weingart

CLASSIC DEFINITION

A strategy of time separation between the administration of a dissociative induction agent and the neuromuscular blocker to allow preintubation optimization.

INTRODUCTION

Delayed sequence intubation (DSI) differs from rapid sequence intubation (RSI), in that it separates the induction and paralysis to allow preintubation procedures such as preoxygenation in patients who are noncompliant (e.g. delirious) (FIGURE 3.1). It can be thought of as procedural sedation where the procedure is preoxygenation. In indicated situations requiring further preoxygenation, DSI is an alternative to precipitous intubation without full paralytic effect or bag-mask ventilation in the sedated and paralyzed patient. Respectively, these two traditional options increase the risk of first-pass failure or the risk of gastric insufflation and passive regurgitation in sick, nonfasted patients. Both options ensure an abbreviated period before critical levels of hypoxemia.

CLASSIC INDICATIONS

- Preoxygenation prior to intubation in a delirious or otherwise uncooperative hypoxemic and/or hypercapnic patient
- Adequate oxygenation but need for further denitrogenation of the lungs and bloodstream in order to prolong the safe apnea period in a delirious or otherwise uncooperative patient

EXTENDED INDICATIONS

- Need for an additional procedure or further optimization of physiologic parameters prior to intubation in a delirious or otherwise uncooperative patient
  - Nasogastric tube placement for a patient with upper gastrointestinal bleed and stomach filled with blood
  - Need to optimize patient's blood pressure secondary to hypotension
  - Need to optimize patient's respiratory and metabolic status secondary to metabolic acidosis

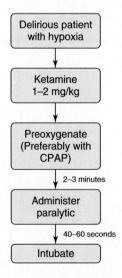

FIGURE 3.1 Delayed sequence intubation algorithm.

CONTRAINDICATIONS

- Need for a "crash" airway
  - ✦ Patient unable to breathe spontaneously
  - ✦ Patient unable to protect his/her own airway
- Relative contraindications—situations in which ketamine would be less than favorable and absence of alternative agents e.g.dexmedetomidate or droperidol
  - ✦ Elderly patients with coronary artery disease
  - ✦ Patients with elevated blood pressure or tachycardia

EQUIPMENT

- Equipment for preoxygenation
  - ✦ Nasal cannula (NC)
  - ✦ Nonrebreather (NRB) mask
  - ✦ Consider methods for positive-pressure ventilation if the patient is exhibiting physiologic shunt
    - ✚ Ventilator and noninvasive ventilation (NIV) mask
    - ✚ Bag-valve mask (BVM) with adjustable positive end-expiratory pressure (PEEP) valve
- Induction medication that maintains ventilatory drive and airway reflexes
  - ✦ That is ketamine (1–2 mg/kg) given over approximately 30 seconds
- Standard equipment and medications for airway management

STANDARD TECHNIQUE

- Administration of induction agents that do not blunt spontaneous ventilations or airway reflexes
  - ✦ Give a dissociative dose of ketamine (1–2 mg/kg) over approximately 30 seconds
  - ✦ Alternative agents
    - ✚ Dexmedetomidine 1 µg/kg over 10 minutes
    - ✚ Droperidol 5 to 10 mg
      - ▪ After intubation, check electrocardiogram (ECG) to determine whether any QT prolongation
      - ▪ For these two latter agents, a separate induction agent should be administered just prior to neuromuscular blocker administration
- Preoxygenation and denitrogenation in standard manner with oxygen saturation >95% for 2 to 3 minutes or at least eight vital capacity (VC) breaths (note: patients who have received a DSI agent cannot take VC breaths)
  - ✦ NRB
  - ✦ Alternatives in patient exhibiting shunt physiology (saturation not improving with increased F_{IO_2})
    - ✚ BVM with PEEP valve
    - ✚ NIV—PEEP/Continuous positive airway pressure (CPAP)
    - ✚ PEEP levels between 5 and 15 cm H_2O
    - ✚ Follow with apneic oxygenation
- Concurrent preparation for definitive airway management in standard manner

EXAMPLE OF PROCEDURE

- Delirious hypoxic patient not tolerating an NRB for preoxygenation
- Ketamine 1 to 2 mg/kg by slow intravenous push
- Preoxygenation and denitrogenation with NRB/NC or NIPPV (Non-Invasive Positive Pressure Ventilation) for 2 to 3 minutes
- Administer NMB (Neuromuscular blockade)
- 45 to 60 seconds of apnea with apneic oxygenation
- Intubate

COMPLICATIONS

Complications from DSI are no different from complications inherent in attempts to intubate hypoxic/hypercapnic, delirious and/or otherwise unstable patients, with the exception being the establishment of a prolonged safe apnea period:

☐ Aspiration
☐ Gastric distention
☐ Emesis with ketamine—occurs after emergence and is a concern if the patient is allowed to emerge from the dissociated state prior to endotracheal intubation

SAFETY/QUALITY TIPS

☐ **Procedural**
   ✦ Administering ketamine as a quick bolus will often cause 15 to 30 seconds of apnea; this can be avoided by pushing ketamine more slowly (over 30 seconds)
   ✦ Application of a NC at high flow, in addition to either a face mask or NIV oxygenation, will optimize oxygenation and facilitate apneic oxygenation after the paralytic is given
   ✦ Avoid very high positive pressure (>15 cm H_2O) when using NIV

☐ **Cognitive**
   ✦ The intubating provider should be at bedside during the entire DSI procedure, prepared to abort DSI at any point and commence with RSI (by giving the paralytic)
   ✦ Although the goal of DSI is to optimize intubating conditions, in some cases, the underlying insult can be adequately addressed during the dissociated period, and intubation avoided. We recommend that a full intubation setup be prepared for every DSI case, however.
   ✦ Current alternatives to ketamine are inferior to ketamine for facilitating DSI; be cautious if using any other agent

Suggested Readings

Delayed sequence intubation. http://www.lifeinthefastlane.com.
Green SM, Roback MG, Kennedy RM, et al. Clinical practice guideline for emergency department ketamine dissociative sedation: 2011 update. *Ann Emerg Med.* 2011;57(5):449–461.
LeCong M. ed. PHARM Podcast 23 – Mr EmCrit and the DSI chronicles. http://www.prehospitalmed.com
Weingart, SD. EMCrit Podcast 40 – Delayed Sequence Intubation (DSI). http://www.emcrit.org.
Weingart, SD. Preoxygenation, reoxygenation, and delayed sequence intubation in the emergency department. *J Emerg Med.* 2011;40(6):661–667.
Weingart SD, Levitan RM. Preoxygenation and prevention of desaturation during emergency airway management. *Ann Emerg Med.* 2012;59(3):165–157.

4

No DESAT: Maximally Aggressive Preoxygenation

J. Michael Guthrie and Scott D. Weingart

INTRODUCTION

- Patients requiring endotracheal intubation in the emergency department (ED) are at a much higher risk for hypoxemia, compared to patients electively intubated in the operating room. Pulmonary disease, anemia, low respiratory drive, decreased ability to protect the airway, and severe illness causing high metabolic demand all contribute to this risk.
- Maximally aggressive preoxygenation, in conjunction with other strategies to prevent desaturation, is required in all ED intubations
- The goal of preoxygenation is to allow the longest apneic time possible before hypoxemia
- Oxygen saturation begins to fall precipitously below 93%. It may take only a few seconds before the saturation drops below 70%, at which point the incidence of dysrhythmias, hypoxic brain injury, and death increase greatly.
- While young healthy patients may remain well oxygenated for 5 minutes or more after preoxygenation, those who are acutely ill with poor lung physiology and high metabolic demands can become hypoxic in seconds regardless of preinduction oxygen saturation. The preoxygenation strategy employed should be tailored to the patient on the basis of their risk of hypoxemia.
- NO DESAT means Nasal Oxygen During Efforts Securing A Tube
- Strategies for oxygenating patients at both low and high risk for desaturation are discussed later

INDICATIONS

- All patients requiring intubation in the ED

CONTRAINDICATIONS

- None

SUPPLIES

- Nasal cannula (NC)
- Bag-valve mask (BVM)
- Positive end-expiratory pressure (PEEP) valve
- Nonrebreather (NRB) mask
- Continuous positive airway pressure (CPAP) machine or ventilator
- Bilevel positive airway pressure (BiPAP)/CPAP mask

> ### General Basic Steps
> - **Preoxygenate using NRB**
> - **Preoxygenate with head of bed elevated**
> - **Preoxygenate for at least 3 minutes or eight vital capacity breaths**
> - **Continue NC at 15 L/min for apneic oxygenation**
> - **For patients with shunt physiology, preoxygenate with positive pressure**
> - **For patients at risk for critical acidosis, continue ventilations during apneic period while waiting for full paralysis**

TECHNIQUE

▢ Place NRB mask with oxygen flow at maximal flow rate
  ✛ Turn oxygen regulator to maximal flow
  ✛ Turn knob counterclockwise till it will turn no further
  ✛ The oxygen flow should be easily audible
  ✛ This will deliver 30 to 60 L/min of oxygen and an F_{IO_2} close to 90%
  ✛ Standard NRB masks set to 15 L/min deliver only around 70% F_{IO_2}
▢ Place an NC on all patients for preoxygenation and apneic oxygenation
  ✛ Place the NC beneath the NRB mask or BiPAP/BVM at 4 to 6 L/min before induction
  ✛ After induction, turn flow rate up to 15 L/min for apneic oxygenation
  ✛ Before induction the NC will bring inspired F_{IO_2} closer to 100%
  ✛ During apneic period, oxygen will flow into alveoli, significantly increasing the time before the patient becomes hypoxic
  ✛ During apnea, oxygen supplied by the NC flows from the nasopharynx to the alveoli because of a slightly subatmospheric pressure in the alveoli. The pressure gradient exists because oxygen moves out of the alveoli faster than CO_2 moves into the alveoli.
  ✛ Apneic oxygenation can be remembered with the mnemonic NO DESAT
▢ Preoxygenate with the head of the bed elevated
  ✛ Set the head of the bed to at least 20 degrees during preoxygenation
  ✛ For immobilized patients, place the bed in reverse Trendelenburg to at least 20 degrees
  ✛ Supine positioning leads to atelectasis, incomplete breaths, and less oxygenation, compared with upright positioning
  ✛ Patients preoxygenated in head-elevated position achieve better preoxygenation and take longer to reach hypoxemia
  ✛ Head-elevated positioning has the added benefit of better laryngeal exposure during laryngoscopy
▢ Preoxygenate for at least 3 minutes
  ✛ Patients should remain on NRB/NC or BiPAP/NC for a full 3 minutes
  ✛ Preoxygenating for 3 minutes ensures full denitrogenation of the residual capacity of the lungs and maximal hemoglobin oxygen saturation
  ✛ In cooperative patients eight vital capacity breaths can achieve similar levels of oxygen saturation and denitrogenation

PREOXYGENATION STEPS FOR PATIENTS AT HIGH RISK FOR DESATURATION

▢ For patients not achieving 100% oxygen saturation after 3 minutes of NRB/NC or with suspected shunt physiology, preoxygenate with noninvasive ventilation or BVM with PEEP valve
  ✛ Place the patient on BiPAP or CPAP with 100% F_{IO_2} and PEEP of at least 5 for 3 minutes Or
  ✛ Allow the patient to spontaneously breathe via BVM with a PEEP valve set to at least 5 for 3 minutes
  ✛ Patients who do not reach 100% oxygen saturation with high F_{IO_2} are likely to have shunt physiology, where alveoli have blood supply but are not receiving oxygen because of alveolar collapse, pulmonary edema, or pneumonia. Positive pressure will open these alveoli, allowing them to be oxygenated.
▢ Continue ventilations after induction and administration of paralytics for patients at high risk for critical acidosis
  ✛ Continue ventilations via ventilator with BiPAP mask or BVM with PEEP valve while awaiting full paralysis
  ✛ Patients who fail to achieve >95% oxygen saturation despite positive-pressure preoxygenation will likely desaturate to critical hypoxemia during the 2 minutes of apneic time required for full muscle relaxation after paralytic administration
  ✛ When using BVM, bag gently with breath delivered slowly over 2 seconds with low tidal volumes (6 cc/kg) and at a rate of 10 to 12 per minute
  ✛ Gentle bagging should decrease risk of gastric insufflation and emesis. Inspiratory pressures <25 mm Hg are unlikely to overcome lower esophageal sphincter.

PULSE OXIMETRY LAG TIME

- Be mindful that the oxygen saturation on the screen does not accurately reflect the patient's current oxygen saturation
- The pulse oximetry value on the screen lags behind the patient's blood oxygen saturation from 30 seconds to 2 minutes
- Sicker patients have longer lag times. Hypothermia, low cardiac output, and vasopressor use may all increase this lag time.

SAFETY/QUALITY TIPS

- **Procedural**
  - Apneic oxygenation requires a patent nasopharyngeal passage. This can be achieved with head elevation: Ear-to-sternal notch, face parallel to ceiling positioning, jaw thrust, and nasal trumpet.
  - The NC for apneic oxygenation will require a third oxygen source
  - Before preoxygenation, discuss the concept of apneic oxygenation with your team and respiratory therapist, as the concept may be new to some and the initial impulse may be to remove the NC after induction
  - A pulse oximetry probe placed on the ear or forehead may reduce lag time as the blood here is closer to the central circulation
  - Avoid the use of cricoid pressure. It has not been shown to prevent emesis and aspiration and may limit preoxygenation and manual ventilation by compressing the trachea. If you decide to use it, release it if there is any difficulty with glottis visualization or tube passage.
- **Cognitive**
  - Patients who are hypoxemic before preoxygenation or who do not achieve a high Spo$_2$ > 95% with NRB/NC likely have shunt physiology and will need positive pressure via CPAP/BiPAP or BVM with PEEP valve for adequate preoxygenation
  - In patients at high risk for desaturation, consider rocuronium over succinylcholine. Paralysis with rocuronium has been shown to lead to longer safe apneic times before hypoxemia, compared to succinylcholine. It is hypothesized that this is due to oxygen consumption from the defasciculation when using succinylcholine.
  - The inflection point of the O$_2$–Hg dissociation curve, where it goes into the steep portion of the curve, is 93%. After this point the patient will desaturate rapidly.

Suggested Readings

Davis DP, Aguilar S, Sonnleitner C, et al. Latency and loss of pulse oximetry signal with the use of digital probes during prehospital rapid-sequence intubation. *Prehosp Emerg Care.* 2011;15(1):18–22.

Davis DP, Hwang JQ, Dunford JV. Rate of decline in oxygen saturation at various pulse oximetry values with prehospital rapid sequence intubation. *Prehosp Emerg Care.* 2008;12(1):46–51.

Weingart SD, Levitan RM. Preoxygenation and prevention of desaturation during emergency airway management. *Ann Emerg Med.* 2012;59(3):165–175.

5

Meconium Aspirator as Airway Suction Device

Kathryn A. Volz and Leon D. Sanchez

INDICATIONS

⊕ To suction/intubate a patient with significant blood, emesis, or secretions within the airway

CONTRAINDICATIONS

⊕ Contraindications to direct laryngoscopy

SUPPLIES

⊕ All necessary supplies for intubation (see Chapter 1)
⊕ Endotracheal tube (ETT) (without stylet, or can use stylet if you have a swivel adapter with a perforated head)
⊕ Neonatal meconium aspirator
⊕ Suction

TECHNIQUE

⊕ **Aspiration without Stylet**
  ✦ Connect meconium aspirator to the end of ETT—see **FIGURE 5.1**
  ✦ Connect suction to meconium aspirator
  ✦ Prepare for intubation (preoxygenate, assess airway, position, prepare medications, etc.)
  ✦ Occluding suction hole of the meconium aspirator with fingertip will allow ETT to function as a large-bore suction device
⊕ **Alternative: Aspiration with Stylet**
  ✦ Connect common swivel adapter with a perforated rubber head (Bodai Swivel, Sontek Medical, Hingham, MA) to the end of the ETT—see **FIGURE 5.2**
  ✦ Connect meconium aspirator to swivel adapter and connect suction to meconium aspirator
  ✦ ETT stylet can be inserted through swivel adapter. See **FIGURE 5.3** for complete setup (Figures 5.1–5.3).

COMPLICATIONS

⊕ Inability to visualize cords
⊕ Inability to intubate without stylet (consider using swivel adapter to allow use of stylet in ETT)
⊕ Clogging of ETT
⊕ Contamination of ETT
⊕ Inability to suction
⊕ Inability to intubate

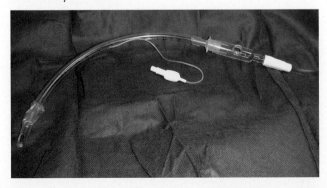

FIGURE 5.1 Meconium aspirator connected to endotracheal tube and wall suction. (Courtesy of Scott D. Weingart and Sabrina D. Bhagwan; used with the permission of Metasin LLC.)

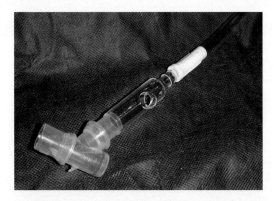

FIGURE 5.2 Swivel adapter attached to meconium aspirator. Stylet can be inserted through perforated rubber head. (Courtesy of Scott D. Weingart and Sabrina D. Bhagwan; used with the permission of Metasin LLC.)

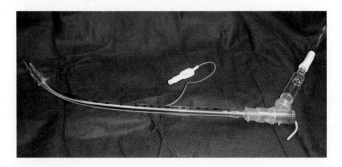

FIGURE 5.3 Complete setup with swivel adapter to allow use of stylet. (Courtesy of Scott D. Weingart and Sabrina D. Bhagwan; used with the permission of Metasin LLC.)

SAFETY/QUALITY TIPS

☐ Procedural

+ Wear personal protective equipment, including facial shield and mask
+ Conscious, vomiting patients should be maintained in an upright position, but unconscious patients with ongoing large emesis/regurgitation should be immediately placed in deep Trendelenburg position so that secretions flow out of the mouth rather than down the trachea.
+ Unconscious patients with very large amounts of emesis in the oropharynx are most effectively cleared by first using the intubator's gloved right hand: with the laryngoscope seated and the tongue controlled, reach deep into the mouth and manually scoop out as much material as possible before initiating suction.

☐ Cognitive

+ An alternative to the meconium aspirator approach is to use *two* Yankauer suction devices, one in the intubator's right hand and the other in the hand of an assistant. Especially if using video laryngoscopy, the assistant can continue to suction as attempts at glottic visualization and tube delivery are continued.
+ Patients with copious secretions are at high risk to desaturate quickly and for laryngoscopy failure. Prepare for a possible surgical airway by having the materials to perform cricothyrotomy at bedside and possibly marking the neck.

Suggested Reading

Weingart SD, Bhagwan SD. A novel set-up to allow suctioning during direct endotracheal and fiberoptic intubation. *J Clin Anesth*. 2011;23(6):518–519.

6

Cricothyroidotomy—Standard and Needle

Jason Imperato and Alden M. Landry

INDICATIONS

- To provide emergent airway access only when a safer, less invasive airway cannot be established or is contraindicated
- For children younger than 12 years, needle cricothyroidotomy is the surgical airway of choice

CONTRAINDICATIONS

- **Absolute**
  - An oral or nasal airway can be established
  - Significant injury or fracture of the cricoid cartilage or larynx (tracheostomy is the procedure of choice)
  - Tracheal fracture or transection
  - Obstruction below the cricothyroid membrane
  - Patients younger than 12 years (needle cricothyroidotomy is the procedure of choice for this age-group)
- **Relative**
  - Neck mass, swelling, or cellulitis
  - Neck hematoma
  - Coagulopathy

LANDMARKS

- The cricothyroid membrane—an elastic membrane located anteriorly and midline in the neck, measuring 9 mm longitudinally and 30 mm transversely. Bordered superiorly by the thyroid cartilage ("Adam's apple") and inferiorly by the cricoid cartilage.
- In children, the larynx is positioned more superiorly than in adults and is relatively smaller in size (FIGURES 6.1 and 6.2)

STANDARD CRICOTHYROIDOTOMY

- **Supplies**
  - Antiseptic solution, drapes, towel clips
  - Lidocaine with epinephrine
  - No. 11 blade scalpel with handle
  - Tracheal hook
  - Trousseau dilator
  - Tracheostomy tube
  - Neck tie or sutures
- **Technique**
  - **Preparation**
    - Hyperextend the neck to more readily identify landmarks, unless the patient has a known or suspected cervical spine injury
    - Preoxygenate the patient by bag-mask ventilation
    - Test the integrity of the balloon on the tracheostomy tube by injecting with 10 mL of air
    - If time permits, apply appropriate antiseptic solution and drape the area with sterile towels
    - If time permits and patient is conscious or responding to pain, infiltrate the skin of anterior neck with 1% lidocaine solution with epinephrine

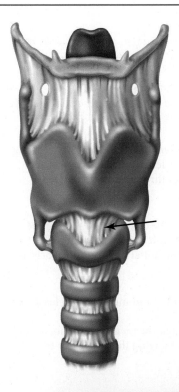

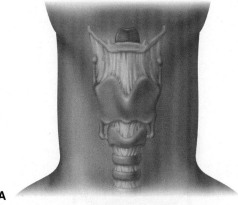

FIGURE 6.1 Anatomy of the larynx. The cricothyroid membrane (*arrow*) is bordered above by the thyroid cartilage and below by the cricoid cartilage. (From Walls RM, Murphy MF. *Manual of Emergency Airway Management*. 4th ed. Philadelphia, PA: Lippincott Williams & Wilkins; 2012:162, with permission.)

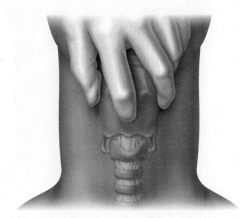

A   B

FIGURE 6.2 A: Surface anatomy of the airway. **B:** The thumb and middle finger immobilize the superior cornua of the larynx; the index finger palpates the cricothyroid membrane. (From Walls RM, Murphy MF. *Manual of Emergency Airway Management*. 4th ed. Philadelphia, PA: Lippincott Williams & Wilkins; 2012:163, with permission.)

☐ **General Basic Steps**
  ✚ **Identify the landmarks**
  ✚ **Stabilize the larynx**
  ✚ **Incise the skin**
  ✚ **Reidentify the cricothyroid membrane**
  ✚ **Incise the cricothyroid membrane**
  ✚ **Insert the tracheal hook**
  ✚ **Insert the trousseau dilator**
  ✚ **Insert the tracheostomy tube**
  ✚ **Inflate the cuff and confirm tube position**
  ✚ **Secure the tracheostomy tube**

▣ **Identify the Landmarks (See Earlier "Landmarks" Section)**

▣ **Stabilize the Larynx**

✚ Grasp both sides of the thyroid cartilage with the thumb and middle finger using the nondominant hand

✚ Palpate the depression over the cricothyroid membrane with the index finger

✚ Control the larynx throughout the procedure by stabilizing it in this manner and reidentify the cricothyroid membrane at any time during the procedure

▣ **Incise the Skin**

✚ Using a no. 11 scalpel blade in the dominant hand, make a *vertical* midline incision through the skin and subcutaneous tissue approximately 2 to 3 cm in length

✚ Care should be taken to extend the incision down to but not through any of the deep structures of the neck

▣ **Reidentify the Cricothyroid Membrane**

✚ Using the index finger of the nondominant hand, reidentify the cricothyroid membrane while maintaining immobilization of the larynx with the thumb and middle finger

✚ If the cricothyroid membrane cannot be palpated, extend the initial incision superiorly and inferiorly and try to palpate again

▣ **Incise the Cricothyroid Membrane**

✚ Using the stabilizing index finger as a guide, incise the cricothyroid membrane at least 1 cm in length in the *horizontal* direction

✚ Note that the skin incision is vertical and the incision through the membrane is horizontal

✚ Place the index finger into the stoma temporarily while exchanging the scalpel for the tracheal hook

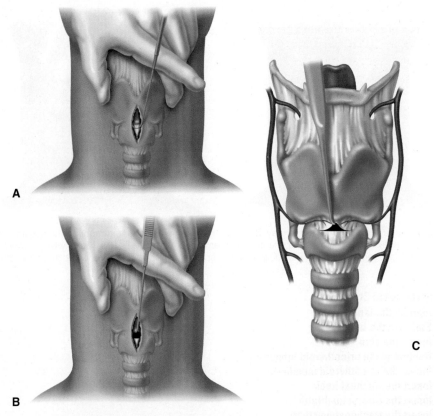

FIGURE 6.3 A: The tracheal hook is oriented transversely during insertion. **B** and **C:** After insertion, cephalad traction is applied to the inferior margin of the thyroid cartilage. (From Walls RM, Murphy MF. *Manual of Emergency Airway Management.* 4th ed. Philadelphia, PA: Lippincott Williams & Wilkins; 2012:166, with permission.)

- ◘ **Insert the Tracheal Hook (FIGURE 6.3)**
  - ✦ Using the dominant hand, insert the tracheal hook into the opening in the cricothyroid membrane
  - ✦ Rotate the handle cephalad while grasping the inferior border of the thyroid cartilage with it
  - ✦ Ask an assistant to apply light upward and anterior traction on the tracheal hook to bring the airway immediately out of the skin incision
- ◘ **Insert the Trousseau Dilator**
  - ✦ Insert the tips of the Trousseau dilator into the opening of the membrane minimally with the blades oriented superiorly and inferiorly, allowing the dilator to open and enlarge the wound in the vertical plane
  - ✦ Using the nondominant hand, rotate the handle of the Trousseau dilator 90 degrees and caudad until the handle is parallel to the neck
- ◘ **Insert the Tracheostomy Tube**
  - ✦ Insert the tracheostomy tube using the dominant hand between the blades of the Trousseau dilator until the flanges rest against the skin of the neck
  - ✦ Keep the thumb on the obturator throughout the procedure
  - ✦ Carefully remove the Trousseau dilator
- ◘ **Inflate the Cuff and Confirm Tube Position**
  - ✦ Remove the obturator and insert the inner cannula
  - ✦ Inflate the balloon
  - ✦ Ventilate the patient
  - ✦ Confirm proper placement by end-tidal carbon dioxide detection, bilateral chest movement, and bilateral breath sounds
- ◘ **Secure the Tracheostomy Tube**
  - ✦ Secure the tracheostomy tube with a circumferential tie around the neck or with sutures
  - ✦ Order a postprocedure portable chest radiography
- ◘ **Complications**
  - ✦ Uncontrolled bleeding
  - ✦ Misplacement of the tube
  - ✦ Subcutaneous emphysema
  - ✦ Pneumothorax
  - ✦ Obstruction of the tracheostomy tube
  - ✦ **Late Complications**
    - ✦ Voice change
    - ✦ Infection
    - ✦ Difficulty swallowing
    - ✦ Subglottic stenosis

SAFETY/QUALITY TIPS

- ◘ **Procedural**
  - ✦ The vertical incision should be generous, longer than your instinct
  - ✦ After the vertical incision is made, the field will be very bloody, and visually identifying landmarks may be impossible—be prepared to base all further steps on palpation rather than on visualization
  - ✦ The cricothyroid membrane is lower than your instinct—in an adult, approximately 3 fingerbreadths above the suprasternal notch
  - ✦ A 6.0 endotracheal tube can be used if a tracheostomy tube is not available
  - ✦ Lubricating the tracheostomy tube/endotracheal tube will facilitate passage through the soft tissues into the trachea
  - ✦ Many variants of the traditional cricothyrotomy technique described above exist; a simpler, recently popular approach is the scalpel–bougie technique, in which, after the horizontal incision, a finger is placed in the trachea, then a bougie alongside the finger. A tracheostomy tube can then be railroaded over the bougie, into the trachea.

NEEDLE CRICOTHYROIDOTOMY

- ⊡ **Supplies**
  - ✦ Antiseptic solution, drapes, towel clips
  - ✦ Lidocaine with epinephrine
  - ✦ Large-bore angiocath (12- to 14-gauge)
  - ✦ 3- or 5-mL syringe and saline
  - ✦ Oxygen supply
- ⊡ **Technique**
  - ✦ **Preparation**
    - ✦ Hyperextend the neck to more readily identify landmarks, unless the patient has a known or suspected cervical spine injury
    - ✦ Preoxygenate the patient by bag-mask ventilation
    - ✦ Attach a large-bore angiocath (12- to 14-gauge) to a 3- or 5-mL syringe filled with 1 to 2 mL of saline
    - ✦ If time permits, apply appropriate antiseptic solution and drape the area with sterile towels
    - ✦ If time permits and the patient is conscious or responding to pain, infiltrate the skin of the anterior neck with 1% lidocaine solution with epinephrine

---

- ⊡ **General Basic Steps**
  - ✦ **Identify the landmarks**
  - ✦ **Palpate the cricothyroid membrane**
  - ✦ **Insert the angiocath**
  - ✦ **Attach the oxygen supply**
  - ✦ **Secure the angiocath**

- ⊡ **Identify the Landmarks (See Earlier "Landmarks" Section)**
- ⊡ **Palpate the Cricothyroid Membrane**
  - ✦ Identify and palpate the cricothyroid membrane using the nondominant hand in a manner similar to the surgical cricothyroidotomy technique
- ⊡ **Insert the Angiocath**
  - ✦ Using the dominant hand, insert the 12- or 14-gauge angiocath through the skin, subcutaneous tissue, and the cricothyroid membrane directed at a 30- to 45-degree angle caudally (see **FIGURE 6.4**)
  - ✦ Aspirate the syringe during advancement of the angiocath. Air bubbles in the syringe confirm that the needle is in the trachea.
  - ✦ Advance the catheter over the needle until the hub is flush with the skin
  - ✦ Remove the needle

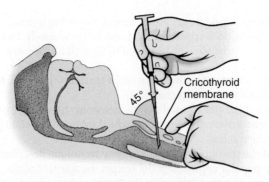

Cricothyroid membrane

45°

FIGURE 6.4 Percutaneous transtracheal catheter ventilation. Insert the needle into the cricothyroid membrane at a 30- to 45-degree angle, directed caudally. (From Simon RR, Brenner BE. *Emergency Procedures and Techniques*. 4th ed. Philadelphia, PA: Lippincott Williams & Wilkins; 2002:100, with permission.)

◻ **Attach the Oxygen Supply**
+ Attach the oxygen supply and begin to ventilate the patient
+ Confirm proper placement by end-tidal carbon dioxide, bilateral chest movement, and bilateral breath sounds. This does not really apply to needle cricothyroidotomy, which hopefully oxygenates, but does not much ventilate.

◻ **Secure the Tube**
+ Secure the tracheostomy tube with a circumferential tie around the neck or with sutures. There is no tracheostomy tube in needle cricothyroidotomy.
+ Order a postprocedure portable chest radiography

◻ **Complications**
+ Uncontrolled bleeding
+ Misplacement of the tube
+ Subcutaneous emphysema
+ Pneumothorax/pneumomediastinum
+ Obstruction/kinking of tube
+ Perforation of the posterior trachea. Most of these does not apply to needle cricothyroidotomy either. This and the preceding section should probably be omitted.

SAFETY/QUALITY TIPS

◻ **Procedural**
+ Needle cricothyrotomy should not be confused with percutaneous cricothyrotomy, in which a Seldinger technique is used to place a tracheostomy tube or small endotracheal tube into the trachea
+ Very little air movement is possible with needle cricothyrotomy; the goal is to oxygenate when all else has failed. Needle cricothyrotomy is generally used when the patient is thought to be too young for conventional open or percutaneous cricothyrotomy.
+ Air can be insufflated into the angiocath using either a specialized transtracheal jet ventilation device or a conventional Ambu bag. A variety of tricks are suggested to allow the bag to be connected to the angiocath; the easiest is using the adaptor on a 3-mm endotracheal tube

◻ **Cognitive**
+ The most important cognitive error around cricothyrotomy is that it is performed too late. You must give yourself permission to cut the neck as soon as intubation and ventilation have failed. An unsuccessful cricothyrotomy performed at the right time is defensible; a successful cricothyrotomy performed too late is indefensible.
+ The materials to perform a cricothyrotomy should be easily accessible at every intubation, preferably at bedside. In higher-risk cases, the sites of the vertical and horizontal incision should be marked on the neck, using a permanent marker. In the highest-risk cases, a double setup should be used with a separate provider standing at bedside with scalpel in hand.
+ Cricothyrotomy is perhaps the most anxiety-provoking procedure in Emergency Medicine. Prepare for it by using simulation, animal, and cadaver labs. Rehearse the procedure mentally so that when the need arises, you are cognitively, emotionally, and spiritually ready.

Suggested Readings

Hebert RB, Base S, Mace SE. Criothyrotomy and percutanous translaryngeal ventilation. In: Roberts RJ, Custalow CB, Thomsen TW, eds. *Roberts and Hedges' Clinical Procedures in Emergency Medicine*. 6th ed. Philadelphia, PA: Elsevier Saunders; 2014:120–133.

Reichman, EF, Freeman CJ. Airway procedures. In: Wolfson AB, ed. *Harwood Nuss' Clinical Practice of Emergency Medicine*. 6th ed. Philadelphia, PA: Lippincott Williams & Wilkins; 2014:12–27.

Vissers RJ, Bair AE. Surgical airway management. In: Walls RM, Murphy MF, eds. *Manual of Emergency Airway Management*. 4th ed. Philadelphia, PA: Lippincott Williams & Wilkins; 2012:193–219.

7

Laryngeal Mask Airway

Czarina E. Sánchez and Matthew Babineau

INDICATIONS

- ⊡ Rescue airway when unable to intubate or difficult ventilation via bag-valve mask (BVM)
- ⊡ Facilitate endotracheal intubation

CONTRAINDICATIONS

- ⊡ **Absolute (When Used as an Airway Rescue Device):** Ability to establish definitive airway with endotracheal intubation
- ⊡ **Relative Contraindications**
  - ✦ High risk of aspiration
    - ✦ Vomiting
    - ✦ Massive hemoptysis or brisk upper gastrointestinal bleeding
  - ✦ Trismus
  - ✦ Laryngeal injuries or tracheal disruption
  - ✦ Recent head and neck radiation
  - ✦ Significant upper airway infection such as epiglottitis
  - ✦ Foreign body in upper airway
  - ✦ Conditions requiring high ventilation pressures (poor pulmonary compliance or increased airway resistance)

LANDMARKS

- ⊡ Insert into oropharynx and advance until mask rests over glottic opening

- ⊡ **General Basic Steps**
  - ✦ **Choose appropriate laryngeal mask airway (LMA) size**
  - ✦ **Deflate and lubricate mask**
  - ✦ **Insert along palate**
  - ✦ **Inflate cuff**
  - ✦ **Confirm placement**
  - ✦ **Secure in place**

TECHNIQUE—STANDARD LARYNGEAL MASK AIRWAY

- ⊡ **Preparation**
  - ✦ Confirm all monitoring equipment is in place and functional, including oxygen saturation probe and cardiac telemetry
  - ✦ Select appropriate LMA size based on estimated patient weight **(TABLE 7.1)**
  - ✦ Assess cuff for air leaks
    - ✦ Inject appropriate amount of air for the selected LMA (Table 7.1)
    - ✦ Deflate while pressing cuff against a flat surface to provide a smooth leading edge for insertion
  - ✦ Apply water-soluble lubricant to distal cuff surface
- ⊡ **Preoxygenation**
  - ✦ Deliver 100% oxygen via nonrebreather mask or BVM ventilation
  - ✦ Administer medications, such as sedatives, if needed

TABLE 7.1. GUIDELINES FOR LARYNGEAL MASK AIRWAY SELECTION AND MASK INFLATION			
LMA size	Weight (kg)	Volume of air inflation (mL)	Maximum ETT size (mm)
1	Neonates/infants <5	4	3.5
1.5	Infants 5–10	7	4.0
2	Infants/children 10–20	10	4.5
2.5	Children 20–30	14	5
3	Children 30–50	20	6.0 cuffed
4	Adults 50–70	30	6.0 cuffed
5	Adults 70–100	40	7.0 cuffed
6	Adults >100	50	7.0 cuffed

LMA, laryngeal mask airway; ETT, endotracheal tube.

Position
+ Use nondominant hand to adjust head position
+ Sniffing position is optimal for nonintubating LMAs
+ May maintain neutral head position if cervical spine immobilization is necessary

Placement
+ Hold LMA in dominant hand like a pencil with index finger placed on airway tube at the tube–mask junction (FIGURE 7.1)
+ Open airway with nondominant hand
+ Insert into oropharynx with aperture facing the tongue (FIGURE 7.2A)
+ Pressing against the hard palate, advance past the posterior border of the tongue
+ Resistance will be noted when the mask rests over the glottic opening (FIGURE 7.2B)
+ Complete insertion by using fingers to push LMA further into the supraglottic region (FIGURE 7.2C)
+ Inflate collar—the increased size will cause LMA to move slightly out of mouth
+ Confirm successful ventilation with end-tidal carbon dioxide ($ETCO_2$) detector and lung auscultation

Protection
+ Secure LMA with tape or tube-securing device

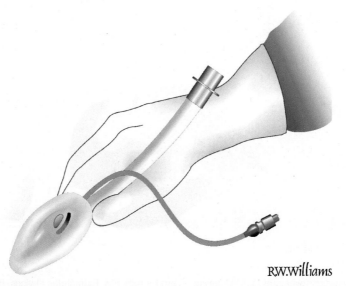

R.W.Williams

FIGURE 7.1 Correct position of the fingers for LMA insertion. From Murphy FM. Extraglottic devices. In: Walls RM, Murphy MF, eds. *Manual of Emergency Airway Management.* 4th ed. Philadelphia, PA: Lippincott Williams & Wilkins; 2012:113–138.

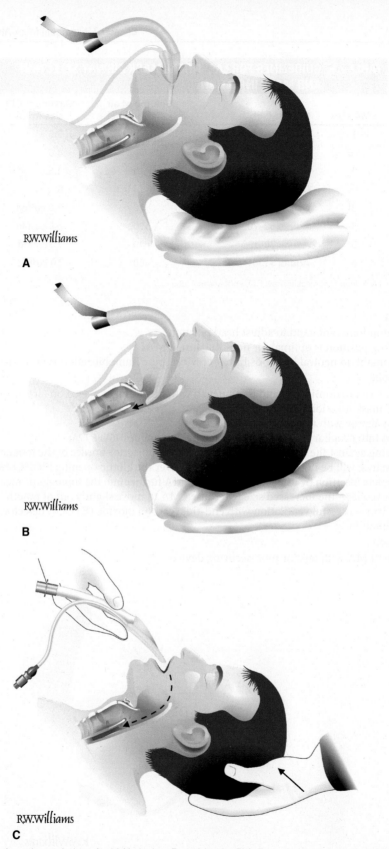

R.W.Williams

A

R.W.Williams

B

R.W.Williams

C

FIGURE 7.2 A–C: Insertion technique for LMA device. From Murphy FM. Extraglottic devices. In: Walls RM, Murphy MF, eds. *Manual of Emergency Airway Management*. 4th ed. Philadelphia, PA: Lippincott Williams & Wilkins; 2012:113–138.

TECHNIQUE—INTUBATING LARYNGEAL MASK AIRWAY

- Ensure integrity of intubating laryngeal mask airway (I-LMA) mask collar and endotracheal tube (ETT) cuff by inflating, then deflating both devices
- Apply lubricant to both I-LMA collar and ETT
- Hold I-LMA by metal handle and insert along the contour of the palate until the device resists further movement (FIGURE 7.3A–C)
- Inflate mask collar
- Connect to BVM and confirm ventilation with $ETCO_2$ detector and auscultation
- Insert ETT through I-LMA lumen with black vertical line facing operator (line indicates correct bevel orientation)
- At the 15-cm mark, ETT is about to emerge from the mask. Advance ETT into trachea while lifting metal handle to improve intubation success (Verghese maneuver; FIGURE 7.4).
- Inflate ETT cuff and confirm tube placement
- Remove I-LMA
  + Deflate I-LMA mask collar
  + Disconnect bag valve from ETT
  + Hold ETT firmly in place with one hand while gently withdrawing the I-LMA. Insert a stabilizer rod into the lumen to prevent dislodgment of the tube.
  + When able to support ETT from inside the mouth, remove the stabilizer rod before fully removing I-LMA
  + Reconnect ETT to continue ventilation

COMPLICATIONS

- **Aspiration**
  + LMA cannot protect against aspiration (main limitation)
  + Gastric inflation from air leak may cause reflux of stomach contents
- **Inadequate Ventilation**
  + Malpositioned device
  + Inappropriate (often too small) LMA size
- **Laryngospasm**
- **Sore Throat**
- **Nerve Damage and Vascular Compression**
  + Although rare, the lingual nerve and blood vessels of the tongue can be compressed by a malpositioned LMA shaft
- **Pulmonary Edema**
  + Reports exist of patients developing negative-pressure pulmonary edema after biting LMA and inhaling against occluded tube

SAFETY/QUALITY TIPS

- **Procedural**
  + Performing a jaw lift while opening the airway may aid LMA insertion. In a sedated patient, a highly effective variant of jaw thrust is reaching into the mouth to grab the mandible and pulling it open and anteriorly.
  + Avoid cricoid pressure during placement
  + If leading edge of LMA is kinking as it is advanced into the oropharynx, insert with mask partially inflated
  + If unable to advance LMA past the tongue, invert device so aperture is facing the palate and rotate into position when LMA has reached the posterior oropharynx
  + If regurgitation occurs, do not remove LMA until after suctioning around mask and into trachea
  + If an I-LMA is not available, a standard LMA can sometimes be used to facilitate blind endotracheal intubation by inserting a gum-elastic bougie through lumen, removing deflated LMA, and passing ETT over bougie into trachea.

(continued)

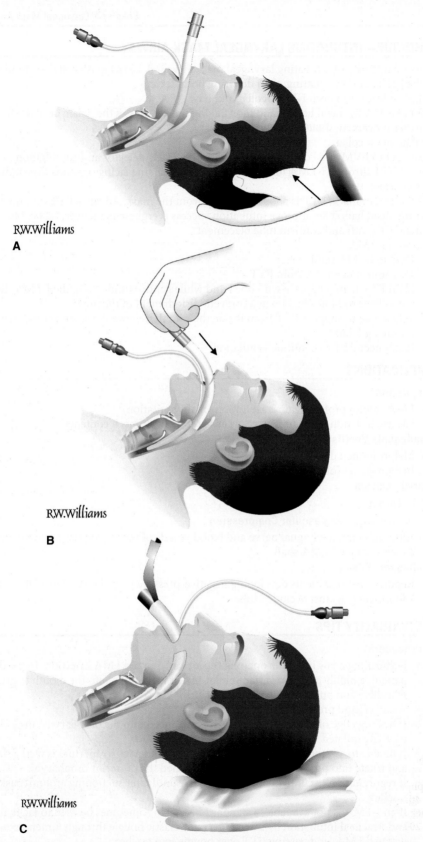

R.W.Williams

A

R.W.Williams

B

R.W.Williams

C

FIGURE 7.3 A–C: Insertion technique for I-LMA device. From Murphy FM. Extraglottic devices. In: Walls RM, Murphy MF, eds. *Manual of Emergency Airway Management*. 4th ed. Philadelphia, PA: Lippincott Williams & Wilkins; 2012:113–138.

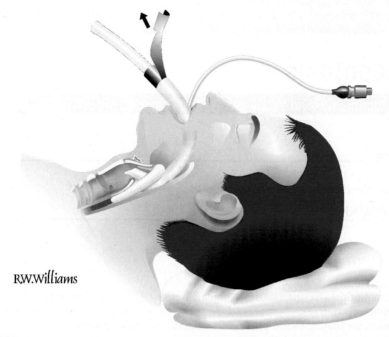

R.W.Williams

FIGURE 7.4 Verghese maneuver in I-LMA insertion. From Murphy FM. Extraglottic devices. In: Walls RM, Murphy MF, eds. *Manual of Emergency Airway Management*. 4th ed. Philadelphia, PA: Lippincott Williams & Wilkins; 2012:113–138.

✚ Cognitive

- ✚ If the patient is in between LMA sizes, select the larger one, which will provide a better seal
- ✚ After placement, avoid aggressive BVM, which can lead to gastric insufflation and aspiration
- ✚ If LMA is being used as a rescue airway device, the operator should simultaneously prepare for surgical airway in the event of LMA failure
- ✚ After placement, the practitioner should consider steps to secure a definitive airway, since LMA devices do not protect from aspiration
- ✚ Ensure adequate sedation and utilize bite block to prevent tube occlusion
- ✚ If the patient desaturates during I-LMA placement, restore normal oxygenation before attempting tracheal intubation
- ✚ If concerned about dislodging ETT with I-LMA removal, I-LMA can be left in place

✚ Acknowledgment

Thank you to prior author Evan Bloom and Lara Kulchycki.

Suggested Readings

Brain AI, Verghese C, Addy EV, et al. The intubating laryngeal mask. II: a preliminary clinical report of a new means of intubating the trachea. *Br J Anaesth*. 1997;79(6):704–709.

Hagberg CA. Layngeal mask airway. In: *Benumof and Hagberg's Airway Management*. 3rd ed. Philadelphia, PA: Saunders; 2013:443–465.

Murphy FM. Extraglottic devices. In: Walls RM, Murphy MF, eds. *Manual of Emergency Airway Management*. 4th ed. Philadelphia, PA: Lippincott Williams & Wilkins; 2012:113–138.

Pollack CV. The laryngeal mask airway: a comprehensive review for the Emergency Physician. *J Emerg Med*. 2001;20(1):53–66.

8

Thoracentesis

Sarah W. Tochman, David W. Callaway, and Daniel C. McGillicuddy

INDICATIONS

- Diagnostic: Acquisition of pleural fluid for analysis
- Therapeutic: Relief of respiratory distress caused by pleural fluid

CONTRAINDICATIONS

- **Absolute**
  - Traumatic hemo- or pneumothorax (tube thoracostomy is more appropriate)
- **Relative**
  - Platelet count <50,000
  - Prothrombin time (PT)/partial thromboplastin time (PTT) >2 × normal
  - Cutaneous infection (e.g., herpes zoster)
  - Mechanical ventilation (small pneumothorax can become a tension)
  - Uncooperative or agitated patient
  - Effusion contralateral to a prior pneumonectomy side

RISKS

Generally an elective procedure. Informed consent is required.

- Injury to lung (tube thoracostomy may be required if a pneumothorax develops)
- Infection (sterile technique will be utilized)
- Injury to liver or spleen
- Pain (local anesthesia will be given)
- Local bleeding

LANDMARKS

- Posterior approach is most common
  - Identify the midscapular line and mark the site one to two rib spaces below the superior portion of the effusion
  - Intercostal neurovascular bundle runs along the inferior portion of the rib. The needle should be inserted superiorly **(FIGURE 8.1)**.
- Hemidiaphragm changes level with respiration. A thoracentesis should not be performed below the eighth intercostal space, given the risk for splenic or hepatic injury.

TECHNIQUE

- **General Basic Steps**
  - **Preparation**
  - **Identify site**
  - **Sterilize**
  - **Analgesia**
  - **Needle insertion**
  - **Aspiration**

- Preparation
  - Place the patient on oxygen
  - Place the patient in upright (most common), lateral decubitus, or supine position
  - Arrange materials on a sterile towel **(FIGURE 8.2)**

Ext. intercostal muscle

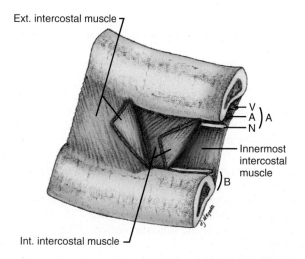

V
A) A
N

Innermost
intercostal
muscle

) B

Int. intercostal muscle

FIGURE 8.1 Relations of structures within an intercostal space **(A)**. Intercostal vessels and nerves are shown in **(B)**. Collateral vessels are shown. *A*, artery; *V*, vein; *N*, nerve.

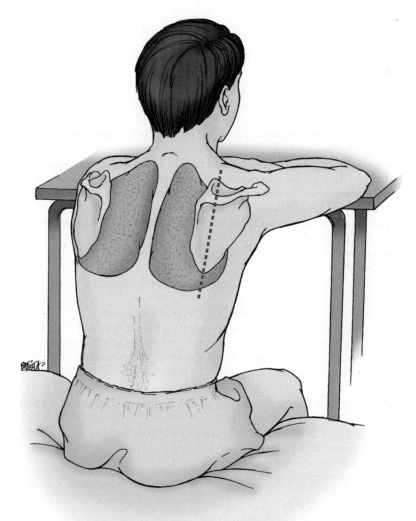

FIGURE 8.2 Landmarks for the posterior approach.

☐ **Identify the Thoracentesis Site**
  ✦ Dullness to percussion, decreased breath sounds, and decreased tactile fremitus can be used to identify the superior margin of the effusion
  ✦ Ultrasound is more accurate than physical examination for identifying effusions
  ✦ Mark needle insertion site one to two rib spaces below the superior margin of the effusion
☐ **Sterilize**
  ✦ Sterilize a wide area surrounding the insertion site
  ✦ Drape the area with sterile towels
  ✦ Observe sterile technique for the remainder of the procedure
☐ **Analgesia**
  ✦ Use lidocaine with epinephrine (1% lidocaine is 10 mg/mL of solution). Usually 5 to 10 mL is required.
  ✦ Inject the subcutaneous tissue with a small-bore (25-gauge) needle and raise a wheal at the superior margin of the selected rib in the midscapular or posterior axillary line
  ✦ Alternating between aspiration and injection, advance to the superior portion of the posterior rib and anesthetize the periosteum
  ✦ Gently advance the needle over the superior portion of the rib while infiltrating with lidocaine
  ✦ Slowly advance the needle while aspirating, until pleural fluid is aspirated. Withdraw the needle 1 to 2 mm and inject 2 to 4 mL of lidocaine to anesthetize the parietal pleura. Though the visceral pleura are not innervated with pain fibers, the parietal pleura are quite sensitive.
  ✦ Mark the depth of the chest wall by grasping the needle at the level of the skin with either your thumb and index finger or a Kelly clamp and withdraw the needle
☐ **Needle Insertion**
  ✦ Make a stab incision parallel to the rib at the marked site for easier insertion of the thoracentesis needle
  ✦ Attach a 60-mL syringe to the catheter-clad needle. Insert the thoracentesis needle, with the bevel inferiorly, through the skin over the selected rib.
  ✦ Advance the needle over the superior portion of the posterior rib, aspirating until pleural fluid is encountered
  ✦ As the catheter enters the pleural space, angle the needle caudally and push the catheter off the needle into the pleural space
  ✦ Occlude the lumen of the catheter (FIGURE 8.3)
☐ **Drain Pleural Fluid**
  ✦ Attach the three-way stopcock to the catheter hub. Set the stopcock valve to occlude the catheter port.
  ✦ Attach the 60-mL syringe to one port of the three-way stopcock
  ✦ Turn the stopcock valve to connect the syringe with the catheter and withdraw fluid from the pleural space. Turn the stopcock to connect the syringe to the intravenous tubing and empty the syringe into the collection bag or bottle. Continue this procedure until no further fluid drainage is desired.
☐ **Postprocedure**
  ✦ When no further fluid can be withdrawn, ask the patient to hum/exhale while the catheter is removed
  ✦ Cover the insertion site with a sterile dressing or adhesive bandage (Band-Aid)
  ✦ Send a Red-top specimen tube (for Gram staining and culture) and a Purple-top specimen tube (for cell count) to the laboratory
  ✦ Indications for chest radiography are:
    + Aspiration of air
    + Hemodynamic instability
    + Shortness of breath during the procedure
    + Multiple needle passes
    + Prior chest radiation therapy
    + Prior thoracentesis
  ✦ Hemodynamic and respiratory monitoring for 1 to 2 hours is recommended

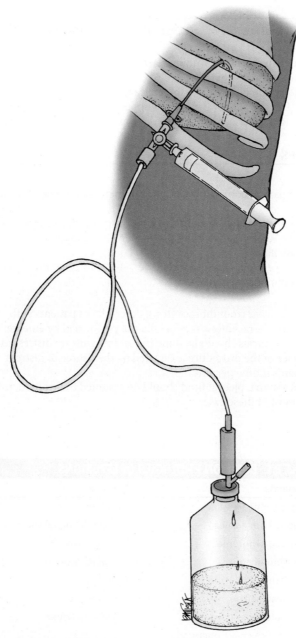

FIGURE 8.3 Needle insertion.

COMPLICATIONS

- Pneumothorax
- Hemopneumothorax
- Lung laceration
- Intra-abdominal injuries
- Diaphragmatic tear
- Hypotension from removal of massive amounts of fluid
- Chest wall bleeding from lacerated intercostal artery
- Reexpansion pulmonary edema
- Development of empyema

FLUID ANALYSIS

The goal of fluid analysis is to identify the etiology of the effusion **(TABLE 8.1)**.

- ☐ Light Criteria
    - ✦ Presence of more than one of the findings is 98% sensitive for exudates
        - ✦ Pleural fluid to serum protein ratio >0.5
        - ✦ Pleural fluid to serum lactate dehydrogenase (LDH) ratio >0.6
        - ✦ Pleural fluid LDH >200 or two-thirds of upper limit of normal serum LDH
    - ✦ Meeting zero of Light criteria is the standard for excluding an exudative effusion

SAFETY/QUALITY TIPS

- ☐ Procedural
    - ✦ Failure to sit the patient completely upright can increase the risk of hepatic or splenic injury
    - ✦ Failure to maintain sterile technique can cause postprocedure empyema
    - ✦ Ultrasound is very useful in detecting the proper needle insertion site, thereby reducing complications **(FIGURE 8.4)**
    - ✦ Therapeutic thoracentesis should not remove >1,000 to 1,500 mL to reduce likelihood of postexpansion pulmonary edema
- ☐ Cognitive
    - ✦ Complications can arise from thoracentesis, especially in patients with underlying lung disease. Diagnostic thoracentesis is generally not performed by emergency physicians. Therapeutic thoracentesis should be done in patients who are distressed by large pleural effusions; the pace of the procedure is dictated by the degree of distress. Do not hesitate to involve consultants if time permits.
    - ✦ In the setting of trauma, pleural fluid should be assumed to be blood; tube thoracostomy is indicated in most of these cases

TABLE 8.1. COMMON ETIOLOGIES OF EFFUSIONS

Transudate	Exudate
Congestive heart failure	Infection
Cirrhosis with ascites	Bacterial pneumonia
Nephrotic syndrome	Lung abscess
Hypoalbuminemia	Tuberculosis
Myxedema	Neoplasm
Peritoneal dialysis	Primary lung
Glomerulonephritides	Mesothelioma
Superior vena cava obstruction	Metastases
Pulmonary embolus	Lymphoma
	Connective tissue disease
	Miscellaneous
	Pulmonary infarct
	Uremia
	Chylothorax

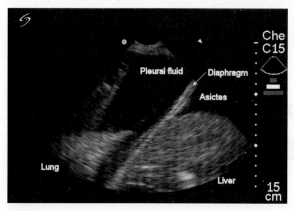

FIGURE 8.4 Ultrasound imaging of pleural effusion.

Acknowledgment

Thank you to prior author David Feller-Kopman.

Suggested Readings

Collins TR, Sahn SA. Thoracentesis. Clinical value, complications, technical problems, and patient experience. *Chest.* 1987;91:817.

Colt HG, Brewer N, Barbur E. Evaluation of patient-related and procedure-related factors contributing to pneumothorax following thoracentesis. *Chest.* 1999;116(1):134–138.

Feller-Kopman D. Ultrasound-guided thoracentesis. *Chest.* 2006;129:1709–1714.

Light RW. Pleural effusion. *N Engl J Med.* 2002;346(25):1971–1977.

Petersen WG, Zimmerman R. Limited utility of chest radiograph after thoracentesis. *Chest.* 2000;117(4):1038–1042.

9

Cardiac Pacing

Christopher K. Hansen

INDICATIONS

- **Hemodynamic instability (presyncope, angina, altered mentation, pulmonary edema) secondary to:**
  - Bradydysrhythmias:
    - Sinus bradycardia
    - Sinus node dysfunction
    - Atrioventricular (AV) node conduction blocks (second and third degree)
    - Acute myocardial infarction with bifascicular block, alternating bundle branch block, new left bundle branch block (LBBB), escape rhythm <40 bpm
    - Malfunctioning permanent pacemaker
    - Electrolyte/metabolic disturbances (i.e., hyperkalemia) if medical therapies fail or are unavailable
    - Post–cardiac surgery (i.e., valve replacement)
    - Thoracic trauma (i.e., cardiac contusion)
    - Other (i.e., lyme carditis, endocarditis)
  - Tachydysrhythmias (overdrive pacing, typically transvenous only):
    - Supraventricular tachycardia (SVT)
    - Ventricular tachycardia (VT)
- **Transvenous Pacing**—same as above, but also including:
  - Failure or nontolerance of transcutaneous pacing
  - Bridge to permanent pacemaker placement
  - High risk of progression to complete heart block
  - Overdrive pacing

CONTRAINDICATIONS

- **Absolute**
  - Asymptomatic, stable rhythms (i.e., first-degree AV block)
  - Prosthetic tricuspid valve (transvenous only)
- **Relative**
  - Severe hypothermia (may be physiologic bradycardia; can induce fibrillation)
  - Brady-asystolic arrest >20 minutes
  - Drug-induced dysrhythmias (although can be utilized as last resort if antidote fails)

TRANSCUTANEOUS PACING PROCEDURE

- **Landmarks**

Pacer pads should preferentially be placed over the precordium anteriorly and in the interscapular paraspinous region posteriorly. Anterolateral pad placement is also acceptable.

- **Supplies**
  - Cardiac monitor with pacemaker capabilities (if electrocardiogram [ECG] monitor is not part of the pacer unit, a separate monitor and adaptor will be required)
  - Adhesive pacing pads
  - ECG electrodes
  - Safety razor

�‌ Technique
✛ **Preparation**
+ In conscious patients, reassurance and explanation of the procedure, including expectations for discomfort, are extremely important
+ Remove excess hair if time permits
+ Continuous cardiac and pulse oximetry monitoring, intravenous access, and bedside capability for resuscitation, including airway management, defibrillation, and arrhythmia treatment, should be at the bedside before initiation
✛ **Pacer/Electrode Placement**
+ Pads are placed as shown in **FIGURE 9.1**
+ Anterior chest pacing pad (negative charge electrode) is placed over the point of maximal impulse
+ If access to the posterior chest wall is limited or difficult, posterior pacer pad may also be placed in cardiac apex/base position (identical to electrical cardioversion placement)
+ ECG electrodes should be placed in limb lead positions for monitoring
✛ **Pacing**
+ Identify pacemaker mode on equipment and turn to "on"
+ Set heart rate to 70 bpm
+ Place and maintain one hand in pulse-check position (radial, femoral, or carotid) or observe noninvasive or invasive blood pressure response
+ In bradyasystole and unconscious patients, set current to 150 to 200 mA and lower in 10-mA decrements; set current at the lowest level that will consistently achieve mechanical capture
+ In stable and conscious patients, set current to 10 mA and raise in 10-mA increments until mechanical capture is achieved
+ Observe cardiac monitor for pacemaker spikes and electrical capture—"electrical capture" refers to narrow pacemaker spikes followed by typically wide ventricular complexes
+ Monitor constantly for "mechanical capture"—a palpable arterial pulse induced by pacemaker discharges or perfusing blood pressure by noninvasive or invasive blood pressure monitoring
+ Titrate sedation/analgesia/anxiolysis to allow for tolerance of ongoing pacing Failure to achieve mechanical capture should prompt immediate preparation for transvenous pacer placement

◌ Complications
+ Unrecognized ventricular fibrillation
+ Local discomfort
+ Cutaneous injury

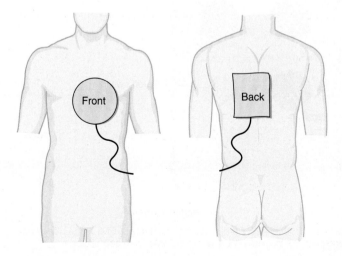

FIGURE 9.1 Proper placement of transcutaneous pacing electrodes. (From Morton PG, Fontaine DK. *Critical Care Nursing.* 10th ed. Philadelphia, PA: Wolters Kluwer Health; 2012.)

SAFETY/QUALITY TIPS

▣ **Procedural**
+ The most common causes of failure to capture in transcutaneous pacing are improper electrode placement or large patient size
+ For many patients, adequate amperage will not be possible without aggressive sedation/analgesia

▣ **Cognitive**
+ Compared to transvenous pacing, transcutaneous pacing is painful and ineffective. Transcutaneous pacing should be thought of as a brief bridge to transvenous pacing or correction of the underlying disorder.
+ Electrical capture is not mechanical capture, and mechanical capture is what counts. Once electrical capture occurs, mechanical capture must be immediately verified using pulses, invasive arterial pressure monitoring, ultrasound, or (most conveniently) pulse oximetry.
+ Be careful not to mistake ventricular fibrillation or tachycardia for a paced rhythm

TRANSVENOUS PACING PROCEDURE

▣ **Landmarks**
+ The **right internal jugular** and **left subclavian** approaches have the advantage of anatomic proximity and directional ease in accessing the superior vena cava

▣ **Supplies**
+ **Pacing Generator** (FIGURE 9.2) contains the following:
  + On/off switch
  + Rate switch (numerical): **70 bpm**

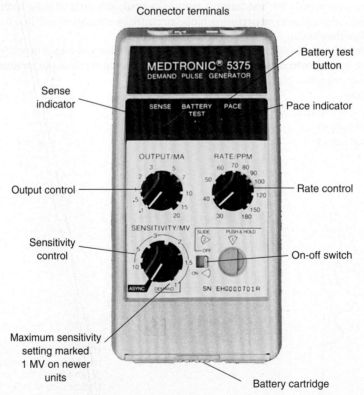

FIGURE 9.2 Medtronic cardiac pacer. (From Kelly KP, Altieri MF. Cardiac pacing. In: Henretig FM, King C. *Textbook of Pediatric Emergency Procedures*. Philadelphia, PA: Williams & Wilkins; 1997:303, with permission.)

+ Demand versus asynchronous switch (detection–sensitivity modes):
    - In "demand" mode, the pacemaker will sense intrinsic cardiac depolarizations and pace only when the intrinsic rate falls below the set rate
    - In "asynchronous" mode, the pacemaker will discharge at the set rate regardless of intrinsic activity. (Some generator units will have an additional numerical sensitivity setting, typically from 20 to 0.5 mV. **Higher** numerical settings cause **less sensitive** detection of intrinsic impulses, while **lower** numerical settings cause **more sensitive** detection.)
+ Output switch (numerical): Determines energy output (mA) per discharge
+ Sense indicator light: Flashes with each detected intrinsic impulse
+ **Flexible Pacing Catheter** (typically 3–5 French, ~100 cm in length) contains the following:
    + Negative and positive terminals at the proximal end
    + Distal balloon (test inflate with 1.5 mL of air)
    + Electrode at the distal tip (delivers the current stimulus)
+ Central venous cannulation equipment—choose an "introducer" sheath **one size larger than the size of the pacing catheter**
+ ECG monitoring
+ If available, an ultrasound unit

Technique
+ **Patient Preparation**
    + Patient should be reassured and the procedure fully explained if possible
    + Physician should wear mask, sterile gown, and sterile gloves
    + Sterile technique should be fully maintained throughout
    + Continuous cardiac and pulse oximetry monitoring should be placed
    + Trendelenburg position is preferred for central venous dilation
+ **Pacemaker Catheter Insertion**
    + Obtain central venous access using the introducer sheath
    + Choose one of three common methods:
        - ECG monitor-assisted
        - Unassisted or blind catheter positioning (for low-flow states)
        - Ultrasound-guided
+ **Electrocardiogram Monitor-Assisted**
    + Attach the **negative terminal** at the proximal end of the pacemaker catheter into the V_1 lead on the ECG monitor, if adaptable (an alligator clamp may be necessary to make the connection)
    + Inflate the balloon with 1.5 mL of air in a container of sterile saline to assess balloon integrity (the presence of bubbles in the saline indicates a balloon leak)
    + Insert the catheter through the introducer sheath into the vein while noting depth
    + After a **10-cm insertion depth**, inflate the balloon with 1.5 mL of air
    + While advancing the catheter, monitor P waves and QRS complexes to determine the location of the catheter tip
    + P wave and QRS morphology correlates with catheter position (**FIGURE 9.3**) as follows:
        - Subclavian/internal jugular vein: P wave and QRS are small, negative
        - Superior vena cava: Larger P wave, QRS unchanged
        - High right atrium: Very large P wave, QRS unchanged
        - Low right atrium: Large positive P wave, larger negative QRS
        - Right ventricle: Small positive P wave, large negative QRS
        - Abutting the right ventricular wall: Injury pattern (ST elevation)
        - Pulmonary artery: P wave negative, QRS becomes smaller
        - Inferior vena cava: P wave positive, QRS negative, both smaller
    + If the catheter is in the pulmonary circulation or inferior vena cava, withdraw 3 to 5 cm until typical right ventricular morphology appears, rotate catheter 90 degrees in either direction, advance again
    + Begin pacing as described in "Pacing" section below.

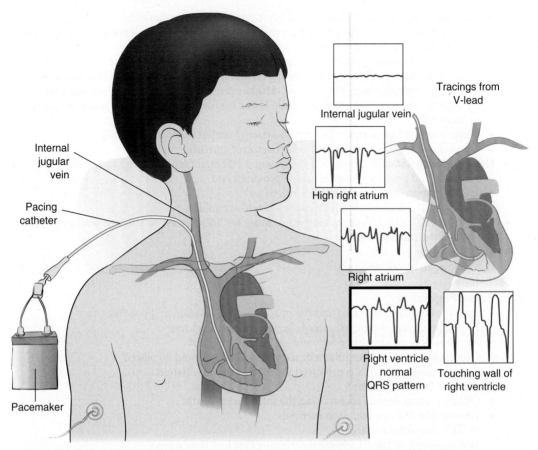

FIGURE 9.3 Transvenous pacemaker placement via the right internal jugular vein. (From Kelly KP, Altieri MF. Cardiac pacing. In: Henretig FM, King C. *Textbook of Pediatric Emergency Procedures.* Philadelphia, PA: Williams & Wilkins; 1997:304, with permission.)

+ **Unassisted or Blind Catheter Positioning in Low-Flow States**
  + Connect the pacemaker catheter to the generator by both electrodes and turn to "on"
  + Set to **Asynchronous mode, 100 bpm, maximal** output
  + If a balloon-tipped pacemaker is used, test balloon integrity as explained earlier
  + Insert the catheter through the introducer sheath into the vein while noting depth
  + After 10-cm insertion depth, inflate the balloon with 1.5 mL of air and lock in place
  + Advance the pacing wire, blindly, until electrical and mechanical capture are attained, as noted by ECG tracing on cardiac monitor and hemodynamic response (capture should be expected approximately 30 cm from the right internal jugular vein site)
  + If ventricular capture is not successful within 10 cm, withdraw the catheter 10 cm, rotate it 90 degrees, and readvance. Repeat until capture is successful.
+ **Ultrasound-Guided Catheter Positioning**
  + As above in "Blind Catheter Positioning," plus the following:
  + Visualize the heart utilizing the **subxiphoid window**
  + Advance the catheter until it is visualized entering the right atrium and right ventricle **(FIGURE 9.4)**
  + Once in the right ventricle, stop advancing the catheter and deflate the balloon
  + Slowly advance until ventricular capture is achieved
+ **Pacing**
  + If utilizing the ECG monitoring technique, disconnect the negative electrode (from the V_1 lead) and reattach to the negative port in the generator

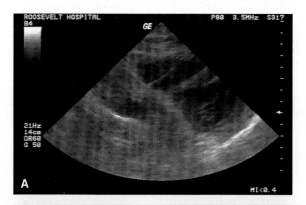

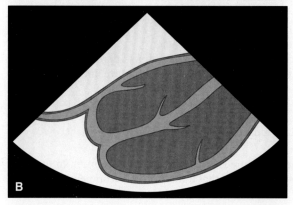

FIGURE 9.4 Subcostal view of the heart with the pacing wire in the right ventricle. **A:** Photograph. **B:** Schematic drawing. (Photograph courtesy of Amir Darvish, MD.)

+ Keep generator on
+ Turn the pacer on (asynchronous mode, 70 bpm, 5-mA energy output)
+ Increase energy output dial until electrical capture (pacing spikes, wide QRS)
+ Check for mechanical capture (corresponding pulses or blood pressure response with each electrical capture)
+ Once mechanical capture is achieved, decrease output until mechanical capture is lost ("threshold point"), and resume at twice the amperage of this point

+ **Testing Threshold**
    + **Threshold** is the minimum current necessary to obtain capture
    + Set the pacer to maximum sensitivity and 5-mA output
    + Reduce output until capture is lost. This amount of current is threshold (usually 0.3–0.7 mA)
    + Increase the output 2.5 times threshold to maintain adequate capture

+ **Testing Sensitivity**
    + **Sensitivity** is the ability of the pacer to detect the intrinsic electrical activity of the heart. In demand mode, the pacemaker will not fire if the patient's ventricular rate is faster than the pacing rate. Decreasing the sensitivity improves the sensing of the pacer.
    + Ensure good capture, then set the rate 10 bpm faster than the intrinsic rate (sensitivity turned all the way up)
    + Decrease the sensing to 3 mV
    + Decrease the pacing rate until the pacer is suppressed by the patient's intrinsic rate. If the pacer does not sense the intrinsic rhythm, turn down the sensing from 3 mV until the pacer is suppressed.

+ **Secure the Pacemaker**
    + Once mechanical capture is achieved, withdraw the introducer sheath, suture the catheter to the chest wall with a 3-0 nylon, and apply sterile dressing

+ **Confirmation**
  + An LBBB pattern should be seen on the 12-lead ECG during pacing
  + Obtain a chest x-ray to confirm right ventricle placement and rule out pneumothorax
  + Bedside ultrasound can also be useful in determining ventricular capture
+ **Complications**
  + Identical to those related to central venous cannulation
  + Right ventricular perforation with diaphragmatic pacing, hemopericardium, and tamponade
  + Displacement or fracture of the electrode, causing loss of capture or dysrhythmias
  + Ventricular dysrhythmias (rare)
  + Left ventricular pacing from atrial septal defect (ASD) or ventricular septal defect (VSD)

SAFETY/QUALITY TIPS

+ **Procedural**
  + Use the introducer that comes with the pacer wire, if available
  + Remember to test the balloon prior to placement of the catheter
  + The right internal jugular or left subclavian veins are the most direct approaches
  + Consider lead fracture if unable to attain electrical or mechanical capture in transvenous pacing after several attempts
  + Suspect septal perforation if increase in pacing threshold or change from LBBB pattern to right bundle branch block (RBBB) pattern noted
  + Always obtain a chest x-ray after placing a pacemaker to confirm lead placement
+ **Cognitive**
  + The most time-consuming part of the procedure is often placing the introducer. In the stable but concerned patient, place the catheter, so that if the patient decompensates, the pacer can be inserted expeditiously.
  + Electrical capture is not mechanical capture, and mechanical capture is what counts. Once electrical capture occurs, mechanical capture must be immediately verified using pulses, invasive arterial pressure monitoring, ultrasound, or (most conveniently) pulse oximetry.
  + Be careful not to mistake ventricular fibrillation or tachycardia for a paced rhythm

+ **Acknowledgment**

Thank you to prior author Oscar Rago and Richard Lanoix.

Suggested Readings

Birkhahn R, Gaeta TJ, Tloczkowski J, et al. Emergency medicine-trained physicians are proficient in the insertion of transvenous pacemakers. *Ann Emerg Med*. 2004;43:469–474.

Holger JS, Lamon RP, Minnigan HJ, et al. Use of ultrasound to determine ventricular capture in transcutaneous pacing. *Am J Emerg Med*. 2003;21:227.

Roberts J, Hedges J. *Clinical Procedures in Emergency Medicine*. 4th ed. Philadelphia, PA: WB Saunders; 2004.

10

Emergency Pericardiocentesis

Jason D'Amore and Hiral H. Shah

INDICATIONS

- Pericardial tamponade with hemodynamic decompensation
- Pulseless electrical activity with clinical suspicion of tamponade or with ultrasonographic evidence of pericardial effusion

CONTRAINDICATIONS

- None for the unstable patient
- Coagulopathy is a relative contraindication

RISKS/CONSENT

- In the emergent situation no consent is required. Consent is implied.
- For risks, see "Complications" section below

LANDMARKS

- **Anatomic Approaches**
  - Subxiphoid
    - Needle is inserted between the xiphoid process and the left costal margin in a 30- to 45-degree angle to the skin
    - Recommendations regarding needle aim vary widely, including right shoulder, sternal notch, and left shoulder
  - Parasternal approach (more common with bedside ultrasonography)
    - Needle is inserted perpendicular to the skin in the left fifth intercostal space immediately lateral to the sternum
  - Ultrasound-guided approach
    - Place a 3.5- to 5.0-MHz probe in the subcostal position to directly visualize both the area of maximal effusion and location of vital structures
    - Insert needle in the left chest wall using a parasternal approach where the largest pocket of fluid is seen

- **General Basic Steps**
  - **Semiupright position**
  - **Local analgesia**
  - **Sterilize local area**
  - **Insert 18-gauge spinal needle**
  - **Aspirate while advancing**

TECHNIQUE

- **Patient Preparation**
  - A 100% oxygen via face mask should be administered if patient is conscious and nonintubated. Consider transiently decreasing tidal volume by 10% to 15% for intubated patients.
  - Ensure continuous cardiac and pulse oximetry monitoring
  - Patient should be placed in the semiupright position (15–30 degrees) if possible to pool pericardial fluid dependently

+ If the patient is awake, local analgesia should be utilized
+ Sterilize locally with chlorhexidine or povidone–iodine solution, and use sterile gloves and universal precautions

Procedural Steps

+ Attach an 18-gauge spinal needle to a 10- to 30-mL syringe
+ Attach an alligator clip to the base of the needle and the other end to the precordial (V) lead of the electrocardiogram (ECG) machine to monitor for ST elevations indicating penetration of the myocardium (**FIGURES 10.1–10.3**)
+ Using either a subxiphoid or parasternal approach (see "Landmarks" section above for details), insert and advance the spinal needle while gently aspirating the syringe, preferably with ultrasonographic assistance

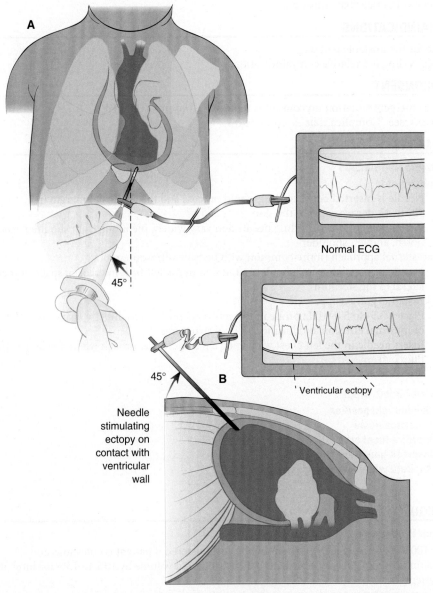

Normal ECG

45°

45° B

Ventricular ectopy

Needle
stimulating
ectopy on
contact with
ventricular
wall

FIGURE 10.1 Attaching an ECG lead to the pericardiocentesis needle will allow you to identify when the needle contacts the ventricular wall. (From Reeves SD. Pericardiocentesis. In: Henretig FM, King C, eds. *Textbook of Pediatric Emergency Procedures.* Philadelphia, PA: Williams & Wilkins; 1997:780, with permission.)

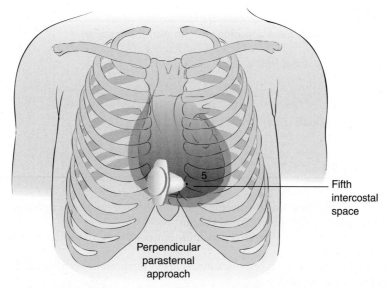

FIGURE 10.2 Pericardiocentesis in adolescent using parasternal approach. (From Reeves SD. Pericardiocentesis. In: Henretig FM, King C, eds. *Textbook of Pediatric Emergency Procedures.* Philadelphia, PA: Williams & Wilkins; 1997:780, with permission.)

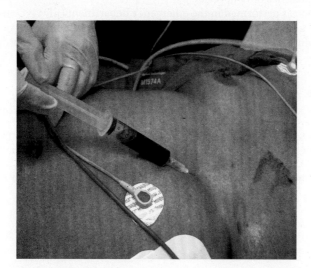

FIGURE 10.3 Emergency pericardiocentesis. (From Wiler J. Pericardiocentesis. In: Greenberg MI, Hendrickson RG, Silverberg M, et al. *Greenberg's Text-atlas of Emergency Medicine.* Philadelphia, PA: Lippincott Williams & Wilkins; 2005:29, with permission.)

- ✛ Pericardium should be reached at approximately 6 to 8 cm below the skin in adults
- ✛ Stop advancing once the fluid is aspirated
- ✛ Remove as much fluid as possible
- ✛ Remove the needle when done
- ✛ If the patient is successfully resuscitated, check for pneumothorax with portable (preferably upright) chest x-ray (CXR) and bedside sonographic lung sliding sign
- ▣ **Confirmation**
  - ✛ Aspiration of blood may indicate cardiac puncture or hemorrhagic pericardial fluid
  - ✛ Clotting of blood does not confirm intracardiac aspirate (brisk bleeding can cause hemorrhagic pericardial fluid to clot)
  - ✛ Nonclotting blood confirms a pericardial source (defibrinated)
  - ✛ Nonbloody fluid confirms a pericardial source

COMPLICATIONS

- Dry tap (no fluid aspirated, more common without ultrasonography)
- Pneumothorax
- Myocardial or coronary vessel injury
- Hemopericardium
- Air embolism
- Dysrhythmias
- Cardiac arrest and/or death (rare)
- Liver injury

SAFETY/QUALITY TIPS

- **Procedural**
  - A common error is inserting the needle below the xiphoid process as opposed to between the xiphoid process and the left costal margin
  - We recommend ultrasound-guided pericardiocentesis over the landmark approach whenever possible
  - Pneumothorax is a common complication; rule out pneumothorax after either a successful or unsuccessful procedure
- **Cognitive**
  - Most complications occur in patients who have no pericardial effusion; use ultrasound to confirm the presence of tamponade
  - Pericardiocentesis performed in the emergency department (ED) is generally a temporizing measure, and most patients will need a more definitive procedure such as a pericardial window. Cardiothoracic surgery involvement is always appropriate.

Suggested Readings

Alan Heffner. Emergency pericardiocentesis. *Uptodate*.com http://www.uptodate.com/contents/emergency-pericardiocentesis#H1617332

Mallemat HA, Tewelde SZ. Pericardiocentesis. In: Roberts JR, Custalow CB, Thomsen TW, et al., eds. *Roberts & Hedges' Clinical Procedures in Emergency Medicine*. 6th ed. Philadelphia, PA: WB Saunders; 2013.

Markovchick VJ. Pericardiocentesis. Rosen P, Chan T, Vilke G, et al. *Atlas of Emergency Procedures*. 5th ed. Maryland Heights, MO: Mosby; 2001.

11

Bedside Echocardiography

Lindsey Lawrence and Daniel Lakoff

INDICATIONS

- ✚ Identifying the presence or absence of cardiac activity in cardiac arrest
- ✚ Identifying the presence or absence of pericardial effusion and differentiating from pleural effusion
- ✚ Identifying the presence or absence of cardiac tamponade
- ✚ Assessing regional wall motion abnormalities in the diagnosis of myocardial infarction
- ✚ Assessing right ventricular size and function in cases suspicious for pulmonary embolism

CONTRAINDICATIONS

- ✚ None: No contrast or radiation involved

PROBE SELECTION AND IMAGING

- ✚ Use a standard 2.0- to 5.0-MHz microconvex or phased-array probe
- ✚ At least two of the four views of the heart are required for diagnosis and billing
- ✚ Orient the probe marker to the top left of the screen
- ✚ Methods of enhancing image acquisition include the following:
  - ✦ Keep the complete ultrasound probe in contact with the chest wall and angle, rotate, and tilt the ultrasound probe as necessary
  - ✦ Use an adequate amount of gel during bedside echocardiography
  - ✦ Try alternative cardiac echocardiography views
  - ✦ Turn the patient in the left lateral decubitus position to bring the heart closer to the anterior chest wall

LANDMARKS: FOUR STANDARD VIEWS

- ✚ **Subxiphoid (Sx) View:** (FIGURE 11.1)
  - ✦ Place the probe in Sx position of abdomen, facing toward the patient's left shoulder, with the probe marker toward the patient's right
  - ✦ If the heart is not adequately viewed, move the probe to the patient's right using the liver as an acoustic window. Asking the patient to take a deep breath will push the heart inferior toward the probe
  - ✦ A moderate amount of pressure may be required for optimal viewing; however, this view is limited by body habitus and pain
  - ✦ This view's utility is predominantly to assess for cardiac activity or pericardial effusion in the setting of trauma (as a part of the focused abdominal sonography for trauma [FAST] examination)
- ✚ **Parasternal Long (PSL) View:** (FIGURE 11.2)
  - ✦ Place the probe just left of the sternum in the third/fourth intercostal space and directed toward the patient's heart, with the probe marker directed toward the patient's left elbow
  - ✦ This view should be your main view—other views can be obtained by slight changes in probe positioning from here
  - ✦ A proper PSL view requires the apex of the left ventricle (LV), the mitral valve, and the aortic valve to be in view
  - ✦ Just deep to the posterior pericardium is the descending aorta
  - ✦ In this view you can assess regional wall motion, valve function, septal movement, and proximal aorta size, and differentiate pericardial effusion from pleural effusion
- ✚ **Parasternal Short-Axis (PSA) View:** (FIGURE 11.3)
  - ✦ From a PSL view, rotate the probe 90 degrees clockwise (toward the patient's right hip)

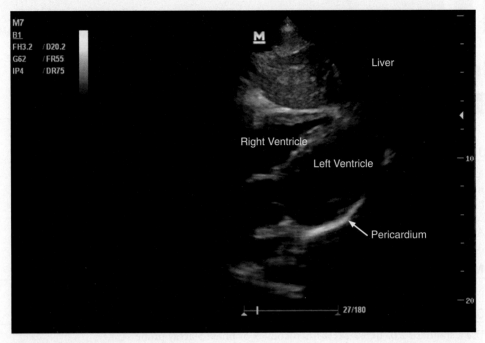

FIGURE 11.1 Subxiphoid view.

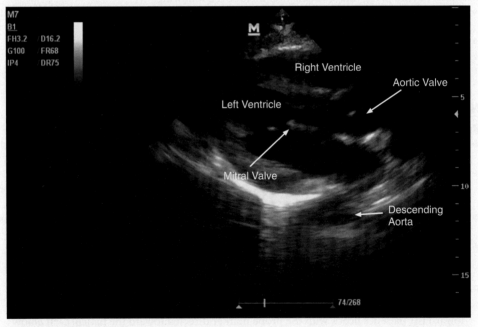

FIGURE 11.2 Parasternal long view.

+ A near circular view of the LV should be visualized
+ Sliding the probe laterally toward the apex demonstrates different regions of the LV from the mitral valve to the apex
+ More precise determination of regional wall motion abnormality can be identified by making an imaginary point in the center of the circular LV and observing all walls moving symmetrically toward that point during systole

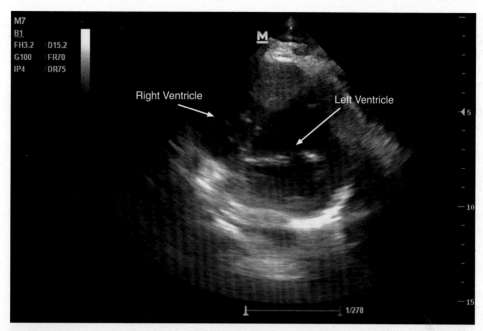

FIGURE 11.3 Parasternal short-axis view.

▣ **Apical Four-Chamber (A4C) View:** (FIGURE 11.4)
- ✦ From a PSA view, slowly move the probe toward the left ventricular apex while flattening the probe to the chest wall until the four chambers come into view
- ✦ Alternatively, place the probe at the presumed point of maximal impulse (PMI), with the probe marker aimed toward the right hip
- ✦ Use an adequate amount of gel for this view
- ✦ In this view you can compare atrial and ventricular sizes as well as assess valvular and septal wall movement

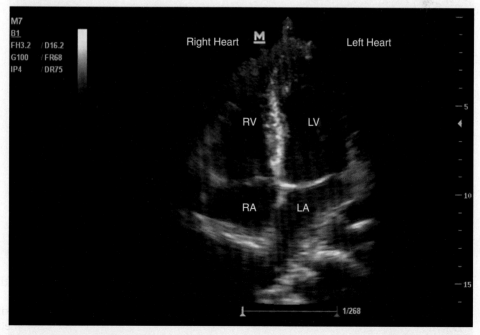

FIGURE 11.4 Apical four-chamber view. LA, left atrium; LV, left ventricle; RA, right atrium; RV, right ventricle.

SONOGRAPHIC SIGNS TO IDENTIFY IN EMERGENCY BEDSIDE ECHOCARDIOGRAPHY

- ☐ **Pericardial Effusion:** (FIGURE 11.5)
  - ✦ Anechoic (dark) fluid collection between the parietal and visceral pericardium
  - ✦ Anterior to the descending aorta on PSL view
  - ✦ An anechoic region anterior to the heart may be an anterior fat pad and may lead to a false-positive study. Closely evaluate for circumferential fluid.
- ☐ **Cardiac Tamponade:** (FIGURE 11.6)
  - ✦ Large amount of pericardial fluid collection with the following:
    - ✦ Right ventricular collapse (indenting the ventricular wall)
    - ✦ Inferior vena cava (IVC) ultrasound should also be performed, which would show a plethoric IVC
- ☐ **Pulmonary Embolism:** (FIGURE 11.7)
  - ✦ Bowing of the right ventricle (RV) into the LV (seen on A4C and PSL views)
  - ✦ Right ventricular dilatation: RV:LV greatest diameter greater than 1:1 (as seen on A4C view)
  - ✦ Right ventricular hypokinesis

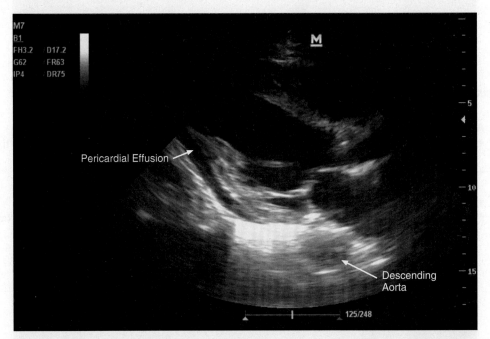

FIGURE 11.5 Parasternal long view with pericardial effusion (identify descending aorta).

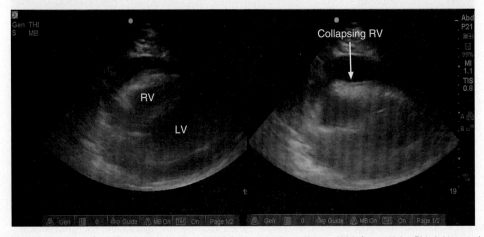

FIGURE 11.6 Subxiphoid view with tamponade with right ventricular collapse. LV, left ventricle; RV, right ventricle.

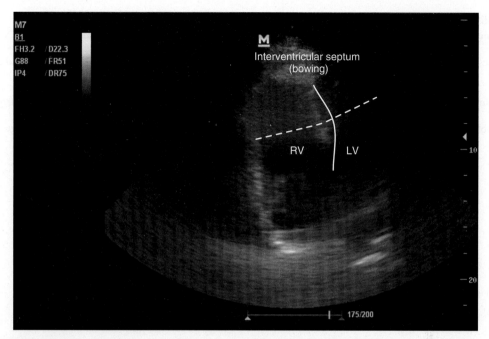

FIGURE 11.7 Apical four-chamber view with enlarged right ventricle and septal bowing. LV, left ventricle; RV, right ventricle.

☐ **Myocardial Ischemia** (visible in real time on both PSL and PSA views):
  ✦ Abnormal wall motion and abnormal ventricular emptying or relaxation
    ✦ Hypokinesis (reduced wall thickening and motion)
    ✦ Akinesis (absent wall thickening and motion)
    ✦ Dyskinesis (paradoxical motion of wall; outward movement of wall during systole)
  ✦ Increased left ventricular size
  ✦ Reduction of left ventricular ejection fraction

SAFETY/QUALITY TIPS

☐ **Procedural**
  ✦ During cardiac arrest, briefly stop ventilations for echocardiography. Motion caused by positive-pressure ventilation can be mistaken for cardiac motion.
  ✦ Patients with subcutaneous emphysema, pneumopericardium, and large anterior–posterior girth can be difficult to image
  ✦ Fluid will appear anechoic. However, a blood clot may be echogenic initially with an anechoic stripe at the borders. Viewing other windows may assist in finding fluid in other areas of the pericardium.
  ✦ In most instances where cardiac sonographic view is inadequate, windows will be improved by turning the patient to the left lateral decubitus position
☐ **Cognitive**
  ✦ Video clips are superior to still images for consultation, educational, and QA (quality assurance) purposes
  ✦ An anterior pericardial fat pad or pleural effusion is commonly mistaken for pericardial effusion
  ✦ In patients with large pericardial effusions, diastolic collapse of the RV indicates emergent pericardial drainage. The sonographic appearance of the RV in these cases has been compared to "a man jumping on a trampoline."
  ✦ Echocardiography may raise or lower the probability of pulmonary embolism, but is not sufficiently accurate to rule in or rule out the disease in the face of contrary evidence
  ✦ Identification of regional wall motion abnormalities is only an accurate indicator of acute myocardial ischemia if the abnormalities are known to be new

Suggested Readings

American College of Emergency Physicians. Policy statement. *Emergency Ultrasound Guidelines*. Dallas, TX: American College of Emergency Physicians; 2008.

Dresden S, Mitchell P, Rahimi L, et al. Right ventricular dilatation on bedside echocardiography performed by emergency physicians aids in the diagnosis of pulmonary embolism. *Ann Emerg Medicine*. 2014;63(1): 16–24.

Mandavia DP, Hoffner RJ, Mahaney K, et al. Bedside echocardiography by emergency physicians. *Ann Emerg Med*. 2001;38(4):377–382.

Noble V, Nelson BP. *Manual of Emergency and Critical Care Ultrasound*. 2nd ed. New York, NY: Cambridge University Press; 2011.

12

Bedside Aorta Ultrasonography

George Lim and Amy Sanghvi

INDICATIONS

- Clinical suspicion of abdominal aortic aneurysm (AAA)
  - Unexplained abdominal, back, or flank pain, particularly in the older patient
  - Unexplained hypotension
  - Syncope in the setting of abdominal pain
  - Palpable and/or pulsatile abdominal mass

CONTRAINDICATIONS

- **None:** No contrast or radiation involved

LANDMARKS

- The proximal aorta is located in the subxiphoid area
- The aorta bifurcates into the iliac vessels at the level of the umbilicus
- On the *ultrasound display* (FIGURE 12.1), first locate the vertebral body. The transverse proximal aorta is located above (anterior to) the vertebral body, to the right of the inferior vena cava (IVC), and below (posterior to) the superior mesenteric artery

TECHNIQUE

- Apply ultrasond gel on the patient's abdomen, from the xiphoid process to just distal to the umbilicus
- Using a standard 3.5- to 5.0-MHz probe with the selection marker to the patient's right, identify the proximal aorta in the epigastric area (FIGURE 12.2)
- Once the aorta is identified, scan the entire length of the vessel to the iliac bifurcation at the umbilicus

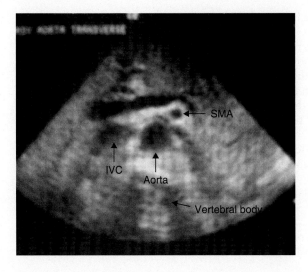

FIGURE 12.1 Transverse proximal aorta anatomy. IVC, inferior vena cava; SMA, superior mesenteric artery. (Courtesy of David Riley, MD.)

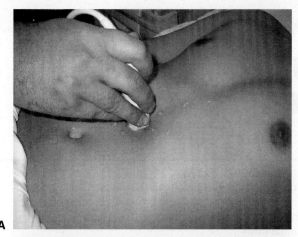

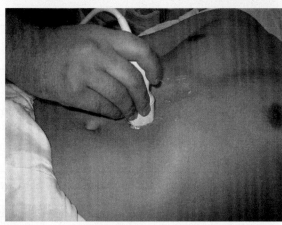

FIGURE 12.2 Ultrasound technique.

▣ Measure the vessel diameter from outer wall to outer wall to avoid underestimation
▣ Vessel measurement in the following views permits adequate screening for AAA (**FIGURE 12.3**):
  ✦ Transverse proximal aorta
  ✦ Transverse middle aorta
  ✦ Transverse distal aorta
  ✦ Transverse view of iliac arteries at the bifurcation
  ✦ Longitudinal aorta
▣ If an aneurysm is detected (**TABLE 12.1**), its relation to the renal arteries and aortic bifurcation should be documented if possible (i.e., proximal, distal)
▣ If the aorta is not readily identified, try the following techniques:
  ✦ Apply gentle downward pressure with the probe to displace bowel gas
  ✦ Increase the depth of penetration on the ultrasound display
  ✦ Reimaging after several minutes may permit improved visualization as intestinal peristalsis displaces bowel
  ✦ Place the patient in the right or left lateral decubitus position
  ✦ Approach para-midline by directing the probe toward the spine to avoid bowel gas
  ✦ Image coronally through the liver
  ✦ Image inferiorly to the umbilicus and direct the probe cephalad

COMPLICATIONS

▣ Delay in definitive surgical treatment in order to perform study. Computed tomography (CT) evaluation typically poses a greater time delay.

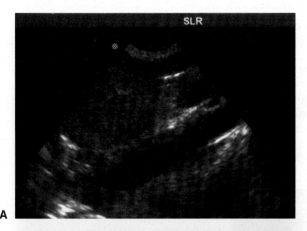

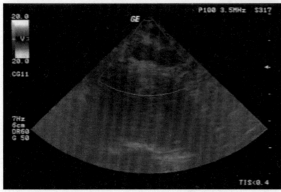

FIGURE 12.3 A: Longitudinal aorta. **B:** Transverse image of the common iliac bifurcation. (Images courtesy of David Riley, MD.)

TABLE 12.1. SONOGRAPHIC SIGNS OF ABDOMINAL AORTIC ANEURYSM
Aortic diameter ≥3 cm
Common iliac artery diameter ≥1.5 cm

SAFETY/QUALITY TIPS

☐ **Procedural**
+ Large body habitus and air, commonly from overlying bowel gas, may prevent adequate visualization. Try increasing probe pressure or repositioning patient.
+ Using color Doppler facilitates identification of vascular structures, and in distinguishing arteries from veins (e.g., the IVC). The aorta is pulsatile, thick-walled, and noncompressible, in contrast to the nonpulsatile, thin-walled, compressible IVC.
+ Measure the aorta from outer wall to outer wall; measuring inner wall to inner wall will result in underestimation of aortic diameter; note that the hypoechoic extramural thrombus may occupy a significant portion of the lumen **(FIGURE 12.4)**.
+ Failure to visualize the entire extent of the abdominal aorta and iliac bifurcation is an ultrasonographic pitfall

☐ **Cognitive**
+ All older patients with hypotension of uncertain etiology should receive point-of-care sonography to exclude AAA (along with other causes of hypotension). AAA mortality increases markedly with delays to diagnosis and repair.
+ Consider mycotic aortic aneurysm in intravenous drug abusers

+ Aneurysm diameter >5 cm is an extremely strong risk factor for rupture; 22% of aneurysms >5 cm in diameter will rupture within 2 years. Surgical repair is generally indicated for AAA >5.5 cm.
+ Free fluid in the abdomen may be absent because AAAs commonly rupture into the retroperitoneum. Ultrasound is a poor imaging modality for this area.
+ Renal colic is the leading misdiagnosis for AAA. Be careful attributing hematuria, flank pain, or hydronephrosis to nephrolithiasis in elderly patients. A large AAA can compress the ureter enough to cause hydronephrosis. AAA can also present as lower extremity weakness and/or numbness.

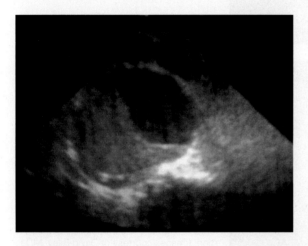

FIGURE 12.4 Large thrombus within the aortic lumen.

▣ Acknowledgment

Thank you to prior author Jessica Paisley and Lekha Ajit Shah.

Suggested Readings

Brewster DC, Cronenwett JL, Hallett JW Jr, et al. Guidelines for the treatment of abdominal aortic aneurysms. *J Vasc Surg.* 2003;37(5):1106.

Nevitt MP, Ballard DJ, Hallet JW Jr. Prognosis of abdominal aortic aneurysms. *N Engl J Med.* 1989;321:1009–1014.

Phalen MP, Emerman CL. Focused aortic ultrasound to evaluate the prevalence of abdominal aortic aneurysm in ED patients with high-risk symptoms. *Am J Emerg Med.* 2006;24(2):227–229.

Rubano E, Mehta N, Caputo W, et al. Systematic review: emergency department bedside ultrasonography for diagnosing suspected abdominal aortic aneurysm. *Acad Emerg Med.* 2011;18(3):227–235.

Tayal VS, Tayal CD, Gibbs MA. Prospective study of accuracy and outcome of emergency ultrasound for abdominal aortic aneurysm over two years. *Acad Emerg Med.* 2003;10:867–871.

13

Induction of Therapeutic Hypothermia

Peter C. England and Ram Parekh

INDICATIONS

⊞ Comatose patients resuscitated from cardiac arrest with restoration of spontaneous circulation (ROSC)

INCLUSION CRITERIA

⊞ Post–cardiac arrest
⊞ ROSC < 30 minutes from the time of EMS arrival
⊞ Time < 6 hours from ROSC
⊞ Comatose (does not follow commands)

EXCLUSION CRITERIA

⊞ **Contraindications**
  + Patients without a pulse
  + Patients responsive to verbal commands
  + Traumatic etiology of arrest
  + Active or intracranial bleeding
  + Patient has DNR, poor baseline status, or terminal illness
  + ROSC >30 minutes from the time of EMS arrival
  + Time of initiation >6 hours from ROSC
  + Pregnancy
  + Age >80 (relative)
  + Asystole as initial rhythm (relative)
  + Severe sepsis/septic shock as cause of arrest (relative)
  + Cryoglobulinemia (relative)

SUPPLIES

⊞ **Temperature Probe**
  + Esophageal
  + Bladder
⊞ **Cooling Methods**
  + Surface cooling with ice packs
  + Surface cooling with blankets or surface heat-exchange device and ice
  + Surface cooling helmet
  + Internal cooling methods using catheter-based technologies
  + Internal cooling methods using infusion of cold fluids
⊞ **Warming Methods**
  + Warm blankets
  + Bair Hugger
  + Room temperature IV fluids

□ **General Basic Steps**
+ **Preparation**
+ **Induction**
+ **Maintenance**
+ **Supportive therapy**
+ **Withdrawal/rewarming**

TECHNIQUE

□ **Patient Preparation**
+ Place definitive airway
+ Completely expose patient
+ Apply cooling blankets or gel pads (if available) with nothing between skin and blankets/pads
+ Place core temperature probe (esophageal preferred)
+ Hook blankets/pads to hypothermia machine, set to 36°C
+ Optimize analgesia and sedation (suggestions below)
    + Analgesia (optimize first): Fentanyl
    + Sedation: Propofol (preferred); alternate: Midazolam
    + Titrate to Richmond Agitation Sedation Scale (RASS) −3/−4 **(TABLE 13.1)**
+ Monitor vital signs and oxygen saturation and place the patient on a continuous cardiac monitor, with particular attention to arrhythmia detection and hypotension

□ **Induction**
+ Keep temperature between 35°C and 36°C
+ If initial temperature >36°C, infuse refrigerated crystalloid at 100 mL/min to maximum initial bolus 30 cc/kg
+ If initial temperature remains >36°C after this amount, wait 15 minutes before giving additional 250-cc boluses every 10 minutes until goal temperature is attained
+ If initial temperature <36°C, allow machine to warm the patient to 35°C
+ Use cold IV fluids or place ice packs on the axilla/groin to reach and maintain target temperature if cooling blankets/pads are unavailable
+ Target temperature should be reached as quickly as possible
+ Start antishivering protocol **(TABLE 13.2)**

TABLE 13.1. RICHMOND AGITATION SEDATION SCALE (RASS)

Score	Term	Description
+4	Combative	Overtly combative, violent, immediate danger to staff
+3	Very agitated	Pulls or removes tube(s) or catheter(s); aggressive
+2	Agitated	Frequent nonpurposeful movement, fights ventilator
+1	Restless	Anxious but movements not aggressive or vigorous
0	Alert and Calm	
−1	Drowsy	Not fully alert, but has sustained awakening
−2	Light sedation	Briefly awakens with eye contact to voice (**<10 seconds**) (eye opening/eye contact) to voice (**≥10 seconds**)
−3	Moderate sedation	Movement or eye opening to voice (**but no eye contact**)
−4	Deep sedation	No response to voice, but movement or eye opening to physical stimulation
−5	Unarousable	No response to voice or physical stimulation

TABLE 13.2. ANTISHIVERING PROTOCOL

Bedside shivering assessment (BSAS) (N. Badjatia. Neurocrit Care 2007)

0 – None—no shivering. Must not have shivering on ECG or palpation.

1 – Mild—localized to neck/thorax. May be noticed only on palpation or ECG.

2 – Moderate—intermittent involvement of upper extremities with or without thorax.

3 – Severe—generalized shivering or sustained upper extremity shivering.

All patients receive:

Acetaminophen 850 mg GT q6h unless allergic and buspirone 30 mg GT q8h (unless pt on MAO inhibitor)

- If BSAS >1, add fentanyl drip
- If BSAS still >1, add propofol drip
- If BSAS still >1, add Bair Hugger device for counterwarming on both of patient's arms
- If BSAS still >1, administer $MgSO_4$ 2 g IVSS (intravenous soluset), then 0.5–1 g/h for target serum Mg 3 mg/dL
- If BSAS still >1, administer dexmedetomidine 1 µg/kg over 10 min, followed by an infusion
- If BSAS still >1, administer ketamine 0.5 mg/kg IVP (intravenous push), may start drip at same dose per hour
- If BSAS still >1 after titration of above meds, add Nimbex 0.15 mg/kg IV q1h PRN

Paralysis after induction should be necessary only under extraordinary circumstances.

ECG, electrocardiography; GT, via gastric tube; MAO, monoamine oxidase; pt, patient.

- **Maintenance**
  + Continue to monitor and maintain body temperature at 36°C for a total of 24 hours
  + If the patient's temperature rises above 36°C, infuse 250-cc boluses of cold crystalloid every 10 minutes until <36°C
  + Remove cold packs or use IV fluids at room temperature if body temperature drops below 34°C (if cooling machine is not employed)
  + Continue medications as needed for sedation, analgesia, and shivering prophylaxis
- **Supportive Therapy**
  + A mean arterial pressure (MAP) goal of more than 80 mm Hg is preferred
  + Norepinephrine with or without dobutamine can be used
  + Practice standard neuroprotective strategies such as placing the head of the bed at 30 degrees
  + Monitor for arrhythmia (most commonly bradycardia) associated with hypothermia
  + If life-threatening dysrhythmia arises and persists, or hemodynamic instability or bleeding develops, discontinue active cooling and rewarm the patient, although this should not occur at current temperature recommendations
  + Do not provide nutrition to the patient during the initiation, maintenance, or rewarming phases of the therapy
  + Consider stress ulcer prophylaxis
  + Consider deep vein thrombosis (DVT) prophylaxis
  + Keep glucose <180 mg/dL (insulin infusion preferred)
  + Keep magnesium at high normal
  + Replete K if <3.4 mEq/L with IV KCl
  + Keep sodium at least 140 mEq/L at all times, 150 mEq/L is preferable
  + Keep ionized calcium at high normal at all times
- **Withdrawal**
  + After 24 hours of hypothermia, remove commercial cooling blanket and begin passive rewarming of the patient with warm blankets and IV fluids at room temperature to raise the body temperature back to normal
  + Rewarm at a rate no faster than 0.5°C per hour
  + Monitor the patient for hypotension secondary to vasodilation related to rewarming
  + Avoid rebound hyperthermia

COMPLICATIONS

- Shivering, cardiac arrhythmia, sepsis, coagulopathy, electrolytes, and metabolic disturbances have been reported with prior hypothermia targets (33°C), but should be infrequently encountered in the updated protocol (36°C target)

SAFETY/QUALITY TIPS

- **Procedural**
  + Set the cooling machine to *automatic mode*, avoiding the need to adjust temperature settings if goal temperature is overshot
  + Placement of an esophageal temperature probe may require a conduit: Use an endotracheal tube in the posterior pharynx to facilitate probe passage. Probe should be advanced to premeasured midsternum.
- **Cognitive**
  + Favorable outcomes from targeted temperature management in post–cardiac arrest care rely on high-quality critical care practices such as lung protective ventilation, assiduous pulmonary toilet, and fluid management
  + Many patients will benefit from postarrest percutaneous coronary intervention (PCI); look for signs of coronary ischemia postarrest (electrocardiography [ECG], echocardiography, biomarkers) and involve a cardiologist in these cases. Hypothermia should be continued during PCI.
  + If a cardiac insult does not appear to be the cause of cardiac arrest, consider subarachnoid hemorrhage and other intracranial catastrophes as an etiology
  + If serum lactate is rising after goal temperature is reached, consider ongoing seizures as an etiology—immediate electroencephalography (EEG) is the test of interest

AUTHOR'S NOTES

- The variables of timing of the initiation of cooling, cooling technique, rate, depth, and length of cooling and rewarming recommended in this chapter are the author's recommendations based on careful analysis of the current literature. At this time, these variables are not well studied and are the focus of several current clinical trials.
- Therapeutic hypothermia initiation, maintenance, and rewarming, followed by subsequent neuroprognostication requires close management and monitoring and presupposes the availability of hospital resources both in the emergency department and in the intensive care unit.

- **Acknowledgment**

Thank you to prior author Alberto Hazan.

Suggested Readings

Bernard SA, Gray TW, Buist MD, et al. Treatment of comatose survivors of out-of-hospital cardiac arrest with induced hypothermia. *N Engl J Med.* 2002;346:557–563.

Badjatia N. Assessment of the metabolic impact of shivering: The Bedside Shivering Assessment Scale (BSAS). *Neurocrit Care.* 2007;6:228

Holzer M, Mortens P, Roine R, et al; for The Hypothermia After Cardiac Arrest Study Group. Mild therapeutic hypothermia to improve the neurologic outcome after cardiac arrest. *N Engl J Med.* 2002;346:549–556.

Nielsen N, Wetterslev J, Cronberg T, et al; for the TTM Trail Investigators. Targeted temperature management at 33°C versus 36°C after cardiac arrest. *N Engl J Med.* 2013;369:2197–2206.

14

Tube Thoracostomy

Chilembwe Mason

INDICATIONS

To evacuate abnormal collections of air or fluid from the pleural space in the following conditions:
- Pneumothorax
- Hemothorax
- Chylothorax
- Empyema
- Recurrent pleural effusion
- Prevention of hydrothorax after cardiothoracic surgery

CONTRAINDICATIONS

- None for unstable injured patients
- **Relative Contraindications**
  + Anatomic abnormalities—pleural adhesions, emphysematous blebs, or scarring
  + Coagulopathy

LANDMARKS

- The fourth or fifth intercostal space at the mid- to anterior axillary line, but multiple sites are possible (**FIGURE 14.1**)
- Intercostal nerve and vessels are located along the inferior margin of each rib; therefore, the tube should pass immediately over the superior surface of the lower rib

SUPPLIES

- Antiseptic solution, drapes, and towel clips
- 1% Lidocaine, 20 mL
- 25- and 22-gauge needles and 10-mL syringe
- No. 10 scalpel blade with handle, Kelly clamps (two), and forceps
- Thoracostomy tube selection
  + Trauma: No. 36–40 French
  + Nontraumatic: No. 24–32 French
  + Children: No. 20–24 French
  + Infants: No. 18 French
- Pleur-evac (collection bottle, underwater seal, suction control)
- Connecting tubing
- Gauze pads, adhesive tape, 4″ × 4″ pads, Xeroform gauze dressing
- 2, 1, or 0 suture (not 2-0 or 1-0), needle driver, and suture scissors

- **General Basic Steps**
  + **Analgesia**
  + **Incision**
  + **Blunt dissection**
  + **Verification**
  + **Insertion**
  + **Securing the tube**
  + **Confirmation**

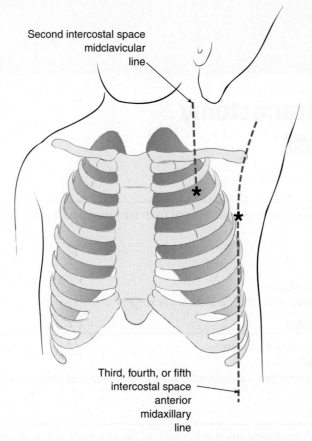

Second intercostal space
midclavicular
line

* *

Third, fourth, or fifth
intercostal space
anterior
midaxillary
line

FIGURE 14.1 Possible sites for chest tube placement. (From Connors KM, Terndrup TE. Tube thoracostomy and needle decompression of the chest. In: Henretig FM, King C, eds. *Textbook of Pediatric Emergency Procedures.* Philadelphia, PA: Lippincott Williams & Wilkins; 1997:399.)

TECHNIQUE

- **Preparation**
  - ✚ Oxygen and continuous pulse oximetry monitoring
  - ✚ If the patient is stable, administer parenteral analgesics or procedural sedation
  - ✚ Elevate the head of the bed to 30 to 60 degrees
  - ✚ Arm on the affected side is placed over the patient's head
  - ✚ Sterilize the area where the tube will be inserted with povidone–iodine or chlorhexidine solution
  - ✚ Drape the area with sterile towels
  - ✚ Assemble the suction-drain system according to manufacturer's recommendations; adjust the suction until a steady stream of bubbles is produced in the water column
- **Analgesia**
  - ✚ Produce local anesthesia using up to 5 mg/kg of 1% lidocaine with epinephrine (1:100,000)
  - ✚ Inject the subcutaneous area with a small-bore (25-gauge) needle
  - ✚ Generously infiltrate the muscle, periosteum, and parietal pleura in the area of the tube's eventual passage using a larger-bore needle
- **Incision**
  - ✚ Using a no. 10 scalpel blade, make at least a 3- to 4-cm transverse incision through the skin and subcutaneous tissue

- One method is to make the incision at an intercostal space lower than the thoracic wall entry site so that the tube may be "tunneled" up over the next rib
- ⊡ **Blunt Dissection**
  - Use a large Kelly clamp or scissor (this often takes considerable force)
  - Track is created over the rib by pushing forward with the closed points and then spreading and pulling back with the points spread
  - Push through the muscle and parietal pleura with the closed points of the clamp until the pleural cavity is entered
  - A palpable pop is felt when the pleura is penetrated, and a rush of air or fluid should occur at this point
- ⊡ **Verification**
  - Once the pleura is penetrated, insert a gloved finger into the chest wall track to verify that the pleura has been entered and that no solid organs are present
  - The finger can be left in place to serve as a guide for tube insertion
- ⊡ **Insertion**
  - It is recommended that the tube be held in a large curved clamp with the tip of the tube protruding from the jaws
  - Pass the tube over, under, or beside the finger into the pleural space
  - The tube is advanced superiorly, medially, and posteriorly until pain is felt or resistance is met; then it is pulled back 2 to 3 cm
  - Ensure that all the holes in the chest tube are within the pleural space
- ⊡ **Securing the Tube (numerous methods are acceptable)**
  - Close the remainder of the incision using a large 0 or 1 silk or nylon suture, keeping the ends long
  - Suture ends are wrapped and tied repeatedly around the chest tube, then knotted securely. The sutures are tied tightly enough to indent the chest tube slightly to avoid slippage.
  - A horizontal mattress (or purse-string) suture is placed approximately 1 cm across the incision on either side of the tube, essentially encircling the tube. This suture helps secure the tube and eventually facilitates closing the incision when the chest tube is removed.
  - Place occlusive dressing of petroleum-impregnated gauze where the tube enters the skin; then cover with two or more gauze pads
  - Wide cloth adhesive tape can be used to hold the tube more securely in place
- ⊡ **Confirmation**
  - Indicators for correct placement are as follows:
    - Condensation on the inside of the tube
    - Audible air movement with respirations
    - Free flow of blood or fluid
    - Ability to rotate the tube freely after insertion
  - Attach tube to previously assembled water seal or suction
    - Observing bubbles in the water seal chamber when the patient coughs is a good way to check for system patency
  - Obtain a chest radiograph

COMPLICATIONS

- ⊡ Hemothorax
- ⊡ Pulmonary edema
- ⊡ Bronchopleural fistula
- ⊡ Empyema
- ⊡ Subcutaneous emphysema
- ⊡ Infection
- ⊡ Contralateral pneumothorax
- ⊡ Subdiaphragmatic placement of the tube
- ⊡ Localized hemorrhage

SAFETY/QUALITY TIPS

▣ **Procedural**

+ The more urgent the chest tube, the less local anesthesia and the more systemic sedation/analgesia, for purposes of speed. In a chest tube required for emergent hemodynamic stabilization, it is reasonable to skip local anesthesia completely and place the chest tube after, for example, a dissociating dose of ketamine.
+ The more urgent the chest tube, the larger the size of the initial skin incision, for purposes of speed
+ Do not use the trocar that comes with many chest tubes. Trocar use is associated with solid organ injury.
+ We recommend inserting the chest tube over a finger that remains in the thorax, to minimize the likelihood of a misdirected chest tube. When a chest tube is advanced blindly through a track, subcutaneous placement is a common complication.
+ Clamp both ends of the tube during insertion to avoid being contaminated by fluid
+ Gently but assertively advance the chest tube completely into the pleural space
+ Avoid causing a contralateral pneumothorax by not directing the tube toward the mediastinum

▣ **Cognitive**

+ Tube thoracostomy for unstable patients, as well as tube thoracostomy for stable patients without complicated lung disease (e.g., primary spontaneous pneumothorax), is well within the domain of emergency medicine. Caution and consultation are advised in placing chest tubes on stable patients with complicated lung disease.
+ Primary spontaneous pneumothorax can and often should be managed with less invasive strategies such as placement of a pigtail catheter, needle aspiration, or, in some cases, observation alone
+ Stable patients (especially older patients or patients with underlying lung disease) thought to have pneumothorax may benefit from computed tomography imaging, as blebs can mimic the appearance of pneumothorax on plain film
+ For a pneumothorax, direct the tube superiorly and anteriorly. For hemothorax, direct the tube posteriorly.
+ If there is no lung reexpansion after chest tube placement, consider the following: (1) the tube may not be in the pleural cavity; (2) the most proximal hole is outside the chest cavity; and (3) there is a large air leak from the tracheobronchial tree.
+ Immediate drainage of more than 1,000 mL of blood from the pleural cavity or continued output of at least 200 mL/h is an indication for thoracotomy

Suggested Readings

Kirsch TD, Mulligan JP. Tube thoracostomy. In: Roberts JR, Hedges JR, eds. *Clinical Procedures in Emergency Medicine*. 4th ed. Philadelphia, PA: WB Saunders; 2004:187–209.

Simon RR, Brenner BE. *Emergency Procedures and Techniques*. 4th ed. Philadelphia, PA: Lippincott Williams & Wilkins; 2002:172–179.

15

Emergency Department Thoracotomy

Benjamin H. Slovis

INDICATIONS

- **Penetrating Chest Trauma**
  - Traumatic arrest with witnessed signs of life* in the field
  - Persistent hypotension (systolic blood pressure (SBP) <60 mm Hg) despite resuscitative efforts
- **Blunt Trauma**
  - Traumatic arrest that occurs in the emergency department (ED)
  - Persistent hypotension (SBP <60 mm Hg) despite resuscitative efforts
- **Pulmonary Trauma**
  - Chest tube drainage >1,500 mL
  - Persistent hypotension or cardiac arrest with known lung laceration
- **Air Embolism**
  - Persistent signs of hypovolemic shock
  - Hemoptysis and cardiac arrest after intubation and ventilation
- **Nontraumatic Hypothermic Cardiac Arrest**
  - In settings where cardiopulmonary bypass is not immediately available
- **Goals**
  - Relief of cardiac tamponade
  - Support of cardiac function with open massage, cross-clamping the aorta, and/or internal cardiac defibrillation
  - Control of hemorrhage
  - Diagnosis and management of air embolism
  - Mediastinal irrigation and rewarming (for hypothermic cardiac arrest)

CONTRAINDICATIONS

- No signs of life and prehospital cardiopulmonary resuscitation (CPR) performed:
  - >15 minutes after penetrating trauma
  - >10 minutes after blunt trauma
- Multisystem blunt trauma
- Severe head injury
- Asystole as an initial rhythm without tamponade
- Inability to provide definitive care after procedure

RISKS/CONSENT ISSUES

- This is an emergent procedure and does not require written consent

LANDMARKS (FIGURE 15.1)

- Left-sided supine anterolateral approach over the 5th rib, in the fourth intercostal space
  - In males incise below the nipple
  - In females below the inframammary fold

---

*Signs of life should include pupillary reflexes, extremity movement, cardiac electrical activity, spontaneous ventilation, and palpable blood pressure or pulses.

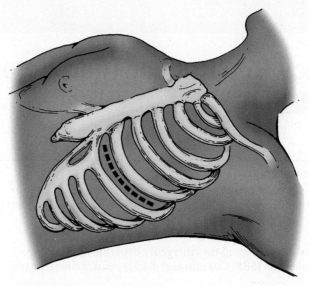

FIGURE 15.1 Thoracotomy landmark.

🔲 **General Basic Steps**
  ✛ **Incision**
  ✛ **Dissection and rib spreading**
  ✛ **Pericardotomy**
  ✛ **Cardiac massage**
  ✛ **Hemorrhage control**
  ✛ **Aortic cross-clamping**

TECHNIQUE

🔲 **Patient Preparation**
  ✛ Patient should be intubated and a nasogastric tube should be placed (this should not delay the procedure!)
  ✛ Place towels under the left chest and place left arm above the head
  ✛ Sterilize the incision area with copious povidone–iodine solution
🔲 **Incision**
  ✛ Using a no. 20 blade, incise from the sternal border to the posterior axillary line
  ✛ During the primary incision, cut firmly through subcutaneous tissue to the intercostal muscle
🔲 **Dissection and Rib Spreading**
  ✛ Using scissors, cut the intercostal muscles above the 5th rib to avoid the neurovascular bundle
  ✛ Temporarily stop ventilation just before exposing the pleura to avoid lacerating the lung
  ✛ Insert rib spreader with the ratchet placed toward the axilla and handlebar down
  ✛ Use a Gigli saw, Lebsche knife, or trauma shears to cut the sternum for right-sided exposure
🔲 **Pericardiotomy**
  ✛ Hold the pericardium with forceps, and use scissors to cut from the cardiac apex to the aortic root (FIGURE 15.2)
  ✛ The incision should be made anterior and lateral, avoiding the left phrenic nerve
  ✛ Evacuate blood and clots from the pericardium
  ✛ Deliver the heart from the pericardium if cardiac repair is required

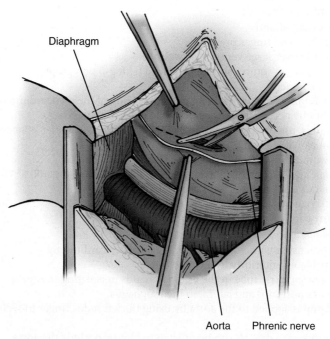

Diaphragm

Aorta   Phrenic nerve

FIGURE 15.2 Pericardium.

Cardiac Massage

+ The left hand is placed over the right ventricle while the right hand supports the surface of the left ventricle (**FIGURE 15.3**)
+ Avoid fingertip pressure and apply the compression force perpendicular to the septum
+ Avoid direct pressure on coronary arteries and allow for relaxation in diastole
+ To defibrillate, apply internal paddles anteriorly and posteriorly. Deliver shocks between 10 and 50 J.

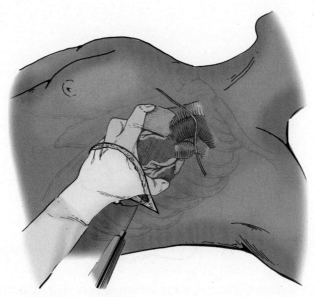

FIGURE 15.3 Internal cardiac massage.

Control of Hemorrhagic Wounds

- Ventricular cardiac wounds
  - Initially apply direct finger pressure
  - Use staples to repair large ventricular wounds
  - Horizontal mattress sutures should be placed with 2-0 polypropylene or 3-0 monofilament
  - The use of Teflon pledgets may help prevent tearing of the myocardium (FIGURE 15.4)
  - Consider briefly occluding cardiac inflow to control hemorrhage
- For atrial wounds, use occlusion clamps or 20-French Foley catheter (FIGURE 15.5) for temporary control of bleeding
- Great vessel wounds
  - Hemorrhage can be controlled using clamps or digital pressure (FIGURE 15.6)
  - Aortic wounds can be closed with 3-0 prolene
  - Both subclavian arteries can be cross-clamped as needed
  - Laparotomy pads can be used to tamponade hemorrhage

Aortic Cross-clamping

- Persistent hypotension with SBP <70 mm Hg after pericardiotomy
- The aorta is palpated anteriorly to the vertebrae
- Palpation of a nasogastric tube in the esophagus aids in isolating the aorta
  - The aorta lies posterior and lateral to the esophagus
- A vascular clamp is applied to the aorta by using the left index finger to secure the clamp (FIGURE 15.7)
  - Aortic compression devices can be utilized to blindly occlude the aorta
- Adjust the clamp until brachial SBP is <120 mm Hg

Management of Air Embolism

- The patient is placed in Trendelenburg position to avoid cerebral emboli
- Consider mainstem intubation of the contralateral lung
- Rinse the hemithorax with sterile saline to isolate bronchovenous fistulas
  - Repeat on the contralateral side if unsuccessful
- Cross-clamp the hilum and repair fistula and aspirate the left ventricle and aorta for remaining emboli
- Consider pressors or cross-clamping the aorta to maintain SBP

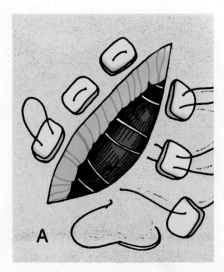

FIGURE 15.4 A: Ventricular septal defect resulting from a penetrating injury. Penetrating communications can often be closed by simple pledgeted mattress sutures. (From Simon RR, Brenner BE. *Emergency Procedures and Techniques.* 4th ed. Philadelphia, PA: Lippincott Williams & Wilkins; 2002:166, with permission.)

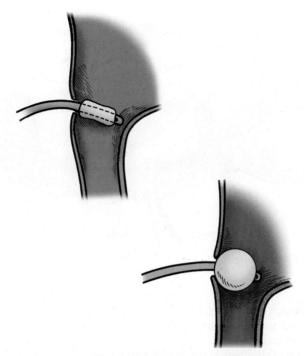

FIGURE 15.5 Place a Foley catheter tip into the wound. Inflate the balloon and pull back the catheter to control bleeding. Then proceed with more definitive repair. (From Simon RR, Brenner BE. *Emergency Procedures and Techniques*. 4th ed. Philadelphia, PA: Lippincott Williams & Wilkins; 2002:167, with permission.)

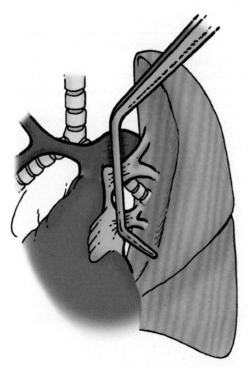

FIGURE 15.6 Occlusion of the pulmonary hilum with a Satinsky clamp. (From Simon RR, Brenner BE. *Emergency Procedures and Techniques*. 4th ed. Philadelphia, PA: Lippincott Williams & Wilkins; 2002:170, with permission.)

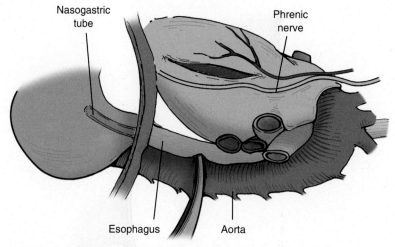

FIGURE 15.7 Aortic clamp.

🔲 **Mediastinal Irrigation**
  ➕ Warm sterile saline to approximately 40°C
  ➕ Irrigate over heart and thorax
  ➕ Attempt to obtain cardiac bypass for further rewarming

AFTERCARE

🔲 Patients should be transported to the operating room immediately for definitive care
🔲 Provide sedation, blood products, fluids, and pressors as needed
🔲 Broad-spectrum antibiotics

COMPLICATIONS

🔲 Injury to healthcare workers associated with sharps or rib fractures
🔲 Neurovascular bundle injury during cutting
🔲 Phrenic nerve transection during pericardotomy
🔲 Myocardial or coronary artery injury secondary to open cardiac massage
🔲 Aortic or esophageal injuries due to cross-clamping
  ➕ Inferior pulmonary vein injury when dissecting to the aorta
🔲 Distal hypoperfusion during aortic cross-clamping
  ➕ Unclamp the aorta for 30 to 60 seconds every 10 minutes
🔲 Wound infection and/or sepsis
  ➕ Antiseptic preparation should not delay the procedure

SAFETY/QUALITY TIPS

▢ **Procedural**
+ Be careful to avoid provider injury from broken ribs or sharps
+ Do not make the incision too small: It is acceptable to incise past the posterior axillary line
+ Start the incision 2 cm lateral to the sternal edge to avoid the internal mammary arteries
+ Cut along the top of the 5th rib to avoid the intercostal neurovascular bundle
+ Rib spreader handle should point down; otherwise does not allow for extension of incision to right chest
+ Open the pericardium. Myocardial injuries cannot be excluded without direct visualization.
+ Be mindful of the phrenic nerve; it runs vertically on the anterior pericardial surface

▢ **Cognitive**
+ Indications for ED thoracotomy are controversial and continue to be debated. It is important to know your institutional policies when considering this procedure. When indicated, it should be done without delay.
+ Severe head trauma is associated with poor outcomes in ED thoracotomy and is generally regarded as a contraindication to ED thoracotomy
+ Survival rate is predicted to be 2% for blunt trauma and 16% for penetrating trauma, but this depends on many variables, and the decision to proceed should be made on a case-by-case basis
+ Consider performing tube thoracostomy to identify potential right-sided injuries, if not extending the thoracotomy to the right side
+ Hyperbaric oxygen therapy can improve outcomes up to 36 hours after vascular air embolism, though within 6 hours is preferred
+ Mediastinal irrigation can achieve rewarming rates up to 8°C per hour
+ Go slow: Healthcare worker injuries have been reported at a high rate during ED thoracotomy. Take universal precautions and wear personal protective equipment.

▢ **Acknowledgment**

Thank you to prior author Oscar Rago and Barbara Kilian.

Suggested Readings

Burlew CC. *Western Trauma Association critical decisions in trauma: resuscitative thoracotomy. J Trauma Acute Care Surg.* 2012;73(6):1359.

Marx JA (ed), *Rosen's emergency medicine concepts and clinical practice.* 8th ed. Philadelphia, PA: Elsevier/ Saunders, 2013.

Reichman EF, ed. *Emergency Medicine Procedures.* 2nd ed. New York, NY: McGraw-Hill; 2013.

Roberts JR, Custalow CB, Thomsen TW, et al. *Roberts & Hedges' Clinical Procedures in Emergency Medicine.* 6th ed. Philadelphia, PA: WB Saunders; 2013.

16

Diagnostic Peritoneal Lavage

Jessica H. Leifer and Joshua Quaas

INDICATIONS

A sensitive way to evaluate for intra-abdominal injury in the trauma patient

- ⊡ **In Blunt Trauma**
  - ✛ Unexplained hypotension
  - ✛ Concern for injury but no obvious indication for laparotomy and serial abdominal examinations are not practical (i.e., unconscious or under anesthesia)
  - ✛ Equivocal focused abdominal sonography for trauma (FAST) examination and concern for an intra-abdominal injury
  - ✛ Patient unsuitable for computed tomography (CT) in whom there is concern for intra-abdominal injury
  - ✛ Concern for mesenteric or hollow viscous injury not seen on CT
- ⊡ **In Penetrating Trauma**
  - ✛ Anterior abdominal stab wound and evidence of fascial penetration in the stable patient with no obvious indication for laparotomy
  - ✛ To evaluate for hollow organ or diaphragmatic injury in the stable patient

CONTRAINDICATIONS

- ⊡ **Absolute Contraindications**
  - ✛ Indication for an emergent laparotomy
- ⊡ **Relative Contraindications**
  - ✛ Prior abdominal surgery
  - ✛ Second or third trimester of pregnancy—consider open technique with supraumbilical approach
  - ✛ Morbid obesity
  - ✛ Significant ascites
  - ✛ Coagulopathy

- ⊡ **General Basic Steps**
  - ✛ **Prepare patient**
  - ✛ **Analgesia**
  - ✛ **Technique**
    - ✛ **Open**
      - ▬ **Incision**
      - ▬ **Dissection**
      - ▬ **Incise fascia, then peritoneum**
      - ▬ **Place dialysis catheter**
    - ✛ **Closed**
      - ▬ **Needle into abdomen**
      - ▬ **Thread guidewire**
      - ▬ **Small skin incision**
      - ▬ **Thread dialysis catheter**
  - ✛ **Aspirate**
  - ✛ **Lavage/Drainage of fluid**
  - ✛ **Analysis of fluid**

LANDMARKS

The incision should be made in the midline, one-third of the way between the umbilicus and pubic symphysis. In the pregnant patient or the patient with a pelvic fracture, the incision should be made in the midline, just above the umbilicus **(FIGURE 16.1)**.

SUPPLIES

- 1% Lidocaine with epinephrine, 20 mL with 25-gauge needle, 10-mL syringe
- Sterile towels or drapes, sterile gown and gloves, mask, and eye protection
- Povidone–iodine (Betadine) solution or chlorhexidine
- 11-Blade scalpel
- Syringe and needle (for closed technique)
- Flexible guidewire (for closed technique)
- Two clamps and two retractors (for open technique)
- Peritoneal catheter
- 1 L warm saline for infusion (for lavage)
- Tubing to let lavage fluid drain
- Suture (for open technique)

TECHNIQUE

- **Preparation**
  + Place a Foley catheter (unless contraindicated)
  + Place a nasogastric tube (unless contraindicated) to suction to decompress the stomach
  + Gather all instruments and sterile gown/gloves
  + Sterilize the abdomen from costal margin to pubis and from flank to flank with povidone–iodine solution (Betadine) or chlorhexidine
  + Drape the area with sterile towels or drapes

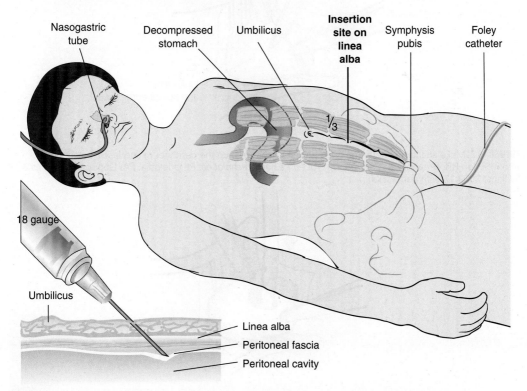

FIGURE 16.1 Anatomical landmarks for diagnostic peritoneal lavage. (From VanDevander PL, Wagner DK. Diagnostic peritoneal lavage. In: Henretig FM, King C, eds. *Textbook of Pediatric Emergency Procedures.* Philadelphia, PA: Williams & Wilkins; 1997:358, with permission.)

⬚ **Analgesia**
+ Using 1% lidocaine with epinephrine (1:100,000), generously anesthetize the skin and subcutaneous tissue where the incision or puncture will be made

⬚ **Access the Peritoneal Cavity (via open or closed technique)**
+ **Open Technique**
    + Using an 11-blade scalpel, make a 2- to 4-cm vertical incision in the midline just below the umbilicus **(FIGURE 16.2)**
    + Using a retractor to hold open the skin, dissect tissue down to the fascia
    + Using clamps, grasp the fascia, elevate it, and incise sharply
    + Grasp the peritoneum with two clamps and incise sharply
    + Insert a peritoneal dialysis catheter into the abdomen, directing it gently toward the pelvis **(FIGURE 16.3)**
    + At the conclusion of the procedure (after the catheter is removed), the fascial incision should be closed with no. 0 or no. 1 PDS or nylon suture. The skin can be closed with staples.
+ **Closed Technique (FIGURE 16.4)**
    + Elevate the skin on either side of the needle insertion site, between clamps
    + Insert an 18-gauge needle attached to a syringe through the skin, soft tissue, and fascia. There will be some resistance followed by a release when the needle is in the peritoneal cavity. Advance the needle about 1 cm further into the abdomen.

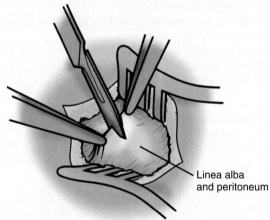

Linea alba
and peritoneum

FIGURE 16.2 Make an incision between two hemostats that pick up the peritoneum and fascia as shown. (From Simon RR, Brenner BE. *Emergency Procedures and Techniques*. Philadelphia, PA: Lippincott Williams & Wilkins; 2002:17, with permission.)

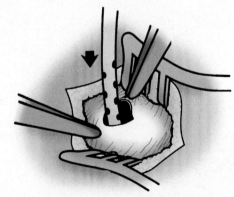

FIGURE 16.3 Pass a catheter through a 2-cm incision and direct it toward the pelvis. (From Simon RR, Brenner BE. *Emergency Procedures and Techniques*. Philadelphia, PA: Lippincott Williams & Wilkins; 2002:17, with permission.)

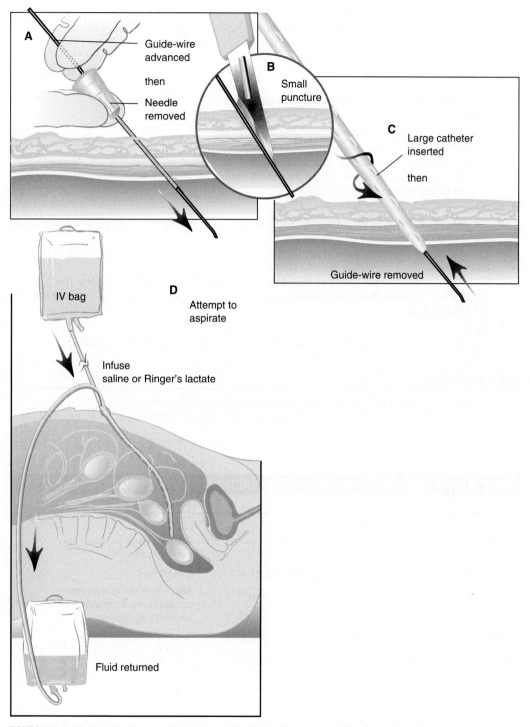

FIGURE 16.4 A: Guidewire advanced through needle. **B:** Small puncture with scalpel. **C:** Lavage catheter advanced into the peritoneal cavity over the guidewire. **D:** An initial attempt is made to aspirate blood from the peritoneal cavity; 10 to 15 mL/kg normal saline or Ringer lactate is infused via the lavage catheter; the bag is dropped to a level below the abdomen and the fluid is recovered by gravity. (From VanDevander PL, Wagner DK. Diagnostic peritoneal lavage. In: Henretig FM, King C, eds. *Textbook of Pediatric Emergency Procedures*. Philadelphia, PA: Williams & Wilkins; 1997:362, with permission.)

+ Thread a flexible guidewire through the needle. Stop if resistance is met or when about 5 cm of wire remains outside the abdomen.
+ Leaving the wire in place, remove the needle
+ Using an 11-blade scalpel, make a small (stab) incision at the site of the wire
+ Thread a dialysis catheter over the wire into the abdomen. Direct the catheter toward the pelvis.
+ Remove the wire while leaving the catheter in place

☐ **Aspiration**
  + Connect the dialysis catheter to a syringe and aspirate
    + If 10 mL of gross blood is aspirated, the diagnostic peritoneal lavage (DPL) is positive and the patient should undergo immediate laparotomy
    + If bile, enteric contents, or food particles are aspirated, the DPL is positive and the patient should undergo immediate laparotomy

☐ **Lavage**
  + If aspiration yields <10 mL of blood, instill up to 1 L (15 mL/kg in children) of warm normal saline into the abdomen through the catheter
  + Try to shift the abdomen/patient gently (i.e., change positioning) to allow the fluid to move and allow the fluid to remain for 5 to 10 minutes
  + Place the empty infusion bag or container on the floor below the patient to allow the fluid to drain. The container should be vented to promote drainage of the fluid. Drain at least half of the infused fluid.

☐ **Analysis**
  + Send a sample of 20 mL of fluid to the laboratory for cell count (red blood cell and white blood cell)

COMPLICATIONS

☐ Local wound complications such as infection, dehiscence, and hematoma
☐ Intraperitoneal injury to solid organs, bowel, bladder, and vasculature (more common with the percutaneous technique)
☐ Pain

TABLE 16.1. INTERPRETATION AND APPROPRIATE ACTION BASED ON LAVAGE FINDINGS

Findings	Interpretation	Action
>100,000 RBC	Positive for **blunt** trauma	Laparotomy
20,000–100,000 RBC	Indeterminate for **blunt** trauma	Consider further imaging; correlate clinically
>10,000 RBC	Positive for **penetrating** trauma	Laparotomy
<10,000 RBC	<2% chance of missed injury	May still need to evaluate for diaphragmatic injury in penetrating trauma
>500 WBC	Positive	Laparotomy

RBC, red blood cells; WBC, white blood cells.

SAFETY/QUALITY TIPS

◻ **Procedural**
+ False-positives may occur in the presence of pelvic fractures
+ Procedure is painful; use sufficient anesthetic and analgesia in the stable patient
+ If resistance is encountered when placing the catheter or infusing fluid, stop and check the catheter position. If the catheter is preperitoneal, DPL can be reattempted.
+ If adequate fluid cannot be siphoned, the catheter may be obstructed and can be gently manipulated. Gently changing the patient's position or shifting the abdomen may release compartmentalized fluid.

◻ **Cognitive**
+ The role of emergency physician-performed DPL has waned with the rise of point-of-care ultrasound. In general, stable trauma patients with concern for serious injury are best evaluated by CT, and unstable patients are best evaluated by FAST ultrasound. The primary role of DPL in modern emergency practice is in the unstable patient with concern for both serious pelvic/retroperitoneal bleeding and abdominal/peritoneal bleeding, when FAST is inadequate or unavailable. In these cases, the result of DPL determines whether the patient moves to angiography or the operating room.
+ DPL does not evaluate the retroperitoneum. CT should be used in the stable patient.
+ Insert a gastric tube and urinary catheter prior to DPL so that the stomach and bladder are decompressed
+ If the initial aspirate is positive, do not attempt the lavage; this is an indication for laparotomy
+ A positive DPL does not mandate laparotomy in the stable patient. These patients may be candidates for nonoperative management.
+ Infusion of fluid can confound future CT and ultrasonography findings **(TABLE 16.1)**

◻ **Acknowledgment**

Thank you to prior author Laura Withers and Raymond Wedderburn.

Suggested Readings

Runyon MS, Marx JA. Peritoneal procedures. In: Roberts, JR, Hedges JR, eds. *Clinical Procedures in Emergency Medicine*. 5th ed. Philadelphia, PA: WB Saunders; 2010:852–861.

Sandeep Johar, Umashankar Lakshmanadoss. Chapter 66. Diagnostic peritoneal lavage. In: Reichman EF, ed. *Emergency Medicine Procedures*. 2nd ed. New York, NY: McGraw-Hill; 2013.

17

Lateral Canthotomy

Joseph Scofi

INDICATIONS

Orbital compartment syndrome (OCS) is an ocular emergency that is characterized by increased intraocular pressure (IOP). If untreated, optic nerve ischemia will develop, resulting in irreversible vision loss in as little as 90 to 120 minutes. Immediate vision saving treatment via lateral canthotomy and cantholysis is required. OCS is most commonly a result of retrobulbar hemorrhage secondary to trauma, but can also be iatrogenic, due to infection or inflammation.

- **Primary Indications**
  - Retrobulbar hemorrhage with the following:
    - Acute loss of visual acuity
    - IOP >40 mm Hg
    - Severe proptosis
    - Marked periorbital edema
    - An unconscious or uncooperative patient with an IOP >40 mm Hg
- **Secondary Indications**
  - Suspected retrobulbar process with the following:
    - Associated afferent pupillary defect
    - Ophthalmoplegia
    - Resistance to retropulsion
    - Cherry-red macula
    - Optic nerve head pallor
    - Severe eye pain

CONTRAINDICATIONS

- Suspected ruptured globe

LANDMARKS

- The lateral canthal tendon is a combined tendon–ligament that provides structural fixation of the lids (tarsal plates) and orbicularis oculi muscle to the inner aspect of the bony lateral orbital wall (zygoma) just posterior to the orbital rim
- The tendon has an inferior and superior crux
- The point at which the tendon attaches is called *Whitnall tubercle*
- Eisler pocket, a small pocket of orbital fat, lies anterior to the lateral canthal tendon

---

- **General Basic Steps**
  - **Position—supine**
  - **Prep and drape**
  - **Anesthetize lateral canthus**
  - **Straight clamp**
  - **Cut skin, then inferior crux of lateral canthus**
  - **Check IOP**
  - **Cut superior crux of lateral canthus if necessary**
  - **Topical antibiotic ointment**

TECHNIQUE (FIGURE 17.1)

- ⊕ **Positioning is critical.** The patient must be supine and be able to cooperate throughout the procedure. Unexpected head movement may lead to iatrogenic globe injury.
- ⊕ The lateral canthus should be prepped and draped in a sterile manner
- ⊕ Irrigate the eye with normal saline to remove surrounding debris
- ⊕ **Anesthetize** the lateral canthus with approximately 1 mL of 1% or 2% lidocaine with epinephrine to obtain both local anesthesia and hemostasis
- ⊕ A **straight clamp** is advanced horizontally across the lateral canthus until the orbital rim is encountered
- ⊕ Leave the clamp in place for 1 to 2 minutes to compress tissues and achieve hemostasis
- ⊕ Release the clamp, leaving an impression for where the incision is to be made
- ⊕ Use a pair of forceps to elevate the skin around the lateral orbit
- ⊕ **Use scissors and cut** a horizontal incision in the tissue, starting at the lateral corner of the eye and extending 1 to 2 cm laterally. This will open the skin, orbicularis muscle, orbital septum, and palpebral conjunctiva, and exposes the Eisler pocket of fat.
- ⊕ **Retract the lid down** and away from the lateral orbit, separating the conjunctiva and the skin
- ⊕ Palpate the inferior portion of the lateral canthal tendon by using your finger or the tip of the scissors. The tendon should be under tension.
- ⊕ With the scissors pointed inferoposteriorly toward the lateral orbital rim (pointing away from the globe), dissect and **cut the inferior crux of the lateral canthal tendon.** This critical incision is approximately 1 to 2 cm in depth and length.

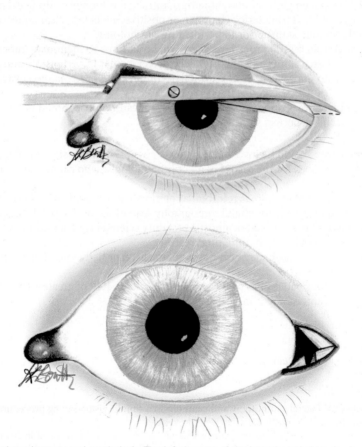

FIGURE 17.1 Lateral canthotomy and cantholysis. The inferior arm of the lateral canthal tendon has been incised to release the globe. (From Knoop KJ, Dennis WR. Eye trauma. In: Wolfson AB, ed. *Harwood-Nuss' Clinical Practice of Emergency Medicine.* 4th ed. Philadelphia, PA: Lippincott Williams & Wilkins; 2005:952, with permission.)

- Upon cutting the inferior crux, the lower lid loses its structural fixation to the lateral orbital wall and becomes lax, releasing the increased IOP from the eye
- Repeated IOP measurement should be below 40 mm Hg
- If the IOP is still elevated, dissect superiorly and cut the superior crux of the lateral canthal tendon
- Apply topical antibiotic ointment to the area

COMPLICATIONS

- Iatrogenic globe injury
- Excessive bleeding
- Local infection or abscess formation
- Improper direction of scissors superiorly may lead to injury to the levator aponeurosis, resulting in ptosis
- Injury to the lacrimal gland and lacrimal artery, which lie superiorly; care must be taken to avoid these structures
- Loss of adequate lower-lid suspension and ectropion (can be repaired at a later date by the ophthalmologist)

SAFETY/QUALITY TIPS

- **Procedural**
  - IOP testing with any instrument that compresses the eye (e.g., Tono-Pen) is contraindicated in patients with suspected ruptured globe. Specifically assess for globe rupture (misshapen globe or enophthalmos, intraocular foreign body, uveal prolapse, irregular pupil, shallow anterior chamber, or positive Seidel test: clear aqueous humor parting fluorescein stain) prior to performing canthotomy.
  - Shortly after a successful procedure, there will be an improvement of extraocular movements, visual acuity, afferent pupillary defect, ocular hypertension, and eye pain. If vision fails to improve, operative orbital decompression or hematoma evacuation is required.
  - A sterile procedure is optimal; however, emergent canthotomy should not be unduly delayed to achieve perfect sterility
- **Cognitive**
  - Ophthalmology should be involved as soon as possible, but this sight-saving procedure must not be delayed for the arrival of an ophthalmologist who cannot be immediately present
  - If it is unclear whether there is retrobulbar hemorrhage or another ocular process occurring, an emergent computed tomography scan of the orbits may be helpful to clarify the diagnosis. The additional diagnostic certainty offered by advanced imaging must be weighed against the delay in initiating treatment.
  - Retrobulbar hemorrhage may occur atraumatically, especially in patients with coagulopathy
  - If an unconscious patient has periorbital edema and an IOP of greater than 40 mm Hg or a firm globe, canthotomy is indicated

- **Acknowledgment**

Thank you to prior author Dean Jared Straff.

Suggested Readings

McInnes G, Howes DW. Lateral canthotomy and cantholysis: a simple, vision saving procedure. *Can J Emerg Med*. 2002;4(1):49–52.

Reichman EF. eds. *Emergency Medicine Procedures. 2nd ed*. New York, NY: McGraw-Hill; 2013.

Rosen P, Barkin R. *Emergency Medicine: Concepts and Clinical Practice*. St Louis, MO: Mosby; 2002:910.

Titinalli JE, Kelen GD, Strapczynski JS. *Emergency Medicine: A Comprehensive Study Guide*. 6th ed. American College of Emergency Physicians, New York, NY: McGraw-Hill; 2004:1458.

Vassallo S, Hartstein M, Howard D, et al. Traumatic retrobulbar hemorrhage: emergent decompression by lateral canthotomy and cantholysis. *J Emerg Med*. 2002;22(3):251–256.

18

Bedside FAST Ultrasonography: Focused Assessment with Sonography for Trauma

Andreana Kwon and David Riley

INDICATIONS

- ⊡ Yes or No: Is there intra-abdominal fluid or fluid around the heart?
- ⊡ The assessment of blunt thoracoabdominal trauma with significant mechanism of injury
- ⊡ The assessment of penetrating torso trauma if operative management is not immediately indicated

CONTRAINDICATIONS

- ⊡ The FAST examination should never delay a patient's transport to the operating room when operative management is clearly indicated

RISKS/CONSENT ISSUES

- ⊡ The only theoretical risk is allergy to the ultrasound gel

ADVANTAGES

- ⊡ Noninvasive and no sedation required
- ⊡ Can be performed at the bedside while resuscitative efforts are simultaneously being performed
- ⊡ Can be performed at the bedside on patients too unstable for the computed tomographic imaging suite
- ⊡ Can be repeated serially along with changes in symptoms or hemodynamic stability

LANDMARKS

- ⊡ Subcostal
  - ✦ Probe placed in the subxiphoid region pointed toward the heart detects fluid in pericardial sac
- ⊡ Hepatorenal
  - ✦ Probe placed in the right midaxillary line between the 8th and 11th ribs detects fluid in the hepatorenal space (Morison pouch)
- ⊡ Splenorenal
  - ✦ Probe placed in the left posterior axillary line between the 8th and 11th ribs detects fluid in the splenorenal recess
- ⊡ Suprapubic
  - ✦ Probe placed 2 cm superior to the symphysis pubis detects fluid in the retrovesical or retrouterine space

TECHNIQUE

The standard four FAST views: Subcostal, hepatorenal pouch (Morison), splenorenal, and suprapubic (FIGURE 18.1)

- ⊡ Subcostal/Subxiphoid View (FIGURE 18.2)
  - ✦ With the probe in the transverse plane, place it in the subxiphoid area and aim toward the patient's left shoulder to see a four-chambered view of the heart
  - ✦ Sweep the probe anteriorly and posteriorly to view the entire pericardium
  - ✦ Unclotted blood will appear as an anechoic black "stripe" within the hyperechoic pericardial sac (FIGURE 18.3)

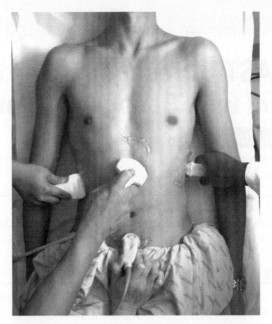

FIGURE 18.1 The four views of the FAST examination.

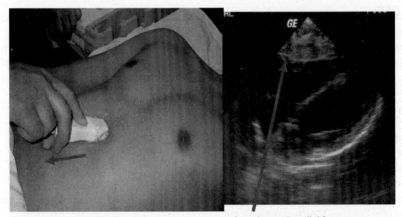

Keep probe parallel to the abdomen.
Bring knees up to relax the
abdominal wall

Anterior pericardial fat
and clotted blood can
look gray

FIGURE 18.2 Subcostal view.

- **Hepatorenal Pouch (of Morison) View (FIGURE 18.4)**
    - With the indicator pointed toward the patient's right axilla, place the probe in the midaxillary line between the 8th and 11th ribs
    - Hold the probe in a longitudinal or an oblique plane to aid visualization through rib spaces
    - Unclotted blood or fluid will appear as an anechoic black stripe in the space between the liver and the right kidney **(FIGURE 18.5)**

- **Splenorenal View (FIGURE 18.6)**
    - With the indicator pointed toward the patient's left axilla, place the probe in the left posterior axillary line between the 8th and 11th ribs, also at an oblique plane
    - Turn the probe longitudinally to enhance your view

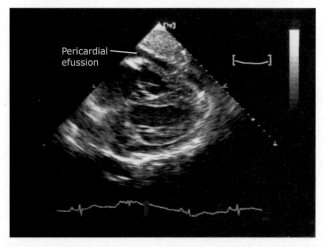

FIGURE 18.3 Ultrasound image taken from the subxiphoid transducer position demonstrating fluid in the pericardial space. (Reprinted with permission from Cosby KS, Kendall JL. *Practical Guide to Emergency Ultrasound*. Philadelphia, PA: Lippincott Williams & Wilkins, 2005.)

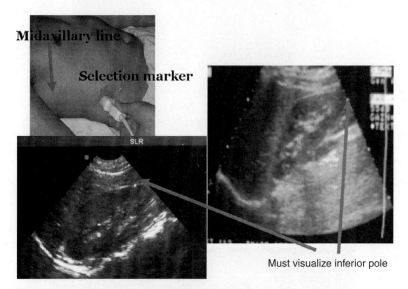

FIGURE 18.4 Hepatorenal pouch (of Morison) view.

✦ Unclotted blood or fluid will appear as an anechoic black stripe in the space between the spleen and left kidney **(FIGURE 18.7)**

▫ **Suprapubic View (FIGURE 18.8)**
✦ This view is facilitated by a full bladder
✦ With the indicator pointing toward the patient's head, place the probe 2 cm superior to the symphysis pubis along the midline
✦ Aim the probe caudally into the pelvis
✦ Rotate the probe 90 degrees counterclockwise for transverse images
✦ Look for anechoic blood adjacent to the bladder and anterior peritoneum **(FIGURES 18.9 and 18.10)**

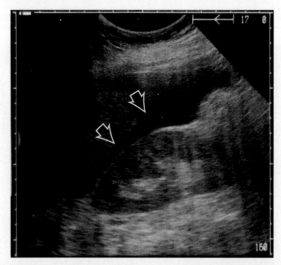

FIGURE 18.5 Intraperitoneal fluid. This image demonstrates free fluid within the peritoneal cavity. Fluid is seen as a black anechoic stripe in Morison pouch (*arrows*), which is the potential space between the liver and the kidney. (Reprinted with permission from Harwood-Nuss A, Wolfson AB, et al. *The Clinical Practice of Emergency Medicine*. 3rd ed. Philadelphia, PA: Lippincott Williams & Wilkins; 2001.)

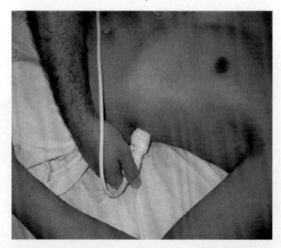

FIGURE 18.6 Location of probe for splenorenal view.

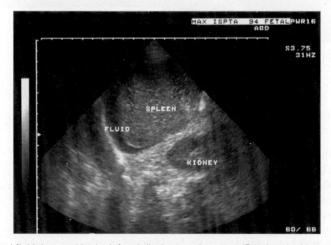

FIGURE 18.7 Peritoneal fluid detected in the left subdiaphragmatic space. (Reprinted with permission from Cosby KS, Kendall JL. *Practical Guide to Emergency Ultrasound*. Philadelphia: Lippincott Williams & Wilkins, 2005.)

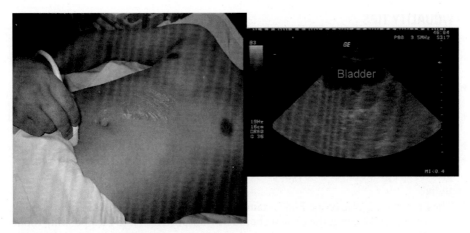

FIGURE 18.8 Suprapubic view.

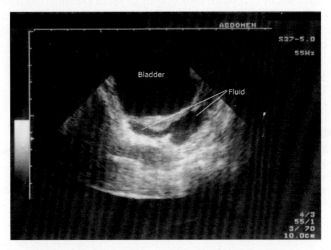

FIGURE 18.9 Sonographic appearance of fluid collecting posterior to the bladder in male patients with the transducer in the transverse orientation. (Reprinted with permission from Cosby KS, Kendall JL. *Practical Guide to Emergency Ultrasound*. Philadelphia: Lippincott Williams & Wilkins, 2005.)

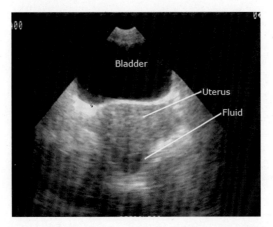

FIGURE 18.10 Ultrasound image of free fluid located posterior to the uterus with the transducer in the transverse orientation. (Reprinted with permission from Cosby KS, Kendall JL. *Practical Guide to Emergency Ultrasound*. Philadelphia: Lippincott Williams & Wilkins, 2005.)

SAFETY/QUALITY TIPS

⬚ **Procedural**

+ Placing the patient in Trendelenburg position makes the examination of the right upper quadrant (RUQ) and left upper quadrant (LUQ) more sensitive
+ Examination may be obscured by obese body habitus, subcutaneous air, pregnancy, preexisting peritoneal fluid, or increased bowel gas
+ The inferior pole of both kidneys must be visualized to avoid missing early fluid/blood accumulation
+ If the subxiphoid view does not adequately image the heart, use an alternate cardiac view
+ Fresh unclotted blood will appear anechoic, but fibrin formation during the clotting process can produce variable echoes

⬚ **Cognitive**

+ The fundamental role of the FAST examination is to determine, in a critically bleeding trauma patient, whether the patient should be transported first to the operating room or to angiography
+ Important abdominal hemorrhage is not ruled out by sonography. In a stable patient, bleeding is ruled out by computed tomography or serial examinations/blood counts.
+ Sensitivity of the FAST examination depends on the experience of the sonographer, position of the patient, equipment used, and the number of serial examinations performed
+ The FAST examination should not be used for the following:
  + Detecting contained solid organ injuries
  + Detecting bowel injuries
  + Detecting blood in the retroperitoneum or pelvis

Suggested Readings

Blackbourne LH, Soffer D, McKenney M, et al. Secondary ultrasound examination increases the sensitivity of the FAST exam in blunt trauma. *J Trauma*. 2004;57:934–938.

Ma OJ, Mateer JR. *Emergency Ultrasound*. 3rd ed. New York, NY: McGraw-Hill; 2013.

Ma OJ, Mateer JR, Ogata M, et al. Prospective analysis of a rapid trauma ultrasound examination performed by emergency physicians. *J Trauma*. 1995;38:879–885.

19

Bedside EFAST Ultrasonography: Extended Focused Assessment with Sonography for Trauma

Allegra Georgian Long and Resa E. Lewiss

INDICATIONS

- To assess for the absence of lung sliding, suggestive of a pneumothorax, in the following conditions:
  - Blunt thoracoabdominal trauma
  - Penetrating thoracoabdominal trauma
  - Unexplained hypotension
- To assess for the presence of pleural fluid, suggestive of a hemothorax, in the following conditions:
  - Blunt thoracoabdominal trauma
  - Penetrating thoracoabdominal trauma
  - Unexplained hypotension

CONTRAINDICATIONS

- If the EFAST examination delays a patient's transport to the operating room
- Theoretical allergy to the ultrasound gel

ADVANTAGES

- Noninvasive
- No sedation required
- Performed at the bedside amidst simultaneous resuscitative efforts
- Does not require transportation to the radiology suite
- Serial examinations may be performed with changes in symptoms or hemodynamics

LANDMARKS

- **Anterior Thorax**
  - The apical midclavicular line in the sagittal plane; transducer marker positioned cephalad
- **Lateral Thorax**
  - The lateral thorax in the axillary region; transducer marker positioned obliquely and cephalad
- **Pleural (Right: Hepatorenal and Left: Splenorenal)**
  - Transducer placed in the axillary line in the coronal plane at the level of 8th and 11th ribs; anterior axillary line on the right and posterior axillary line on the left, with the diaphragm as a landmark; transducer marker positioned toward the axilla.

TECHNIQUE

- The EFAST standard views in addition to the basic FAST examination:
  - Bilateral anterior thorax
  - Bilateral lateral thorax
  - Bilateral pleural spaces

🔲 **Anterior Thorax**
  ✚ Place the transducer in the second or third intercostal space in the midclavicular line
  ✚ The indicator should be cephalad
  ✚ **Identify the bat sign:** The upper rib–pleural line–lower rib profile **(FIGURE 19.1)**
  ✚ Normal lung findings
     ✚ B-mode: Visible sliding (shimmering or twinkling) at the level of the pleura
     ✚ **B-mode: Comet tails**—vertical reverberation artifacts arising from the pleural line **(FIGURE 19.2)**
     ✚ **M-mode: Seashore sign** **(FIGURE 19.3)**
  ✚ Pneumothorax
     ✚ B-mode: Loss of pleural sliding, as there is loss of contact between the visceral and the parietal pleura
     ✚ B-mode: Absence of comet tails
     ✚ **M-mode: Stratosphere sign** or **bar-code sign** **(FIGURE 19.4)**
     ✚ **Lung point:** Transition between collapsed and normally expanded lung; 100% specific for pneumothorax when identifiable
  ✚ **TABLE 19.1** compares the signs suggestive of normal lung with those of pneumothorax

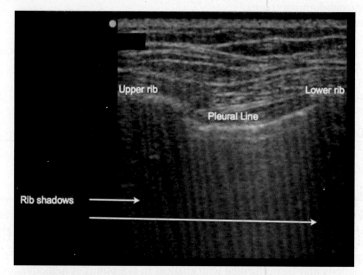

FIGURE 19.1 The bat sign (rib shadow, pleura, rib shadow).

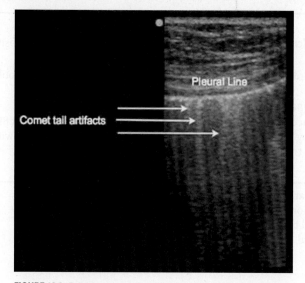

FIGURE 19.2 Bright white pleural line with comet-tail artifacts.

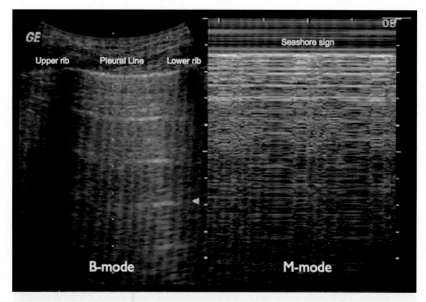

FIGURE 19.3 M-mode demonstrates the seashore sign seen in normal lung.

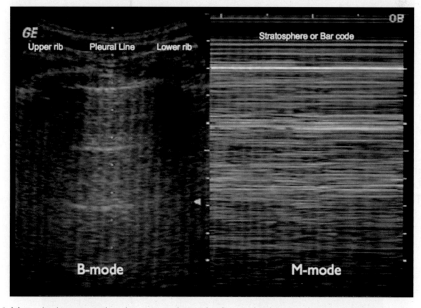

FIGURE 19.4 M-mode demonstrating the stratosphere sign/bar-code sign consistent with pneumothorax. (Courtesy of Dr. Marina Del Rios.)

- **Lateral Thorax**
  - Place the transducer in the second or third intercostal space in the midaxillary line
  - The indicator should be positioned obliquely and cephalad
- **Pleural Spaces**
  - With the indicator pointed toward the patient's axilla, place the transducer in the midaxillary line at the level of 8th and 11th ribs
  - Slide the transducer 1 or 2 spaces superiorly to visualize the space above the diaphragm
  - Normal lung findings
    - **"Mirror imaging"** of the liver or spleen above the hemidiaphragm **(FIGURE 19.5)**
    - **Nonvisualization of spine shadows above the diaphragm**

TABLE 19.1. SIGNS SUGGESTIVE OF NORMAL LUNG VERSUS THOSE OF PNEUMOTHORAX USING ULTRASONOGRAPHY	
Normal lung	**Pneumothorax**
Lung sliding	Absence of lung sliding
Comet-tail artifact	Absence of comet tails
Seashore sign	Stratosphere/bar-code sign lung point

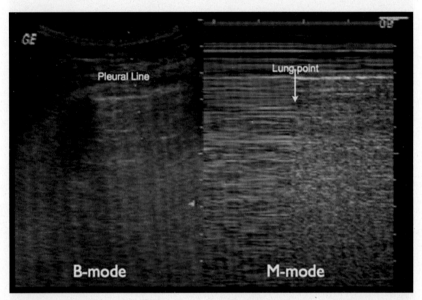

FIGURE 19.5 Right pleural–hepatorenal space. "Mirror imaging" (evidence against the presence of pleural fluid) is demonstrated.

+ Pleural fluid
  + **Loss of mirror imaging:** Anechoic "stripe" above the diaphragm **(FIGURE 19.6)**
  + **Thoracic spine sign:** Visualization of the thoracic spine shadows above the diaphragm

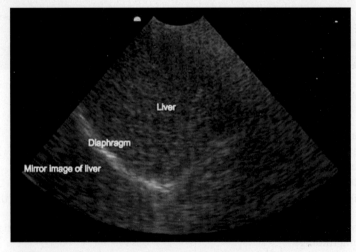

FIGURE 19.6 Right pleural–hepatorenal space with pleural fluid.

SAFETY/QUALITY TIPS

▢ **Procedural**

✦ Rotate the probe obliquely toward the back if rib shadows prevent full evaluation in pleural–hepatorenal and pleural–splenorenal views

✦ If poor views: Add more gel, reposition the patient, try a different probe, try a different ultrasound operator

▢ **Cognitive**

✦ Lung sliding may be absent in:
  + Patients who are not spontaneously breathing
  + Complete atelectasis
  + The presence of blebs
  + Pleural scarring
  + Intubation on the opposite side

✦ Pleural fluid:
  + Fresh blood is anechoic; clotted blood has different echogenicities
  + Mirror imaging can be difficult to detect
  + Thoracic spine sign may be more reliable

Suggested Readings

Ma OJ, Mateer JR, Kirkpatrick AW. Trauma. In: Ma OJ, Mateer J, Reardon R, et al, eds. *Emergency Ultrasound.* 3rd ed. New York, NY: McGraw-Hill; 2014:61–92.

Silva FR, Mills LD. Pulmonary. In: Ma OJ, Mateer J, Reardon R, et al, eds. *Emergency Ultrasound.* 3rd ed. New York, NY: McGraw-Hill; 2014:169–190.

Volpicelli G, Elbarbary M, Blaivas M, et al. International evidence-based recommendations for point-of-care lung ultrasound. *Intensive Care Med.* 2012;38:577–591.

20

Perimortem Cesarean Section

Penelope Chun Lema and Armin Perham Poordabbagh

INDICATIONS

- Gravid patient with a potentially viable fetus of ≥24 weeks' gestational age and imminent maternal death or unresponsive to cardiopulmonary resuscitation (CPR) for 5 minutes

Survival of mother and infant is greatest when the procedure is performed within 5 minutes of maternal arrest.

CONTRAINDICATIONS

- Fetus <24 weeks' gestational age
- Lower limit of fetal viability varies depending on institution and available resources

RISK/CONSENT ISSUES

- Verbal consent from family when possible

TECHNIQUE

- **General Basic Steps**
  - **Maternal patient CPR**
  - **Estimate fetal age**
  - **Incision**
  - **Delivery**
  - **Neonatal resuscitation**
  - **Continue maternal patient CPR**

- **Patient Preparation**
  - Procedure should be performed by the most experienced person available
  - Contact all essential personnel (i.e., neonatology/pediatrics, obstetrics)
  - Continue CPR on maternal patient throughout the entire procedure
  - Estimate fetal age (if unknown from history):
    - Height of uterine fundus reaches the umbilicus at 20 weeks' gestational age and increases 1 cm for each additional week
    - Four fingerbreadths above the umbilicus is approximately 24 weeks' gestational age
- **Incision (FIGURE 20.1)**
  - No. 10 scalpel blade
  - Make a midline vertical incision from just above the symphysis pubis extending to the umbilicus along the linea nigra/linea alba
  - Incise through the abdominal wall to the peritoneal cavity
  - Use retractors to retract abdominal wall and expose the uterus
- **Reflect Bladder Inferiorly**
  - If a full bladder obstructs view of the uterus, decompress bladder with a puncture incision and deflate with either pressure or suction
  - Bladder repair may be done later if mother survives

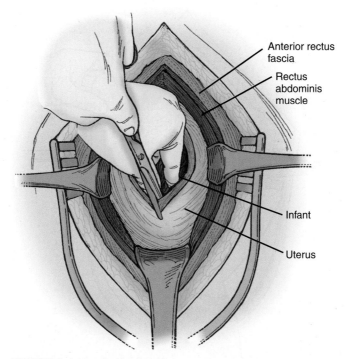

Anterior rectus fascia

Rectus abdominis muscle

Infant

Uterus

FIGURE 20.1 Anatomical landmarks.

- Make a small vertical incision (2 to 5 cm) along the lower uterine segment until amniotic fluid is encountered
    - Be careful not to cause inadvertent injury to the underlying fetus
- Insert index finger into incision and lift the uterus away from the fetus
- Use bandage (blunt-ended) scissors to extend the incision either transversely or vertically
    - Avoid tearing the uterine vessels located along the lateral margins of the uterus when making a transverse incision
    - Incision should be large enough for delivery of the fetal head and body
- **Deliver Baby** (FIGURE 20.2)
    - Place hand into the uterus and gently deliver the infant's head. Check for nuchal cord.
    - If the infant's feet are first encountered, continue as a breech delivery
- Suction the mouth and nares with bulb suction
- Complete delivery of the infant's shoulders and thorax
- Clamp and cut the umbilical cord
- Continue neonatal resuscitation
- Check maternal pulses and continue CPR
    - Relief of aortocaval compression by the uterus improves maternal hemodynamics
    - Cases of maternal survival have been reported

COMPLICATIONS

- Bladder injury
- Bowel injury
- Fetal lacerations and injury
- Neonate with neurologic deficits and/or demise
- Maternal bleeding and infection
- Maternal morbidity and mortality

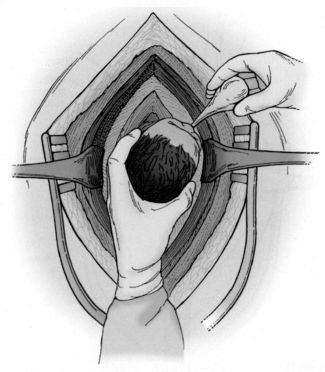

FIGURE 20.2 Delivery through cesarean section.

SAFETY/QUALITY TIPS

Procedural

✦ Assign someone to displace the uterus to the left until the scalpel hits the skin
✦ Ensure incision is sufficiently large for delivery of the fetus
✦ Be careful to prevent inadvertent lacerations and injury to the fetus
✦ Continue CPR throughout procedure and reassess maternal vital signs after delivery. Maternal survival after relief of aortocaval compression has been reported.

Cognitive

✦ Although commonly recommended to initiate the procedure within 4 minutes of arrest, the procedure is primarily for the mother, not the fetus. Any arrested woman pregnant with a fetus near or beyond viability should receive perimortem cesarean section (PMCS) unless maternal and fetal recovery are deemed impossible.
✦ If possible, bring neonatologist/pediatrician and obstetrician to the bedside when PMCS is likely or happening
✦ If there is time to prepare, gather materials necessary to resuscitate the baby (warmer, appropriately-sized airway equipment) and the mother (surgical kit or scalpel, surgical scissors, clamps, towels, clamps for the cord)
✦ If it is unclear whether the baby is a first trimester baby or a "big baby," a very brief assessment by ultrasound may answer this question. Do not focus on whether the baby is 23 or 24 or any particular number of weeks' gestation.
✦ Do not neglect psychological debriefing with the team after the dust settles; PMCS is usually distressing to staff

Suggested Readings

Raja AS, Zabbo CP. Trauma in pregnancy. *Emerg Med Clin N Am.* 2012;30(4):937–948.
Roberts JR, Hedges JR. *Clinical Procedures in Emergency Medicine.* 4th ed. Philadelphia, PA: WB Saunders; 2004:1137–1139.
Wolfson AB. *Harwood-Nuss' Clinical Practice of Emergency Medicine.* 6th ed. Philadelphia, PA: Lippincott Williams & Wilkins; 2014.

21

Retrograde Urethrography

Nicholas D. Caputo

INTRODUCTION

- Retrograde urethrography (RUG) is generally and commonly done in male patients as they have a longer and more complex urethral pathway
- The genitourinary system is divided into the upper urinary tract (kidneys, ureters), the lower urinary tract (bladder, urethra), and external genitalia (penis, scrotum, testes)
- Trauma to the urinary tract accounts for about 10% of all injuries seen in the emergency department
- Early clinical suspicion, appropriate and reliable radiologic studies, and prompt surgical intervention, when indicated, are the keys to successful diagnosis and management

INDICATIONS

- Blood at the urethral meatus
- Abnormal position of the prostate on rectal examination
- Perineal ecchymosis
- Scrotal ecchymosis
- Blood from the introitus/vaginal vault

CONTRAINDICATIONS

- No absolute contraindications exist

LANDMARKS

- The dome of the bladder is covered by peritoneum, and the bladder neck is fixed to neighboring structures by reflections of the pelvic fascia and by true ligaments of the pelvis
- In males, the bladder neck is contiguous with the prostate, which is attached to the pubis by puboprostatic ligaments
- In females, pubourethral ligaments support the bladder neck and urethra
- The body of the bladder receives support from the urogenital diaphragm inferiorly and the obturator internus muscles laterally

EQUIPMENT

- Radiopaque contrast material
- X-ray machine or fluoroscope machine
- 16-French or 18-French Foley catheter
- Catheter tip syringe
- 5-mL syringe to fill the Foley catheter balloon

- **General Basic Steps**
  - **Prepare 10% contrast solution**
  - **Insert syringe or Foley in urethral meatus**
  - **Inject contrast slowly**
  - **X-ray (urethrogram)**

TECHNIQUE

- ☐ Dilute stock contrast solution with saline 1:10 (10% solution)
- ☐ Lay the patient supine
- ☐ Acquire a plain film (kidneys, ureters, and bladder [KUB]) of reference prior to injecting contrast
- ☐ In males, firmly grip the penis with a folded 4 × 4 gauze with your long finger and ring finger of your nondominant hand and stretch the penis in a caudal direction in order to straighten the urethral path to the bladder and prevent urethral folding
- ☐ After sterile preparation, a catheter-tipped Toomey irrigating syringe or a regular 60-cc piston syringe is gently placed inside the urethral meatus until a snug fit is ensured
- ☐ Inject approximately 50 to 60 cc of dilute contrast material slowly under constant pressure for more than 30 to 60 seconds. During the injection of the last 10 cc of contrast material, the x-ray film (urethrogram) is taken.
- ☐ *Alternative technique* **(FIGURE 21.1)**:
  - ✦ Insert a Foley catheter just inside the urethral meatus
  - ✦ Inflate the balloon with 2 cc of sterile water for a snug fit within the fossa navicularis
  - ✦ Inject contrast at a constant rate similar to the technique defined above

FINDINGS

- ☐ Urethral injury is indicated by
  - ✦ Extravasation of contrast material **(FIGURE 21.2)**
    - ✦ Anterior tears will demonstrate extravasation below the urogenital diaphragm
    - ✦ Posterior tears will demonstrate extravasation above the urogenital diaphragm
  - ✦ Failure of contrast material to reach bladder

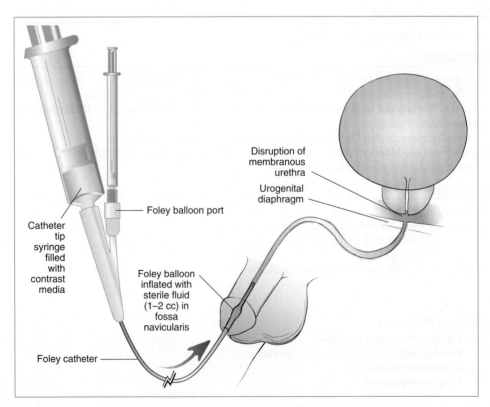

Disruption of membranous urethra

Urogenital diaphragm

Foley balloon port

Catheter tip syringe filled with contrast media

Foley balloon inflated with sterile fluid (1–2 cc) in fossa navicularis

Foley catheter

FIGURE 21.1 The Foley catheter technique for retrograde urethrography. (Reprinted with permission from King C, Henretig FM, King, BR, et al. *Textbook of Pediatric Emergency Procedures.* 2nd ed. Philadelphia, PA: Lippincott Williams & Wilkins, 2008.)

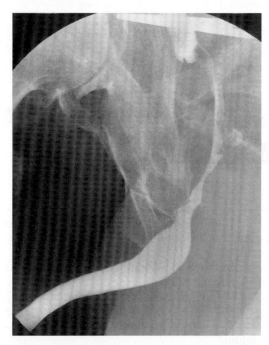

FIGURE 21.2 Retrograde urethrogram with partial tear of membranous urethra. (Reprinted with permission from Wolfson AB, Hendey GW, Ling LJ, et al. *Harwood-Nuss' Clinical Practice of Emergency Medicine.* 5th ed. Philadelphia, PA: Lippincott Williams & Wilkins, 2009.)

◻ If retrograde urethrogram shows injury
  ✚ Do not pass the urethral catheter
  ✚ Obtain a urology consultation

SAFETY/QUALITY TIPS

◻ **Procedural**
  ✚ To prevent contrast extravasation out of the meatus, grasp the distal end of the penis so as to prevent placing pressure proximal to the insufflated Foley balloon
◻ **Cognitive**
  ✚ The most important error is to neglect to perform an RUG when there is an indication, then worsening a urethral injury by attempting to place a Foley catheter
  ✚ Complete tear is indicated by lack of contrast in the bladder; in a partial tear there will be some contrast in the bladder

◻ **Acknowledgment**

Thank you to prior author Michael Rosselli.

Suggested Readings

Carroll PR, McAninch JW. Major bladder trauma: mechanisms of injury and a unified method of diagnosis and repair. *J Urol.* 1984;132(2):254–257.

Corriere JN Jr, Sandler CM. Bladder rupture from external trauma: diagnosis and management. *World J Urol.* 1999;17(2):84–89.

Hoecker C, Ruddy R. Emergent radiologic evaluation of renal and genitourinary trauma. In: Henretig F, King C, eds. *Pediatric Emergency Procedures.* Philadelphia, PA: Lippincott Williams & Wilkins; 1997:429–434.

Schneider R. Urologic procedures. In: Roberts JR, Hedges JR, eds. *Clinical Procedures in Emergency Medicine.* 4th ed. Philadelphia, PA: Saunders; 2004:1107–1112.

22

Femoral Vein—Central Venous Access

Anar D. Shah and Jennifer V. Huang

INDICATIONS

- Emergency venous access for fluid resuscitation, drug infusion, and renal dialysis
- Infusions requiring central venous administration (vasopressors, calcium chloride, hyperosmolar solutions, hyperalimentation)
- Critically ill patients who cannot be placed flat or in Trendelenburg position due to respiratory distress
- Access site for transvenous pacemaker
- Nonemergent venous access due to inadequate peripheral IV sites

CONTRAINDICATIONS

- No absolute contraindications
- **Relative Contraindications**
  - Coagulopathic patients (femoral approach is preferred over the subclavian and internal jugular approaches because it is more easily compressed)
  - Combative or uncooperative patients
  - Overlying infection, burn, or skin damage at puncture site
  - Trauma to the ipsilateral groin or lower extremity
  - Suspected proximal vascular injury, particularly of inferior vena cava (IVC)
  - Ipsilateral renal transplant (risk of venous thrombosis)

RISKS/CONSENT ISSUES

- Pain (local anesthesia will be administered)
- Local bleeding and hematoma
- Infection (sterile technique will be utilized)

- **General Basic Steps**
  - **Vessel localization**
  - **Analgesia**
  - **Insertion**
  - **Seldinger technique**
  - **Dilation**
  - **Catheter placement**
  - **Confirmation**
  - **Flush and secure**

LANDMARK TECHNIQUE

Site of insertion is 2 to 3 cm inferior to the midpoint of inguinal ligament and 1 fingerbreadth medial to the femoral artery (FA) pulse (Figure 22.1). Anatomically, the structures underlying the inguinal ligament, from lateral to medial, are recalled by the mnemonic **NAVEL**.

Femoral **N**erve
Common Femoral **A**rtery
Common Femoral **V**ein
Empty Space
Lymphatics (FIGURE 22.1)

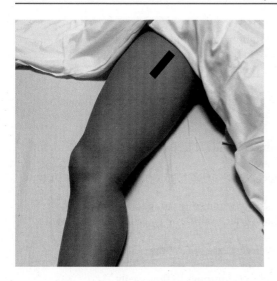

FIGURE 22.1 The thin line represents the pulsatile common femoral artery. The thick line 1 finger-breadth medial to it represents the common femoral vein.

SUPPLIES

- ◘ Central Venous Catheter Kit
  - ✛ Drapes, chlorhexidine prep (2), gauze
  - ✛ Catheter (multiport, cordis, or hemodialysis)
  - ✛ Guidewire within plastic sheath
  - ✛ Lidocaine, anesthesia syringe, and small-gauge needle
  - ✛ Three-inch introducer needle and syringe
  - ✛ Dilator
  - ✛ Scalpel
  - ✛ Suture
  - ✛ Sterile gloves, sterile gown, sterile cap and mask
  - ✛ Sterile drapes
  - ✛ Sterile saline flushes
  - ✛ Sterile port caps
  - ✛ Ultrasound machine (optional)
  - ✛ Sterile ultrasound probe cover with sterile gel (optional)

TECHNIQUE

- ◘ **Patient Preparation**
  - ✛ Cardiac monitoring to detect dysrhythmias triggered by wire advancement into the right ventricle
  - ✛ Supplemental oxygen and continuous pulse oximetry monitoring
  - ✛ Externally rotate the leg and slightly bend the knee to expose the groin
  - ✛ If using ultrasound guidance, evaluate the right and left femoral veins (FVs) before prepping to confirm ideal vein location and compressibility
  - ✛ Sterilize the entire groin with chlorhexidine or povidone–iodine solution
  - ✛ Wear surgical cap, eye protection, mask, sterile gown and gloves
  - ✛ Drape with sterile sheets, covering the body liberally
  - ✛ If using ultrasound guidance, have an assistant place the probe (with gel applied) inside the sterile probe sheath

Note: Unless immediate emergent access is warranted, the physicians attempting the procedure must wear cap, eye protection, and mask, along with sterile gown and gloves.

Vessel Localization

+ If attempting to localize the right FV, use the right hand to hold the introducer needle and syringe. With the left hand, palpate the FA to avoid arterial puncture while guiding needle insertion. If attempting to localize the left FV, reverse hands.

Analgesia

+ Use a small-gauge needle to anesthetize skin and subcutaneous tissue with 1% lidocaine

Insertion

+ Attach a syringe to the introducer needle
+ Using the above landmarks, insert the introducer needle at a 30- to 60-degree angle to skin just medial to the palpated FA pulse
+ Apply negative pressure to the syringe plunger while advancing the needle 3 to 5 cm or until a flash of blood is seen in the syringe
+ If no flash is obtained, withdraw the needle slowly while continuing to aspirate
+ If redirecting the needle, always withdraw the needle to the level of skin before advancing again
+ Once the needle enters vessel, blood will flow freely into the syringe
+ Stabilize and hold the introducer needle
+ Remove the syringe and ensure that venous blood continues to flow easily
+ Use a finger to occlude the needle hub to prevent air embolism

Seldinger Technique

+ Advance the guidewire through the introducer needle. The wire should pass easily. *Do not force it.*
+ Always hold on to the guidewire with one hand. *Never let go of the guidewire.*
+ If resistance is met, withdraw the wire and rotate it, adjust the angle of needle entry, or remove the wire and reaspirate with the syringe to ensure the needle is still in the vessel.
+ When at least half of the guidewire is advanced through the needle, remove the needle over wire. Keep one hand holding the wire at all times.
+ Make a superficial skin incision with the bevel of the scalpel blade angled away from wire
+ Ensure the incision is large enough to allow easy passage for the dilator

Dilation

+ Thread the dilator over the guidewire, always holding on to the wire
+ Advance the dilator through the skin into the vessel with a firm, twisting motion while holding the guidewire with the nondominant hand
+ Remove the dilator, leaving the guidewire in place

Catheter Placement

+ Thread the catheter over the guidewire and retract the guidewire until it emerges from the catheter's port
+ While holding the guidewire, advance the catheter through the skin into the vessel to the desired length
+ Withdraw the guidewire through the catheter
+ Use a syringe to aspirate blood from the catheter to confirm placement in the vein

Confirmation

+ Manometry
+ Blood gas analysis
+ Sonographic confirmation of the catheter in the vein (Figure 22.2)
+ Postprocedure chest x-ray (CXR)
+ Confirm the catheter tip in the superior vena cava just proximal to the right atrium
+ Rule out pneumothorax

Flush and Secure

+ Aspirate, flush, and heplock each central line lumen
+ Suture the catheter to the skin using silk or nylon sutures
+ Cover the skin insertion site with a sterile dressing (bacteriostatic if available) **(FIGURE 22.2)**

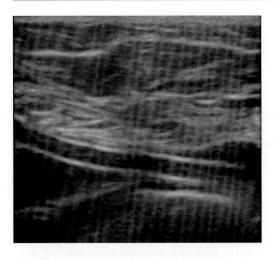

FIGURE 22.2 Longitudinal view of a catheter in the femoral vein.

ULTRASOUND-GUIDED TECHNIQUE

Real-time ultrasound-guided FV catheterization has been shown to:
- Increase success rates
- Decrease the number of attempts
- Decrease skin-to-blood flash time
- Decrease complications
- Help achieve successful cannulation when landmark attempts have failed

SONOGRAPHIC TECHNIQUE

- Use a high-frequency linear probe (5–10 MHz)
- The probe marker should point toward the operator's left so that it corresponds with the marker on the left side of the ultrasound screen
- Identify the FV and FA **(FIGURE 22.3)**
  + Blood vessels are *anechoic* (appear black)
  + Veins are *compressible*. Arteries are not.
  + Veins *do not* have pulsatile flow. Arteries do.
- Evaluate the right and left FVs in the transverse orientation to determine the best site for catheter placement
  + Larger FV diameter improves success
  + Locate an area along the FV where its overlap with the artery is minimal
  + Use gentle compression to assess the patency of the FV. Presence of a noncompressible segment or visible thrombus is a contraindication to catheter placement.

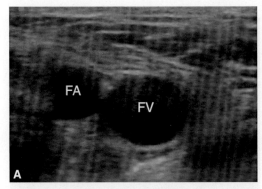
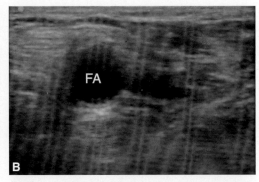

FIGURE 22.3 Sonographic images of the right groin without **(A)** and with **(B)** compression demonstrate the lateral location and noncompressibility of the femoral artery compared to the medial location and compressibility of the femoral vein. FA, femoral artery; FV, femoral vein.

◻ **Sterile Preparation**
- ✚ Follow the steps in the Patient Preparation section as described above
- ✚ Position the ultrasound machine such that the operator's sight, the procedure site, and the screen are in line
- ✚ Have an assistant place the probe (with gel applied) inside the sterile probe sheath **(FIGURE 22.4)**

◻ **Analgesia**
- ✚ Center the probe over the vessel in the transverse orientation. The center of the probe corresponds to the middle of the ultrasound screen.
- ✚ Use a small-bore needle (25 gauge) to anesthetize the skin and subcutaneous tissue with 1% lidocaine just proximal to the probe

◻ **Insertion—Static and Dynamic Techniques**

◻ **Static Ultrasound-guided Technique**
- ✚ Approximate the depth of the vein on the ultrasound screen. If the depth of the vein is 1 cm, the needle should enter the skin approximately 1 cm away from the probe. This will facilitate visualization of the needle as it enters the vein (Figure 22.5).
- ✚ Without moving the probe, insert the needle into the skin 1 cm proximal to the midline of the probe at 30- to 60-degree angle to the skin **(FIGURE 22.5)**
- ✚ Maintain the needle alignment with center of the probe to ensure your needle enters the vessel centered on the ultrasound screen

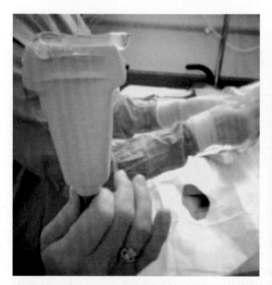
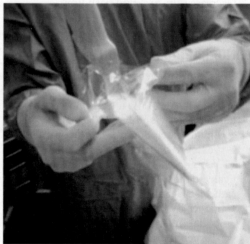

FIGURE 22.4 Sterile probe sheath application. Image courtesy of Mount Sinai Emergency Medicine (http://sinaiem.us/tutorials/peripheral-iv-access).

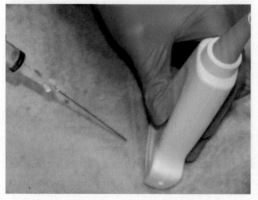
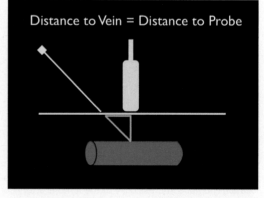

Distance to Vein = Distance to Probe

FIGURE 22.5 Static ultrasound-guided technique.

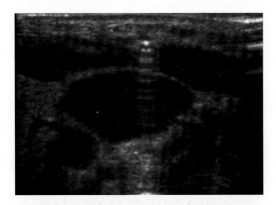

FIGURE 22.6 Ring-down artifact of an echogenic needle.

+ As the needle enters, the subcutaneous tissue distorts. Sometimes the actual needle may not be visualized. To identify the needle location and direction, look for ring-down artifact of the needle and vessel wall tenting **(FIGURE 22.6)**.
+ Apply negative pressure to the syringe plunger and advance the needle until the tip is visualized as it penetrates the superior wall of the vessel or until a flash of blood is seen in the syringe
+ Place the probe on the sterile drape, and stabilize the introducer needle with the nondominant hand
+ Remove the syringe from the introducer needle and confirm that venous blood continues to flow
+ Advance the guidewire through the introducer needle and remove the introducer needle
+ Prior to dilating the vein, use ultrasonography to confirm that the wire is within the vein by using either a transverse or a longitudinal view **(FIGURE 22.7)**
+ Finish placing the catheter using the Seldinger technique as described above

▣ **Dynamic Ultrasound-guided Technique—Track the Needle Tip**
+ Center the probe over the FV in the transverse orientation. The center of the probe corresponds to the middle of the ultrasound screen (Figure 22.3).
+ Without moving the probe, insert the needle 1 to 2 mm proximal to the midline of the probe at a 30- to 60-degree angle **(FIGURE 22.8)**
+ As the needle enters, the subcutaneous tissue distorts and the needle tip should be visualized at the top of the ultrasound screen
+ Once the needle tip is visualized, slide the probe distally along the vein (about 1 cm) until the needle is no longer visualized on the ultrasound screen
+ Advance the needle until it is visualized on the ultrasound screen closer to the vein. Slide the probe distally until the needle is no longer visualized.

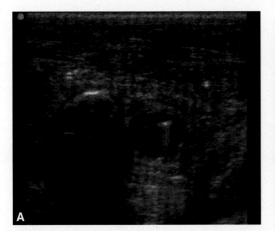

FIGURE 22.7 Transverse **(A)** and longitudinal **(B)** views of the guidewire in the femoral vein.

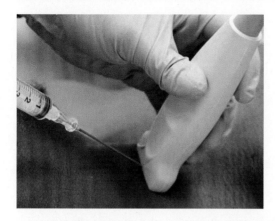

FIGURE 22.8 Dynamic ultrasound-guided technique. Initial needle insertion directly next to the probe with the needle at a 30- to 60-degree angle to the skin.

+ If necessary, redirect the angle of the needle so that it remains centered over the vessel
+ Repeat these steps until the needle is visualized as it penetrates the superior wall of the vessel or until a flash of blood is seen in the syringe **(FIGURE 22.9)**
+ Place the probe on the sterile drape and stabilize the introducer needle with the nondominant hand
+ Remove the syringe from the introducer needle and confirm that venous blood continues to flow
+ Advance the guidewire through the introducer needle and remove the introducer needle
+ Prior to dilating the vein, use ultrasonography to confirm that the wire is within the vein using either a transverse or a longitudinal view (Figure 22.7)
+ Finish placing the catheter using the Seldinger technique as described above

COMPLICATIONS

- Dysrhythmias
- Arterial puncture or cannulation
- Vessel laceration or dissection
- Retroperitoneal hemorrhage due to puncturing of vessel above inguinal ligament
- Guidewire embolism/Lost guidewire
- Air embolism
- Catheter tip embolism
- Catheter malposition
- Venous thrombosis
- Insertion site cellulitis
- Line sepsis
- Local hematoma

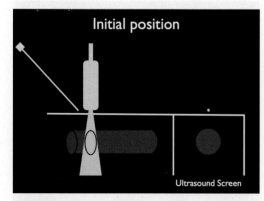
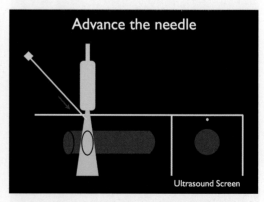

FIGURE 22.9 Dynamic ultrasound-guided technique. Alternate advancing the introducer needle and sliding the probe distally to track the tip of the needle until it is visualized entering the vessel.

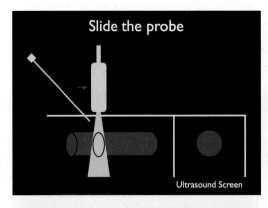

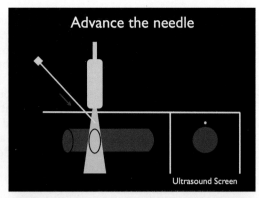

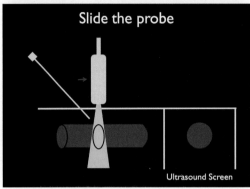

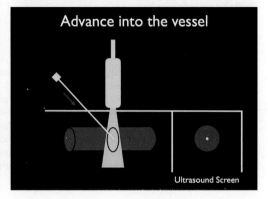

FIGURE 22.9 *(continued)*

SAFETY/QUALITY TIPS

🔲 **Procedural**

✚ Provide adequate local anesthesia and consider using sedation to facilitate the procedure

✚ Never release the guidewire—it must always be secured to prevent its embolism into the vessel

✚ Never force the guidewire or catheter—applying excessive force during insertion or removal can cause vessel injury, wire breakage, or wire embolism

✚ If concerned for wire loss/embolism, immediately clamp the catheter just distal to skin insertion site and seek help

✚ When passing a dilator or catheter over the wire, applying back tension on the wire can prevent the wire from kinking

✚ If the diameter of the FV appears small on ultrasound, lower the foot of the bed 15 to 30 degrees in reverse Trendelenburg or have the patient Valsalva to help dilate the vein

✚ In coagulopathic patients, to prevent inadvertent puncture of the posterior wall of the vein, consider rotating the ultrasound probe 90 degrees to obtain a longitudinal view of the vein to confirm the position of the needle within the FV lumen prior to threading the guidewire

✚ Use a venous confirmation method to verify the wire is in the vein and not in the artery prior to dilating

🔲 **Cognitive**

✚ Ultrasound should be used when feasible, especially in coagulopathic patients, obese patients, or when the landmark technique is unsuccessful

✚ An alternative to the conventional Seldinger technique is to approach the vein with a catheter-over-needle, which comes with most central line kits. Once the needle enters the vein, advance the catheter as you would a peripheral vein. The needle can then be withdrawn, leaving the catheter in the central vein which can be easily transduced or sampled for venous confirmation. Once confirmed, a wire can be passed through the catheter (the catheter transmits the wire better than a needle), the catheter removed, and the procedure proceeds as usual.

+ A common error is to persist with attempts at one site after several failed attempts. It is generally advisable to switch to a different site.
+ Use caution during cardiac arrest to avoid inadvertent cannulation of FA (risk of limb ischemia if infusing vasopressor through artery)
+ Use catheter bundles and a checklist-guided approach to central line placement to minimize the risk of complications

⊡ Acknowledgment

Thank you to prior author Amir Darvish.

Suggested Readings

Balls A, LoVecchio F, Kroeger A, et al. Ultrasound guidance for central venous catheter placement: results from the Central Line Emergency Access Registry Database. *Am J Emerg Med*. 2010;28(5):561–567.

Marik PE, Flemmer M, Harrison W. The risk of catheter-related bloodstream infection with femoral venous catheters as compared to subclavian and internal jugular venous catheters: a systematic review of the literature and meta-analysis. *Crit Care Med*. 2012;40(8):2479–2485.

Miller AH, Roth BA, Mills TJ, et al. Ultrasound guidance versus the landmark technique for the placement of central venous catheters in the emergency department. *Acad Emerg Med*. 2002;9(8):800–805.

Reichman EF, Simon RR. *Emergency Medicine Procedures*. New York, NY: McGraw-Hill; 2004:331–336.

23

Internal Jugular Vein—Central Venous Access

Felipe Teran and Jennifer V. Huang

INDICATIONS

- Emergency venous access for fluid resuscitation and drug infusion
- Infusions requiring central venous administration (vasopressors, hyperosmolar solutions, hyperalimentation)
- Central venous pressure and oxygen monitoring
- Routine venous access due to inadequate peripheral IV sites
- Introduction of pulmonary artery catheter
- Introduction of transvenous pacing wire

CONTRAINDICATIONS

- No absolute contraindications
- **Relative Contraindications**
  - Coagulopathic patients (femoral approach preferred)
  - Combative or uncooperative patients
  - Overlying infection, burn, or skin damage at puncture site
  - Trauma at the cannulation site
  - Penetrating trauma with suspected proximal vascular injury
  - Suspected cervical spine fracture

RISKS/CONSENT ISSUES

- Pain (local anesthesia will be given)
- Local bleeding and hematoma
- Infection (sterile technique will be utilized)
- Pneumothorax or hemothorax and the need for thoracostomy tube

- **General Basic Steps**
  - **Preprocedure ultrasound (if using ultrasound guidance)**
  - **Vessel localization**
  - **Analgesia**
  - **Insertion**
  - **Seldinger technique**
  - **Dilation**
  - **Catheter insertion**
  - **Confirmation**
  - **Flush and secure**

LANDMARK TECHNIQUE

Site of insertion is the apex of the triangle formed by the sternal and clavicular heads of the sternocleidomastoid muscle and the clavicle. This point is lateral to the carotid pulse. The needle is pointed toward the ipsilateral nipple (FIGURE 23.1).

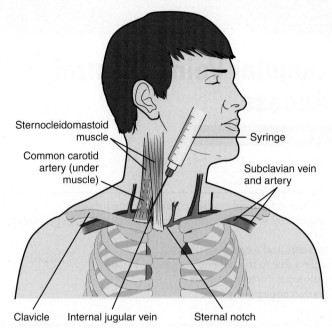

Sternocleidomastoid muscle

Common carotid artery (under muscle)

Syringe

Subclavian vein and artery

Clavicle   Internal jugular vein   Sternal notch

FIGURE 23.1 Landmarks for internal jugular vein central venous catheter placement.

ULTRASOUND-GUIDED TECHNIQUE

Real-time ultrasound-guided internal jugular vein (IJV) catheterization has been shown to:
- Increase success rates
- Decrease the number of attempts
- Decrease skin to blood flash time
- Decrease complications
- Help achieve successful cannulation when landmark attempts have failed

The use of ultrasound to guide the procedure also allows detection of anatomical variants:
- Carotid artery (CA) directly below the IJV instead of lateral
- Small IJV diameter
- Noncompressible IJV, indicating the presence of thrombus

If ultrasound is available for use, placement of the IJV catheter using ultrasound guidance is highly recommended.

SUPPLIES

- Central Venous Catheter (CVC) Kit
  - Drapes, chlorhexidine prep (2), gauze
  - Catheter (multiport, cordis, or hemodialysis)
  - Guidewire within plastic sheath
  - Lidocaine, anesthesia syringe, and a small-gauge needle
  - Three-inch introducer needle and syringe
  - Dilator
  - Scalpel
  - Suture
- Sterile gloves, sterile gown, sterile cap, eye protection, and mask
- Sterile drapes
- Sterile saline flushes
- Sterile port caps
- Ultrasound machine (optional)
- Sterile ultrasound probe cover with sterile ultrasound gel (optional)

TECHNIQUE

Patient Preparation

+ Cardiac monitoring to detect dysrhythmias triggered by the wire being advanced into the right ventricle
+ Supplemental oxygen and continuous pulse oximetry monitoring
+ Rotate the patient's head 30 to 45 degrees away from the side of cannulation
+ Lower the head of the bed to 15 to 30 degrees in Trendelenburg position
+ If using ultrasound guidance, evaluate the right and left IJVs for ideal size and position
+ Sterilize the neck and clavicle area with chlorhexidine or povidone–iodine solution
+ Wear surgical cap, eye protection, mask, sterile gown and gloves
+ Drape with sterile sheets to cover the patient's head and legs
+ If using ultrasound guidance, have an assistant place the probe (with gel applied) inside the sterile probe sheath

Note: Unless immediate emergent access is warranted, the physicians attempting the procedure must wear cap, eye shields, and mask, along with sterile gown and gloves.

Vessel Localization

+ If attempting localization of right IJV, use the right hand to hold the syringe and introducer needle. With the left hand, palpate the CA to avoid arterial puncture while guiding needle insertion. If attempting the left IJV, reverse hands.

Analgesia

+ Use a small-gauge needle to anesthetize skin and subcutaneous tissue with 1% lidocaine

Insertion

+ Using the above landmarks, insert the introducer needle at 30- to 60-degree angle to the skin just lateral to the apex of the triangle just lateral to the carotid pulse (Figure 23.1)
+ Apply negative pressure to the syringe plunger while advancing the needle 3 to 5 cm or until a flash of blood is seen in the syringe
+ If no flash is obtained, withdraw the needle slowly while continuing to aspirate
+ If redirecting the needle, always withdraw the needle to the level of skin before advancing again
+ Once the needle enters the vessel, blood will flow freely into the syringe
+ Stabilize and hold the introducer needle with the nondominant hand
+ Remove the syringe and ensure that venous blood continues to flow easily
+ Use a finger to occlude the needle hub to prevent air embolism

Seldinger Technique

+ Advance the guidewire through the introducer needle. The wire should pass easily. *Do not force the guidewire.*
+ If resistance is met, withdraw the wire and rotate it, adjust the angle of needle entry, or remove the wire and reaspirate with the syringe to ensure the needle is still in the vessel.
+ When at least half of the guidewire is advanced through the needle, remove the needle over the wire. Keep one hand holding the wire at all times. *Never let go of the guidewire.*
+ Make a superficial skin incision with the bevel of the scalpel blade angled away from wire
+ Ensure the incision is large enough to allow easy passage of the dilator

Dilation

+ Thread the dilator over the guidewire, always holding onto the wire
+ While holding the guidewire with the nondominant hand, advance the dilator through the skin into the vessel with a firm, twisting motion
+ Remove the dilator, leaving the guidewire in place

Catheter Insertion

+ Thread the catheter over the wire and retract the wire until it emerges from the catheter's port
+ While holding the guidewire, advance the catheter through the skin into the vessel to the desired depth. Optimal depth depends on patient size and is typically 12 to 18 cm for the right IJV and 15 to 20 cm for the left IJV.
+ Withdraw the guidewire through the catheter
+ Use a syringe to aspirate blood from the catheter to confirm placement in the vein

◻ **Confirmation**
  ✦ Manometry
  ✦ Blood gas analysis
  ✦ Sonographic confirmation of the catheter in the vein
  ✦ Post procedure chest x-ray (CXR)
    ✚ Confirm the catheter tip in the superior vena cava just proximal to the right atrium
    ✚ Rule out pneumothorax
◻ **Flush and Secure**
  ✦ Aspirate, flush, and heplock each central line lumen
  ✦ Suture the catheter to the skin using silk or nylon sutures
  ✦ Cover the skin insertion site with a sterile dressing (bacteriostatic if available)
◻ **Ultrasound-guided Technique**
  ✦ Use a high-frequency linear probe (5–10 MHz)
  ✦ Probe marker on the ultrasound probe should point toward the operator's left so that it corresponds with the marker on left side of the ultrasound screen **(FIGURE 23.2)**
  ✦ Identify the IJV and CA **(FIGURE 23.3)**

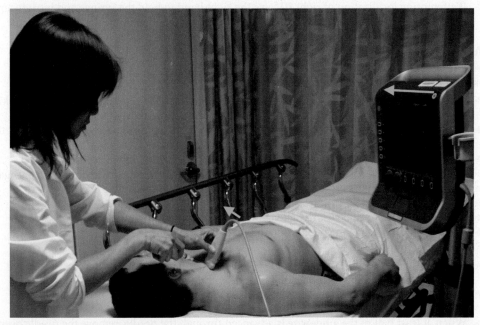

FIGURE 23.2 Correct positioning of the ultrasound machine in line with the operator's sight and procedure site with the probe marker facing the operator's left. (Image courtesy of Mount Sinai Emergency Medicine site, http://sinaiem.us/tutorials/peripheral-iv-access)

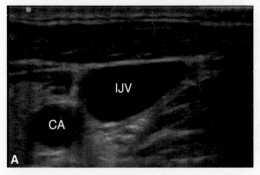
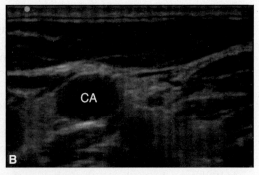

FIGURE 23.3 Sonographic images of the right neck without **(A)** and with **(B)** compression demonstrating the medial location and noncompressibility of the common carotid artery (CA) compared to the lateral location and compressibility of the common internal jugular vein (IJV).

+ Blood vessels are *anechoic* (appear black)
+ Veins are *compressible*. Arteries are not.
+ Veins *do not* have pulsatile flow. Arteries do.
+ Evaluate the right and left IJVs in the transverse orientation to determine the best site for catheter placement
+ Assess the following:
    + IJV diameter >0.7 cm improves successful cannulation
    + Locate an area along the IJV where its overlap with the CA is minimal
    + Use gentle compression to assess the patency of the IJV. Presence of a noncompressible segment or visible thrombus is a contraindication to catheter placement.

Sterile Preparation
+ Follow the steps in the Patient Preparation section as described above
+ Have an assistant place the probe (with gel applied) inside the sterile probe sheath (FIGURE 23.4)

Analgesia
+ Center the probe over the vessel in the transverse orientation. The center of the probe corresponds to the middle of the ultrasound screen.
+ Use a small-bore needle (25 gauge) to anesthetize skin and subcutaneous tissue with 1% lidocaine proximal to the probe

Insertion—Static Technique
+ Approximate the depth of the vein on the ultrasound screen. If the depth of the vein is 1 cm, the needle should enter the skin approximately 1 cm away from the probe. This will facilitate visualization of the needle as it enters the vein (FIGURE 23.5).
+ Without moving the probe, insert the introducer needle 1 cm proximal to the midline of the probe at a 30- to 60-degree angle to the skin (Figure 23.5)
+ Maintain the needle alignment with the center of the probe to ensure your needle enters the vessel centered on the ultrasound screen
+ As the needle enters the skin, the subcutaneous tissue distorts; however, the actual needle may not be visualized. To identify the needle location and direction, look for ring-down artifact of the needle or vessel wall tenting (FIGURE 23.6).
+ Apply negative pressure to the syringe plunger and advance the needle until the tip is visualized as it penetrates the superior wall of the vessel or until a flash of blood is seen in the syringe
+ Place the probe on the sterile drape and stabilize the introducer needle with the nondominant hand

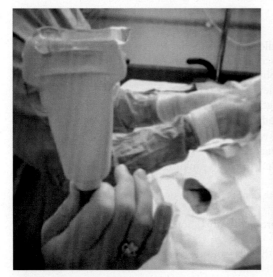 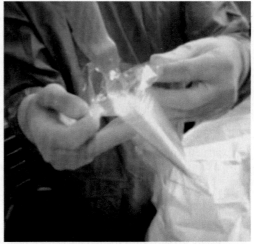

Figure 23.4 Sterile ultrasound probe sheath placement. (Image courtesy of Mount Sinai Emergency Medicine site, http://sinaiem.us/tutorials/peripheral-iv-access)

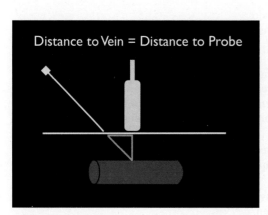
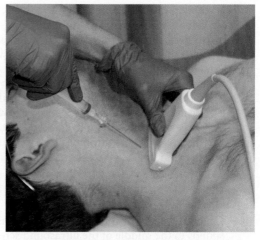

FIGURE 23.5 Static technique: Introducer needle position shown at a 30- to 60-degree angle to the skin.

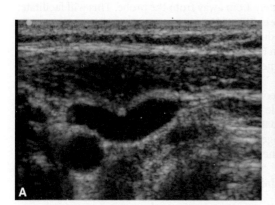
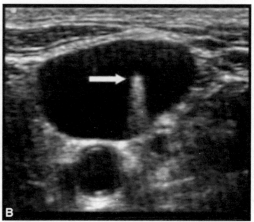

FIGURE 23.6 A: IJV tenting. **B:** Ring-down artifact of the needle within the internal jugular vein. (Image **B** courtesy of Mount Sinai Emergency Medicine site, http://sinaiem.us/tutorials/peripheral-iv-access)

+ Remove the syringe from the introducer needle and confirm that venous blood continues to flow
+ Advance the guidewire through the introducer needle and remove the introducer needle
+ Prior to dilating the vein, use ultrasonography to confirm that the wire is within the vein by using either a transverse or a longitudinal view **(FIGURE 23.7)**
+ Finish placing the catheter using the Seldinger technique as described above

□ **Insertion—Dynamic Technique (Track the Needle Tip)**

+ Center the probe over the vessel in the transverse orientation. The center of the probe corresponds to the middle of the ultrasound screen.
+ Without moving the probe, insert the needle 1 to 2 mm proximal to the midline of the probe at a 30- to 60-degree angle **(FIGURE 23.8)**
+ As the needle enters, the subcutaneous tissue distorts and the needle tip should be visualized at the top of the ultrasound screen
+ Once the needle tip is visualized, slide the probe distally (about 1 cm) until the needle is no longer visualized on the ultrasound screen
+ Advance the needle until it is visualized on the ultrasound screen closer to the vein. Slide the probe distally until the needle is no longer visualized.
+ If necessary, redirect the angle of the needle so that it remains centered over the vessel

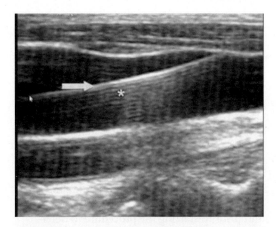

FIGURE 23.7 Long-axis view of the internal jugular vein for the confirmation of wire placement before dilation and catheter insertion. (Image courtesy of Mount Sinai Emergency Medicine site, http://sinaiem.us/tutorials/peripheral-iv-access)

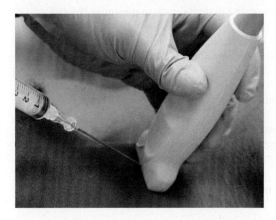

FIGURE 23.8 Dynamic ultrasound-guided technique. Initial needle placement with the needle at a 30- to 60-degree angle to the skin.

+ Repeat these steps until the needle is visualized as it penetrates the superior wall of the vessel or until a flash of blood is seen in the syringe
+ Place the probe on the sterile drape and stabilize the introducer needle with the nondominant hand
+ Remove the syringe from the introducer needle and confirm that venous blood continues to flow
+ Advance the guidewire through the introducer needle and remove the introducer needle
+ Prior to dilating the vein, use ultrasonography to confirm that the wire is within the vein by using either a transverse or a longitudinal view (Figure 23.7)
+ Finish placing the catheter using the Seldinger technique as described above

COMPLICATIONS

- Dysrhythmias
- Arterial puncture or cannulation
- Vessel laceration or dissection
- Pneumothorax or hemothorax
- Thoracic duct injury (left internal jugular [IJ] catheter)
- Guidewire embolism
- Air embolism
- Catheter tip embolism
- Catheter malposition
- Venous thrombosis
- Insertion site cellulitis
- Line sepsis
- Local hematoma

SAFETY/QUALITY TIPS

▢ **Procedural**

+ Provide adequate local anesthesia, and do not neglect sedation if needed to facilitate the procedure
+ Never release the guidewire, for concern of losing the guidewire into the vasculature
+ Never force the guidewire or catheter. Applying excessive force during insertion or removal can cause vessel injury, wire breakage, or wire embolism.
+ If concerned for wire loss/embolism, immediately clamp the catheter just distal to skin insertion site and seek help
+ Always occlude the open hub of the needle to prevent air embolism
+ Sterilize both sides of the neck and clavicle before placing the sterile drapes so that if the first attempted location is unsuccessful, an attempt at the subclavian on the same side can be made
+ Evaluate both sides of the neck with ultrasound prior to starting the procedure to determine the best site for catheter placement
+ When choosing an insertion site, err higher on the patient's neck to minimize the risk of pneumothorax
+ If the diameter of the IJV appears small on ultrasound, lower the head of the bed to increase the degree of Trendelenburg position or have the patient Valsalva to help dilate the vein
+ Unless the patient is in extremis, confirm venous placement of the wire prior to dilation by using manometry, blood gas, or ultrasound to verify that the wire/catheter is properly positioned
+ To prevent inadvertent puncture of the posterior wall of the vein in coagulopathic patients, consider rotating the probe 90 degrees to obtain a longitudinal view of the vein to confirm the position of the needle within the IJ lumen prior to threading the guidewire

▢ **Cognitive**

+ Using ultrasound to guide, IJV access will increase the likelihood of early success and decrease the risk of complications
+ If unsuccessful, do not attempt the opposite side without first obtaining a CXR to avoid bilateral pneumothoraces

▢ **Acknowledgment**

Thank you to prior author Amir Darvish.

Suggested Readings

Beddy P, Geoghegan T, Ramesh N, et al. Valsalva and gravitational variability of the internal jugular vein and common femoral vein: ultrasound assessment. *Eur J Radiol.* 2006;58(2):307–309.

Blaivas M, Adhikari S. An unseen danger: frequency of posterior vessel wall penetration by needles during attempts to place internal jugular vein central catheters using ultrasound guidance. *Crit Care Med.* 2009;37:2345–2349.

Leung J, Duffy M, Finckh A. Real-time ultrasonographically-guided internal jugular vein catheterization in the emergency department increases success rates and reduces complications: a randomized, prospective study. *Ann Emerg Med.* 2006;48(5):540–547.

Miller AH, Roth BA, Mills TJ, et al. Ultrasound guidance versus the landmark technique for the placement of central venous catheters in the emergency department. *Acad Emerg Med.* 2003;9(8):800–805.

Roberts JR, Custalow CB, Thomsen TW, et al. eds. *Roberts & Hedges' Clinical Procedures in Emergency Medicine.* 6th ed. Philadelphia, PA: WB Saunders; 2014.

24

Subclavian Vein—Central Venous Access

George Lim and Jennifer V. Huang

INDICATIONS

- Emergency venous access for fluid resuscitation and drug infusion
- Central venous pressure and oxygen monitoring
- Infusions requiring central venous administration (vasopressors, hyperosmolar solutions, hyperalimentation)
- Routine venous access due to inadequate peripheral IV sites
- Introduction of pulmonary artery catheter
- Introduction of transvenous pacing wire

CONTRAINDICATIONS

- No absolute contraindications
- **Relative Contraindications**
  - Coagulopathic patients (inability to compress)
  - Overlying infection, burn, or skin damage at puncture site
  - Distorted anatomy or trauma at the cannulation site
  - Combative or uncooperative patients
  - Penetrating trauma with suspected proximal vascular injury
  - Pneumothorax on contralateral side (risk of bilateral pneumothoraces)
  - Chronic obstructive pulmonary disease (COPD)

RISKS/CONSENT ISSUES

- Pain
- Local bleeding and hematoma
- Infection
- Pneumothorax/hemothorax (necessitating chest tube)

- **General Basic Steps**
  - **Analgesia**
  - **Insertion**
  - **Seldinger technique**
  - **Dilation**
  - **Catheter insertion**
  - **Confirmation**
  - **Flush and secure**

LANDMARKS

Right subclavian vein (SCV) approach is preferred because (1) pleural dome is lower on the right and (2) thoracic duct is on the left.

- **Infraclavicular Approach** (FIGURE 24.1)
  - Place the left index finger on the suprasternal notch and the thumb on the costoclavicular junction

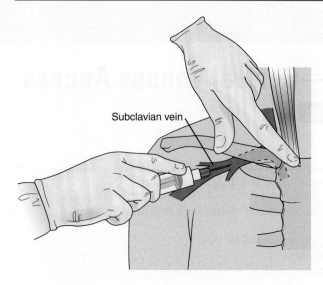

Subclavian vein

FIGURE 24.1 Infraclavicular approach to subclavian vein cannulation. Needle insertion at the bisection of the medial and middle thirds of the clavicle. Aim the needle toward the suprasternal notch.

- ✦ Needle insertion is at the bisection of the medial and middle thirds of the clavicle
- ✦ Aim the needle toward suprasternal notch
- ✦ Needle bevel is oriented inferomedially to facilitate wire entry
- ☐ **Supraclavicular Approach (FIGURE 24.2)**
  - ✦ Needle insertion is just above the clavicle, 1 cm lateral to the insertion of clavicular head of sternocleidomastoid (SCM)
  - ✦ Aim to bisect angle between SCM and clavicle with the needle tip pointing toward the contralateral nipple
  - ✦ Needle bevel is oriented medially

SUPPLIES

- ☐ Central Venous Catheter Kit
  - ✦ Drapes, chlorhexidine prep (2), gauze
  - ✦ Catheter (multiport, cordis, or hemodialysis)
  - ✦ Guidewire within plastic sheath
  - ✦ Lidocaine, anesthesia syringe, and small-gauge needle
  - ✦ Three-inch introducer needle and syringe
  - ✦ Dilator
  - ✦ Scalpel
  - ✦ Suture
- ☐ Sterile gloves, sterile gown, sterile cap and mask
- ☐ Sterile drapes
- ☐ Sterile saline flushes
- ☐ Sterile port caps
- ☐ Ultrasound machine (optional)
- ☐ Sterile ultrasound probe cover with sterile gel (optional)

TECHNIQUE

- ☐ **Patient Preparation**
  - ✦ Cardiac monitoring to detect dysrhythmias triggered by the wire being advanced into the right ventricle
  - ✦ Supplemental oxygen and continuous pulse oximetry monitoring
  - ✦ Lower the head of the bed to 15 to 30 degrees in Trendelenburg position
  - ✦ Place a rolled up towel or sheet in between the patient's shoulder blades to elevate the patient's clavicle and provide better access to the SCV (optional)

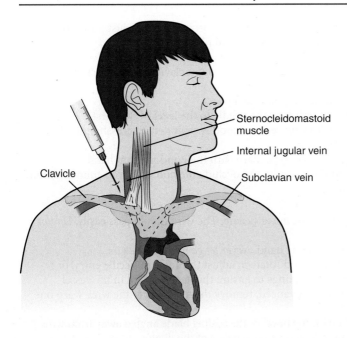

Sternocleidomastoid muscle

Internal jugular vein

Clavicle

Subclavian vein

FIGURE 24.2 Supraclavicular approach to subclavian vein cannulation. Needle insertion is just above the clavicle, 1 cm lateral to the insertion of clavicular head of sternocleidomastoid (SCM). Aim to bisect angle between SCM and clavicle with the needle tip pointing toward the contralateral nipple. The needle tip is pointed 10 degrees above horizontal.

+ Place the ipsilateral arm in abduction
+ Sterilize clavicular insertion site, including ipsilateral neck in case subclavian vascular access fails and internal jugular (IJ) vascular access is necessary
+ Wear surgical cap, eye protection, mask, sterile gown and gloves
+ Drape with sterile sheets to cover the patient's head and legs

Note: Unless immediate emergent access is necessary, the procedure must be performed in full sterile technique (i.e., cap, eye protection, mask, sterile gown, and sterile gloves).

Analgesia
+ Use a small-bore needle (25 gauge) to anesthetize the skin and subcutaneous tissue with 1% lidocaine

Insertion
+ **Infraclavicular Approach**
    + Place the left index finger on the suprasternal notch and the thumb on the costoclavicular junction
    + The needle insertion is at the bisection of medial and middle thirds of the clavicle
    + Aim the needle toward the suprasternal notch with the bevel oriented inferomedially
    + At a shallow angle to the skin, advance the needle just posterior to the clavicle at the junction of middle and medial thirds
    + Apply posterior pressure on the needle to direct it under the clavicle, aiming toward suprasternal notch
    + The needle should be parallel to the bed as it is advanced. Avoid advancing the needle posteriorly into the dome of the lung.
    + Aspirate continuously while advancing the needle
    + If redirecting the needle, always withdraw the needle to the level of skin first
    + Once the vessel is located, free-flowing venous blood is aspirated
    + Stabilize and hold the introducer needle in place with the nondominant hand
    + Gently remove the syringe from the needle and occlude the hub with your thumb to minimize the risk of air embolism
+ **Supraclavicular Approach**
    + The needle insertion is just above the clavicle, 1 cm lateral to the insertion of clavicular head of SCM
    + Aim to bisect the angle between SCM and clavicle with the tip pointing just caudal to the contralateral nipple

- Direct the needle 10 to 15 degrees upward from the horizontal plane, just posterior to the clavicle, again aiming just caudal to the contralateral nipple
- The needle bevel is oriented medially
- Note that the SCV is found more superficially in the supraclavicular approach than in the infraclavicular approach
- Aspirate continuously while advancing the needle
- If redirecting the needle, always withdraw the needle to the level of skin first
- Once the vessel is located, free-flowing venous blood is aspirated. Successful puncture usually occurs at a depth of 2 to 3 cm.
- Stabilize and hold the introducer needle in place with the nondominant hand
- Gently remove the syringe from the needle and occlude the hub with your thumb to minimize the risk of air embolism

Seldinger Technique

- Advance the guidewire through the introducer needle. The wire should pass easily. *Do not force the guidewire.*
- Always hold on to the guidewire with one hand. *Never let go of the guidewire.*
- If resistance is met, withdraw the wire and rotate it, adjust the angle of needle entry, or remove the wire and reaspirate with the syringe to ensure the needle is still in the vessel
- When at least half of the guidewire is advanced, remove the needle over the wire. Keep one hand holding the wire at all times.
- Make a superficial skin incision with the bevel of the scalpel blade angled away from wire
- Ensure the incision is large enough to allow easy passage of the dilator

Dilation

- Thread the dilator over the guidewire, always holding on to the wire
- Advance the dilator through the skin into the vessel with a firm, twisting motion while holding the guidewire with the nondominant hand
- Remove the dilator, leaving the guidewire in place

Catheter Insertion

- Thread the catheter over the wire and retract the wire until it emerges from the catheter's port
- While holding the guidewire, advance the catheter through the skin into the vessel to the desired depth. Optimal depth depends on patient size and is typically 10 to 15 cm for the right SCV and 14 to 19 cm for the left SCV.
- Withdraw the guidewire through the catheter
- Use a syringe to aspirate blood from the catheter to confirm placement in the vein

Confirmation

- Manometry
- Blood gas analysis
- Sonographic confirmation of the catheter in the vein
- Post procedure chest x-ray (CXR)
  - Confirm the catheter tip is in the superior vena cava just proximal to the right atrium
  - Rule out pneumothorax

Flush and Secure

- Aspirate, flush, and heplock all central line lumens
- Suture the catheter to the skin by using silk or nylon sutures
- Cover the skin insertion site with sterile dressing (bacteriostatic if available)

COMPLICATIONS

- Dysrhythmias
- Arterial puncture or cannulation
- Vessel laceration or dissection
- Pneumothorax or hemothorax
- Brachial plexus injury
- Phrenic nerve injury
- Tracheal puncture or endotracheal cuff perforation

- Guidewire embolism
- Air embolism
- Catheter tip embolism
- Catheter malposition
- Venous thrombosis
- Insertion site cellulitis
- Line sepsis
- Local hematoma

ULTRASOUND-GUIDED CENTRAL VENOUS ACCESS

- Use of ultrasound guidance to place IJ and femoral central venous catheters has been shown to increase success rates and decrease complications
- Current literature suggests that the use of ultrasound guidance can be helpful when placing subclavian central venous catheters

SONOGRAPHIC TECHNIQUE

- Place a high-frequency linear probe (5–10 MHz) just inferior to the middle and medial thirds of the clavicle with the probe marker pointed cephalad (a probe with a smaller footprint will allow better visualization of the subclavian anatomy)
- Obtain a transverse view of SCV inferior to the clavicle and superior to the 1st rib. Use color flow and/or Doppler to distinguish the artery from vein (FIGURE 24.3).
- Rotate the probe 90 degrees, visualizing the vein continuously, and obtain a longitudinal view of SCV. Because of the clavicle, the probe may need to be moved laterally to visualize the SCV as it becomes the axillary vein distal to the 1st rib.
- Use color flow and/or Doppler to distinguish the vein from artery (FIGURE 24.4)
- Maintain a longitudinal view of the SCV (stabilize the hand holding the probe on the patient's chest to keep the probe in position)
- Insert the introducer needle at a 30- to 45-degree angle to the skin in line with the long axis of the ultrasound probe
- Note that the probe marker is facing the needle entry site and the needle should enter the skin directly next to the probe (FIGURE 24.5)
- The needle must be parallel to the long axis of the ultrasound probe to be visualized
- This in-plane approach allows direct visualization of the entire needle shaft and tip as it enters the vein and decreases the risk of pneumothorax and arterial puncture

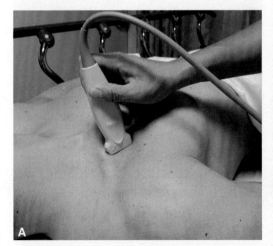
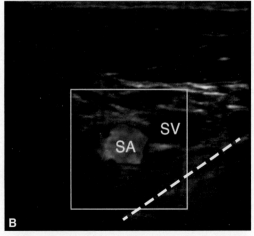

FIGURE 24.3 A: Ultrasound probe inferior to the clavicle with probe marker pointed cephalad. **B:** Subclavian artery (SA, red) and subclavian vein (SCV) with color flow just superior to the 1st rib and pleural line (*dashed line*).

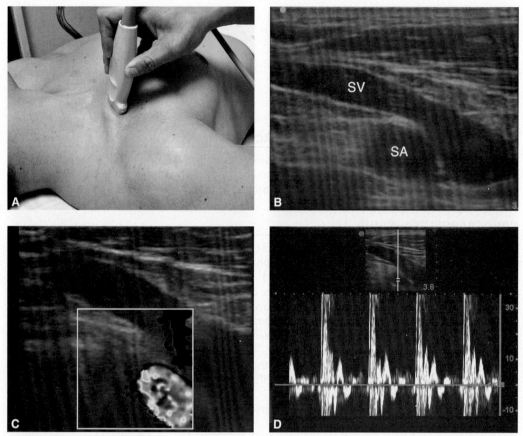

FIGURE 24.4 **A:** Ultrasound probe inferior to the clavicle with probe marker pointed toward the operator. **B:** Longitudinal view of the subclavian vein (SCV) and subclavian artery (SA). **C:** Color flow imaging of the SV and SA. **D:** Doppler illustrating an arterial wave form within the subclavian artery.

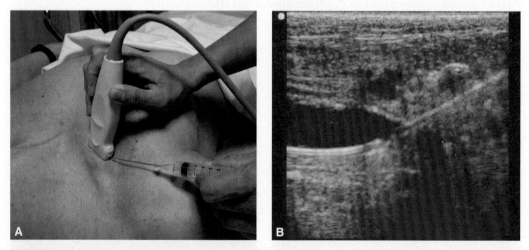

FIGURE 24.5 **A:** Ultrasound probe positioned inferior to the clavicle. The needle path is parallel to the long axis of the probe and the insertion site is directly next to the probe. **B:** Longitudinal view of the axillary vein as the wire is being thread through the introducer needle.

SAFETY/QUALITY TIPS

⬚ **Procedural**

+ Provide adequate local anesthesia and do not neglect sedation if needed to facilitate the procedure
+ Never release the guidewire, for concern of losing the guidewire into the vasculature
+ Never force the guidewire or catheter. Applying excessive force during insertion or removal can cause vessel injury, wire breakage, or wire embolism.
+ If concerned for wire loss/embolism, immediately clamp the catheter just distal to skin insertion site and seek help
+ Always occlude the open hub of the needle to prevent air embolism
+ Sterilize both sides of the neck and clavicle before placing the sterile drapes so that if the first attempted location is unsuccessful, an attempt at the IJ on the same side can be made
+ If the diameter of the SCV appears small on ultrasound, lower the head of the bed to increase the degree of Trendelenburg position or have the patient Valsalva to help dilate the vein
+ Unless the patient is in extremis, confirm venous placement of the wire prior to dilation by using manometry, blood gas, or ultrasound to verify that the wire/catheter is properly positioned

⬚ **Cognitive**

+ The subclavian approach has fallen out of favor because the internal jugular vein (IJV) is so amenable to ultrasound guidance. However, the supraclavicular approach to the SCV and, to a lesser degree, the conventional infraclavicular approach can be imaged with ultrasound.
+ The noncompressible subclavian site is avoided in coagulopathic patients
+ The subclavian approach is also suboptimal in patients with respiratory compromise, as pneumothorax is most likely at the subclavian site
+ If unsuccessful, do not attempt the opposite side without first obtaining a CXR to avoid bilateral pneumothoraces

⬚ **Acknowledgment**

Thank you to prior author Lucy Willis.

Suggested Readings

Balls A, LoVecchio F, Kroeger A, et al. Ultrasound guidance for central venous catheter placement: results from the Central Line Emergency Access Registry Database. *Am J Emerg Med.* 2010;28:561–567.

Fragou M, Gravvanis A, Dimitriou V, et al. Real-time ultrasound-guided subclavian vein cannulation versus the landmark method in critical care patients: a prospective randomized study. *Crit Care Med.* 2011;39:1607–1612.

Mansfield PF, Hohn DC, Fornage BD, et al. Complications and failures of subclavian-vein catheterization. *N Engl J Med.* 1994;331:1735–1738.

Simon RR, Brenner BE. *Emergency Procedures and Techniques.* 4th ed. Philadelphia, PA: Lippincott Williams & Wilkins; 2002:452–469.

Troianos CA, Hartman GS, Glas KE, et al. Guidelines for performing ultrasound guided vascular cannulation: recommendations of the American Society of Echocardiography and the Society of Cardiovascular Anesthesiologists. *J Am Soc Echocardiogr.* 2011;24:1291–1318.

25

Intraosseous Vascular Access

Bret P. Nelson

INDICATIONS

- Used as emergent vascular access for fluid resuscitation and drug infusion when unable to obtain peripheral venous access
- Primarily used in pediatric cardiac arrest—generally a faster access than central line in infants or children
- Used in adult resuscitation if other forms of vascular access cannot be established

CONTRAINDICATIONS

- **Absolute Contraindications**
  - Fracture at the insertion site
- **Relative Contraindications**
  - Previous attempt to place intraosseous (IO) needle on the same bone
  - Osteogenesis imperfecta
  - Osteoporosis
  - Overlying infection, burn, or skin damage at insertion site

RISKS/CONSENT ISSUES

- Pain (local anesthesia can be given)
- Local bleeding and hematoma
- Growth plate injuries or fractures
- Extravasation of fluid or drugs through iatrogenic fracture/puncture site
- Osteomyelitis and cellulitis

- **General Basic Steps**
  - **Sterilize**
  - **Anesthesia**
  - **Place IO**

LANDMARKS

- Standard placement of the IO line is 1 to 2 cm distal to the tibial tuberosity on the anteromedial aspect of the tibia (FIGURE 25.1)
- Alternate sites for placement
  - Medial aspect of the distal tibia approximately 1 to 2 cm proximal to the medial malleolus (FIGURE 25.2)
  - Anterior aspect of the distal femur just proximal to the junction of the femoral shaft and the lateral and medial condyles

TECHNIQUE

- Sterilize the insertion site with povidone–iodine solution, chlorhexidine, or alcohol
- If the patient is awake, administer a local anesthetic to the skin and periosteum
- For manual IO insertion:
  - Grasp the IO needle in the palm of the hand using the index finger and thumb to guide and stabilize the needle

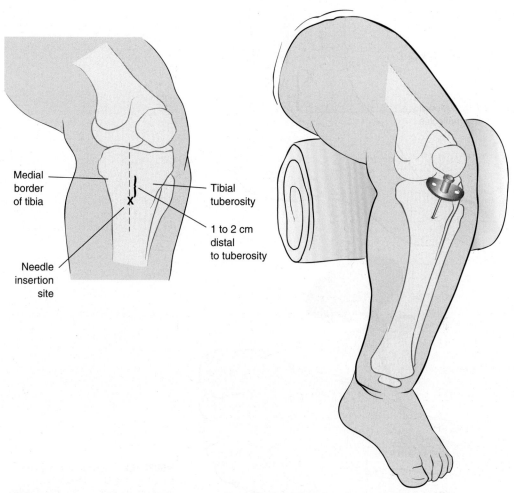

FIGURE 25.1 Entry site at the proximal tibia. (From Hodge D III. Intraosseous infusion. In: King C, Henretig F, eds. *Textbook of Pediatric Emergency Procedures.* Baltimore, MD: Williams & Wilkins; 2008.)

+ Use the nondominant hand to stabilize the leg
+ Insert the IO needle either perpendicular (90 degree) to the tibial surface, or angled 60 to 75 degree caudad to avoid the growth plate. Using firm, constant pressure and a twisting motion, puncture the bone.
- Using a powered (drill) IO insertion device (such as the EZ-IO [Vidacare, San Antonio, TX]):
  + Attach the needle to the drill
  + Grasp the drill in the dominant hand
  + Use the nondominant hand to stabilize the leg
  + Using firm, steady pressure as the drill is powered on, drill the needle until a decrease in resistance is felt
  + Remove the needle from the drill
- Note that the resistance suddenly decreases once the marrow cavity is entered. It is rarely >1 cm from the skin through the cortex. Excessive force may cause puncture through the posterior cortex.
- Remove the stylet
- Use a 5- to 10-mL syringe to aspirate blood for confirmation of placement
- If no aspirate is obtained, carefully infuse 3 mL of normal saline. Palpate the area for any signs of extravasation.
- Secure the needle and immobilize extremity

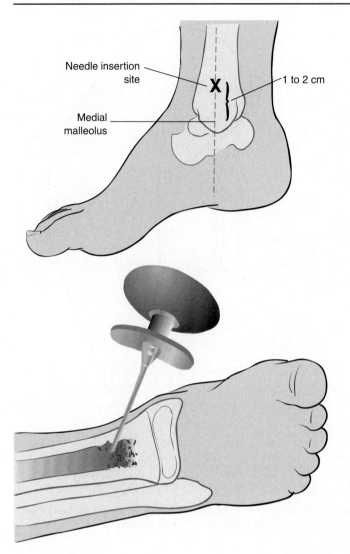

Needle insertion site

1 to 2 cm

Medial malleolus

FIGURE 25.2 Intraosseous infusion. (From Hodge D III. Intraosseous infusion. In: King C, Henretig F, eds. *Textbook of Pediatric Emergency Procedures.* Baltimore, MD: Williams & Wilkins; 2008.)

COMPLICATIONS

- Undetected extravasation of fluid into the surrounding tissue leading to compartment syndrome
- Extravasation of medications into the surrounding skin leading to skin necrosis
- Localized bleeding
- Fat embolization (rare complication only reported in adults)
- Iatrogenic fractures
- Cellulitis and osteomyelitis
- Growth plate injuries possible (no report of permanent growth plate or bone damage reported)

SAFETY/QUALITY TIPS

- **Procedural**
  + Applying excessive force on the needle during insertion can lead to penetration through the posterior cortex; be especially mindful in smaller patients/pediatrics
  + Conversely, especially in obese patients, incomplete insertion of the needle into the bone, not penetrating the marrow space, is a common cause of procedural failure

□ **Cognitive**

+ All medications, as well as crystalloid solutions and blood products, can be given safely through the IO line

+ Blood from the IO access site may be sent for typing and screening and serum chemistries. Complete blood count of marrow aspirate is not a reliable representation of peripheral blood.

+ If unsuccessful, move to opposite leg or alternative site because even if successful with the second attempt, the first puncture site will allow fluid to extravasate into surrounding tissue

+ Infusion rates are three to four times faster with pressure infusions when compared to gravity infusions. Therefore, use a 30- to 60-mL syringe to give fluid boluses or use pressure bags for rapid infusion of fluid or blood products.

+ Blood clots may block the needle opening. Frequent flushing of the line with 3 to 5 mL of saline or use of pressure infusions will prevent this from occurring.

+ Remove the IO line once other vascular access has been established to reduce the risk of infection, extravasation, or dislodgement of needle

□ **Acknowledgment**

Thank you to prior author Kimberly Reagans.

Suggested Readings

Hodge D III. Intraosseous infusion. In: King C, Henretig F, eds. *Textbook of Pediatric Emergency Procedures.* Baltimore, MD: Williams & Wilkins; 2008;281–288.

26

Peripheral Venous Cutdown—Saphenous Vein at Ankle

Raashee Sood Kedia

INDICATIONS

- ⊞ Emergent venous access for fluid resuscitation or drug infusion if alternative peripheral or central access is either unattainable or contraindicated

CONTRAINDICATIONS

- ⊞ **Absolute Contraindications**
  - ✛ Major blunt, long-bone fracture or penetrating trauma proximal to site of cutdown
- ⊞ **Relative Contraindications**
  - ✛ Suspected proximal vascular injury (in the extremity or inferior vena cava)
  - ✛ Overlying infection, burn, or skin damage at the site of cutdown
  - ✛ Coagulopathy

RISKS/CONSENT ISSUES

- ⊞ Pain (local anesthesia can be given)
- ⊞ Local bleeding and hematoma
- ⊞ Infection (sterile technique will be utilized)

- ⊞ **General Basic Steps**
  - ✛ **Analgesia**
  - ✛ **Isolate**
  - ✛ **Stabilize**
  - ✛ **Cannulate**
  - ✛ **Secure**

LANDMARKS

Greater saphenous vein is most easily accessible 1 to 2 cm anterior and 1 to 2 cm superior to the medial malleolus. The vein may be palpable in a nonhypotensive patient (**FIGURE 26.1**).

SUPPLIES

- ⊞ Povidone–iodine or chlorhexidine solution
- ⊞ Anesthetic supplies: 1% lidocaine, 1 vial, 10-mL syringe, 22- or 25-gauge needle
- ⊞ No. 10 and no. 11 scalpel blades
- ⊞ Curved Kelley hemostat
- ⊞ Catheter-over-the-needle, 16 or 18 gauge
- ⊞ Needle driver
- ⊞ Silk sutures (3-0 and 4-0), nylon suture (4-0)
- ⊞ Iris scissors
- ⊞ Intravenous tubing and injectable sterile saline
- ⊞ Wound dressing supplies

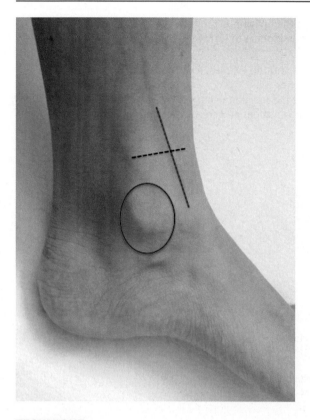

FIGURE 26.1 Saphenous vein runs vertically 2 cm anterior to the medial malleolus of the ankle. The ideal site of cutdown is 2 cm superior to the medial malleolus (*dotted lines*).

TECHNIQUE

☐ **Patient Preparation**
  ✦ Extend and externally rotate lower extremity
  ✦ Immobilize if needed, especially in children
  ✦ Sterilize entire ankle with povidone–iodine solution and drape
Note: Unless immediate emergent access is warranted, universal precautions (cap, eye shields, mask, sterile gown and gloves) should be worn.

☐ **Analgesia**
  ✦ Use 25- or 27-gauge needle to anesthetize skin and subcutaneous tissue with 1% lidocaine

☐ **Isolate: FIGURES 26.2A and B**
  ✦ Make a skin incision *transversely* over saphenous vein landmark
  ✦ Apply traction to skin on either side of the incision to expose subcutaneous tissue
  ✦ Dissect the subcutaneous tissue using a curved hemostat with the tip facing downward, *parallel to the course of the vein*
  ✦ After exposing the vein, pass the hemostat under the vein, turn the tip upward, and spread to isolate the vein above the hemostat

☐ **Stabilize: FIGURE 26.2C**
  ✦ Pass two 3-0 or 4-0 silk suture ties under the vein using the curved hemostat
  ✦ Clamp each tie with hemostats, one proximally and the other distally
  ✦ Distal suture may be tied to ligate the vessel. This decreases bleeding, but also sacrifices the vessel.
  ✦ Apply traction on each tie, thereby lifting the vessel and exposing the anterior surface of the vein

☐ **Cannulate: FIGURES 26.2D and E**
  ✦ With the tip of no. 11 scalpel blade make a flap incision to the anterior surface of the vein, approximately one-third the diameter of the vein
  ✦ A vein pick may be used to elevate the flap

- Carefully advance the catheter through the incision
- Flush the catheter with saline solution and attach to intravenous line

◻ **Secure Catheter:** FIGURE 26.2F

- Tie the proximal suture around the vein and the IV catheter to secure in place
- Cut the ends of the proximal and distal ties
- Suture the catheter to the skin and close the incision using 4-0 nylon sutures
- Cover skin insertion site with antibiotic ointment and sterile dressing

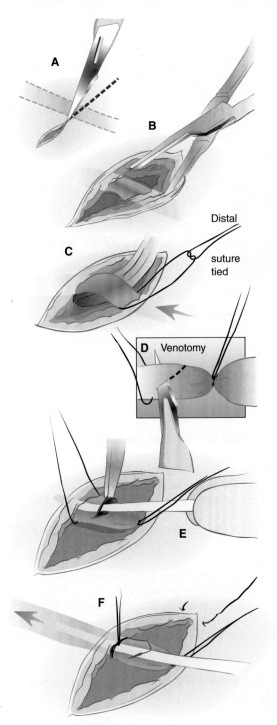

FIGURE 26.2 Procedures for venous cutdown catheterization. **A:** A transverse incision is made 2 cm anterior and superior to medial malleolus. The incision should extend into the subcutaneous tissue but not deep enough to potentially lacerate the vein. **B:** The vein is isolated using blunt dissection. A suture is passed around the vein and cut to give two ligatures. **C:** The distal suture is tied and used to stabilize the vessel. **D:** Venotomy is performed to allow insertion of the catheter. Alternatively the surgeon may choose to insert the catheter over a needle without performing a venotomy, in a manner similar to percutaneous catheterization. **E:** The catheter is inserted into the vein. Placement within the vessel is confirmed by aspirating blood or infusing fluid. **F:** The proximal suture is tied and the wound is closed and dressed. (From Vinci RJ. Venous cutdown catheterization. In: Henretig FM, King C, eds. *Textbook of Pediatric Emergency Procedures.* Philadelphia, PA: Williams & Wilkins; 1997:284, with permission.)

COMPLICATIONS

✢ Injury to surrounding structures such as tibialis anterior tendon and saphenous nerve
✢ Vein transection or laceration without ability to cannulate
✢ Hematoma formation
✢ Phlebitis
✢ Wound infection or dehiscence

SAFETY/QUALITY TIPS

⊡ **Procedural**

✢ Skin incision with scalpel should be superficial to only expose subcutaneous tissue. Deep incision may transect the vein.
✢ The incision on the anterior surface of the vein must be deep enough to fully enter the lumen of the vein. If too large (>½ the diameter of the vein), the vessel may tear completely and cause significant bleeding.
✢ Gently lifting up the proximal tie will help minimize backflow bleeding
✢ Do not tie the proximal suture too tightly around the catheter; this may occlude it
✢ The most difficult and time-consuming aspect is usually threading the catheter into the vein
✢ The vein is very delicate. Do not force the catheter through the vein.

⊡ **Cognitive**

✢ Cut-down vascular access techniques, which are time-consuming and associated with some morbidity, especially in inexperienced hands, have a greatly reduced role in emergency medicine with the rise of intraosseous and ultrasound-guided peripheral intravenous access
✢ Early catheter removal will decrease the incidence of phlebitis and infection

⊡ **Acknowledgment**

Thank you to prior author Amir Darvish.

Suggested Readings

Reichman EF, Simon RR, eds. Peripheral Venous Cutdown. *Emergency Medicine Procedures;New York,* McGraw-Hill; 2013;351–353.
Shockley LW, Butzier DJ. A modified wire-guided technique for venous cutdown access. *Ann Emerg Med.* 1990;19:393.
Vasquez V, Aguilera P. Venous cutdown. In: Roberts JR, Custalow CB, Thomsen TW, et al. eds. *Roberts & Hedges' Clinical Procedures in Emergency Medicine.* 6th ed. Philadelphia, PA: Elsevier Saunders; 2014:432–439.
Vinci R. Venous cutdown catheterization. In: King C, Henretig F, eds. *Textbook of Pediatric Emergency Procedures.* Baltimore, MD: Williams & Wilkins; 2008;273–280.

27

Radial Arterial Cannulation

Ashley Shreves

INDICATIONS

- Direct arterial blood sampling
- Continuous arterial blood pressure monitoring

CONTRAINDICATIONS

- Absolute: None
- **Relative Contraindications**
    + Coagulopathy or recent thrombolysis
    + Overlying infection, burn, or skin damage
    + Severe peripheral atherosclerosis

RISKS/CONSENT ISSUES

- Thrombosis and occlusion of the vessel are common (30%–40%) but almost all resolve spontaneously without requiring intervention, and ischemic complications are rare/case-reportable
- Risk of bleeding and infection are low

- **General Basic Steps**
    + **Position patient**
    + **Locate radial artery**
    + **Anesthetize**
    + **Perform procedure**

LANDMARKS

- Radial artery cannulation site is just medial and proximal to the radial styloid on the volar surface of the wrist

TECHNIQUE

- Position the patient's supinated wrist in 60 degree of extension. Placement of a gauze or towel under the dorsal surface of the wrist and taping the wrist in extension may facilitate positioning.
- Prepare and drape the area in a sterile manner
- Anesthetize the skin over the radial artery with a small wheal of 1% lidocaine
- Open the packaging and remove unit. Remove the protective shield. To ensure proper feeding, advance and retract the spring-wire guide through the needle via the lever. Then retract the wire proximally as far as possible before using.
- Palpate the course of the artery with the middle and index fingers of the nondominant hand. Hold the needle at a 45-degree angle to the skin, pointing cephalad, and puncture the skin. Advance the needle until a flash of bright red blood is seen in the clear hub of the needle.
- Decrease the angle of the needle to 20 degrees and advance the guidewire (via actuating lever) into the artery. Do not force the wire if resistance is encountered.
- Hold the clear transducer needle and advance the catheter forward into the vessel. A rotating motion can be applied to the catheter if resistance is encountered (**FIGURES. 27.1** and **27.2**).
- Holding the catheter in place, remove the introducer needle, guidewire, and feed tube assembly. Pulsatile flow indicates successful cannulation.
- Attach a stopcock and injection tubing to the catheter hub. Suture into place. Apply dressing.

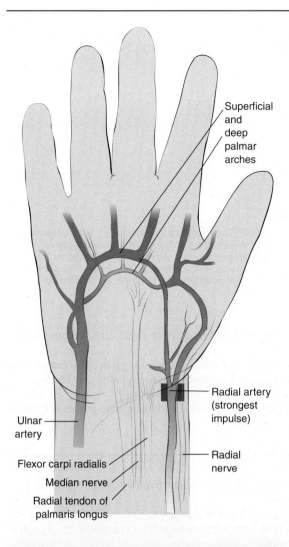

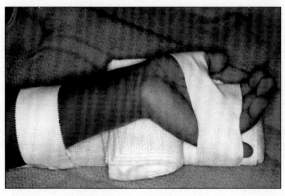

FIGURE 27.1 Radial artery anatomy. (From Torrey SB, Saladino R. *Arterial puncture and catheterization*. In: Henretig FM, King C, eds. *Textbook of Pediatric Emergency Procedures*. Philadelphia, PA: Williams & Wilkins; 1997:784, with permission.)

COMPLICATIONS

➕ Radial artery thrombosis and subsequent occlusion ranges from 4% to 40%, and resolution of thrombosis may take weeks. However, permanent ischemic damage is extremely rare. The Allen test is not a valid predictor of ischemic injury to the hand.

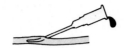

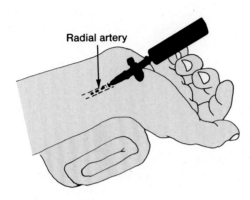

Radial artery

FIGURE 27.2 Radial artery cannulation. Secure the hand and wrist to the arm board, with the wrist placed in extension as shown. (From Simon RR, Brenner BE. *Emergency Procedures and Techniques.* Philadelphia, PA: Lippincott Williams & Wilkins; 2002:505, with permission.)

- Cerebral embolization is theoretically possible and could result from rapid, large-volume, arterial catheter irrigation
- Ecchymoses and minor hematomas at the cannulation site are common (up to 80%) but almost always asymptomatic. If the patient is anticoagulated, compression neuropathy can develop from larger hematomas.
- Infection (line sepsis and cellulitis) is very rare (0.6%), as is pseudoaneurysm formation (0.09%)

SAFETY/QUALITY TIPS

- **Procedural**
  + When arterial pulsations are difficult to palpate (e.g., obesity, hypotensive patients), consider ultrasound-guided catheterization
  + Advancement of wire through resistance can result in damage to the vessel
  + Use of a 20-gauge Teflon catheter has been associated with the least complications. Larger catheters have greater risk for thrombosis.
  + Make sure the target wrist is not rotated as this can shift the location of the vessel
  + Apply a three-way stopcock to the catheter hub to facilitate easy blood gas draws
  + Saline (versus heparin) is sufficient for flushing the catheter, especially during the patient's stay in the emergency department (ED)
- **Cognitive**
  + Venous blood gas analysis is appropriate for most patients who have reliable pulse oximetry. Venipuncture is less painful and associated with fewer complications than arterial puncture.
  + Traditional noninvasive blood pressure monitoring is adequate for the vast majority of patients. Consider invasive monitoring only for critically ill patients, particularly those in shock.

Suggested Readings

Berg K, Riesenberg LA, Berg D, et al. The development of a validated checklist for radial arterial line placement: preliminary results. [Published online ahead of print Jul 11, 2013]. *Am J Med Qual.* 2014;29:242–246. doi: 10.1177/1062860613492189.

Downs JB, Rackstein AD, Klein EF, et al. Hazards of radial-artery catheterization. *Anesthesiology.* 1973;38:283.

Kim HT. Arterial puncture and cannulation. In: Roberts JR, Custalow CB, Thomsen TW, et al. eds. *Roberts & Hedges' Clinical Procedures in Emergency Medicine.* 6th ed. Philadelphia, PA: Elsevier Saunders; 2014;368–384.

Wilkins RG. Radial artery cannulation and ischemic damage: A review. *Anesthesiology.* 1985;40:896.

28

Paracentesis

Maxwell Morrison

INDICATIONS

Paracentesis is the removal of fluid from the peritoneal cavity through the use of a needle for either therapy (to relieve patient symptoms) or diagnosis (to determine causes or complications of ascites). The procedure is generally well-tolerated and simple to perform, especially with the general availability of bedside ultrasound.

DIAGNOSTIC

- To analyze abnormal fluid collection in peritoneal space to determine etiology or pathologic conditions (e.g., infection). Most commonly for diagnosis of spontaneous bacterial peritonitis (SBP).

THERAPEUTIC

- To evacuate ascites for symptomatic relief, usually of shortness of breath and discomfort from abdominal distention. Paracentesis decreased in-hospital mortality 24% when done early (within 24 h of admission) as opposed to later in one large study (Orman ES et.al).

CONTRAINDICATIONS

- Absolute Contraindications
  + Disseminated intravascular coagulopathy
- Relative Contraindications
  + Intra-abdominal adhesions
  + Abdominal wall cellulitis
  + In second or third trimester pregnancy, an open supraumbilical or ultrasound-assisted approach is preferred
  + Exercise caution in coagulopathic or renal failure patients.

- General Basic Steps
  + **Prepare patient**
  + **Anesthesia**
  + **Ultrasound**
  + **Perform procedure**
  + **Send for fluid analysis**

LANDMARKS

- Preferred approach: 3 cm superior and medial to the anterior superior iliac spine
- Stay lateral to the rectus sheath to avoid the inferior epigastric artery. The abdominal wall is also thinner in this location.
- Alternative approach: 2 cm below the umbilicus in the midline. Avoid if the patient has a midline surgical scar.

TECHNIQUE

☐ **Supplies**
   + Bedside ultrasound machine, if available
   + Culture bottles and tubes for cell count, Gram stain, and albumin
   + Have a low threshold to send a cell count with differential, even if the tap is being performed for primarily therapeutic purposes.
   + Commercial paracentesis kits containing rigid plastic sheath cannula, if available
☐ If a kit is not available, then the following supplies should be obtained:
   + Iodine or chlorhexidine swabs
   + Sterile 4 × 4 gauze
   + Sterile towels or fenestrated drape
   + Sterile and nonsterile gloves
   + Sterile 60-cc syringes for collecting fluid sample
   + 10-cc syringe for anesthesia
   + 1% to 2% lidocaine (preferably with epinephrine)
   + Skin anesthesia needles
      + 25- or 27-gauge 1.5-inch needle (local anesthesia)
      + 20- or 22-gauge 1.5-inch needle (local anesthesia)
      + 18-gauge needle (inoculating specimen tubes)
   + Paracentesis needles
      + 22-gauge needle for diagnostic taps, 18-gauge needle for therapeutic taps
      + 1.5 inch should be sufficient, may need 3.5 inch (spinal needle) for obese patients
   + Adhesive bandage
☐ **Patient Preparation**
   + Direct the patient to urinate or empty the bladder via urinary catheterization
   + Ultrasonography (preferred, but not essential). Bedside ultrasonography is used to verify that the chosen site has a large fluid pocket with no bowel adhesions.
   + Sterilize the area where the needle will be inserted with copious povidone–iodine solution or similar surgical prep
   + Drape the area with sterile towels or sterile fenestrated drape
☐ **Patient Positioning**
   + If there is a large amount of ascites, the patient may be placed in a supine position with the head of the bed slightly elevated
   + Patients with lesser amounts of ascites may be placed in a lateral decubitus position for optimal pooling of fluid. Left lateral decubitus may be ideal, as this is generally the most fluid-rich area.
☐ **Analgesia**
   + Produce local anesthesia using up to 5 mg/kg of 1% lidocaine with epinephrine
   + Raise a subcutaneous wheal with a small-bore (25- or 27-gauge) needle, and then generously infiltrate the deeper tissues in the area of the paracentesis needle's eventual passage using a longer, larger-bore needle
   + Anesthetize to the depth of the peritoneum
☐ **Needle Insertion**
   + Standard-sized (1.5-inch) metal needle will be sufficient in most cases
      + A longer (3.5-inch) spinal needle may be necessary in obese patients
      + For diagnostic taps, a smaller-gauge (22–20 gauge) needle should be utilized to decrease the chance of postprocedural fluid leak
      + For therapeutic taps, a larger (18 gauge) needle may be used to hasten fluid evacuation
   + Attach needle to a 60-mL syringe
   + Advance the needle in slow, controlled 5-mm increments with continuous gentle aspiration of the syringe. A "Z-tract" method may be employed to decrease the risk of postprocedural fluid leak (FIGURE 28.1).
      + Overlying skin is pulled by an assistant or by the non–needle bearing hand 2 cm in the caudal direction

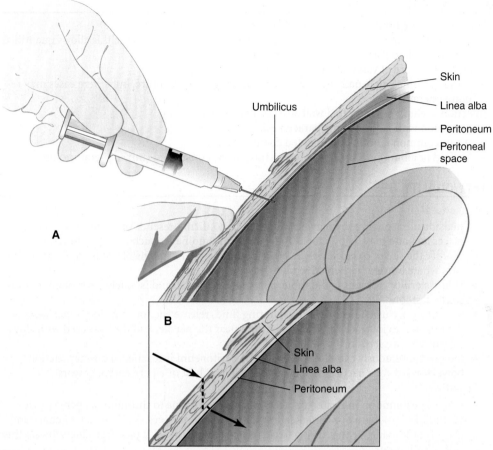

FIGURE 28.1 Z-track formation and controlled removal of ascetic fluid. **A:** Needle insertion with caudal traction on overlying skin. **B:** Z-track formation after release of skin and removal of needle. (From Lane NE, Paul RI. Paracentesis. In: Henretig FM, King C, eds. *Textbook of Pediatric Emergency Procedures*. Philadelphia, PA: Williams & Wilkins, 1997:924, with permission.)

+ After penetrating the peritoneum and obtaining fluid return, the skin is released
+ Upon removal of the needle, skin will slide and return to original positioning, sealing the needle tract

◻ **Fluid Drainage**
  ✛ Metal needles should be stabilized to the patient's skin with a thick stack of commercial tube sponges or with 4-inch gauze pads secured with tape. Metal needles may be left in place for 1 hour without significant risk of injury.
  ✛ If the flow ceases, the needle should be gently rotated and/or advanced in 1-mm increments
  ✛ IV tubing and a three-way stopcock may be attached to facilitate drainage of larger quantities
  ✛ Vacuum bottles may be utilized to facilitate drainage
  ✛ Use caution because the continuous suction provided may attract bowel or omentum to the end of the paracentesis needle with resultant occlusion

◻ **Ascitic Fluid Analysis**
  ✛ Order the following standard tests (see Safety/Quality Tips for additional tests). Generally, 1 to 2 mL of fluid is needed for each tube.
    + Culture and sensitivity
    + Gram stain
    + Cell count
    + Albumin level

COMPLICATIONS

- Persistent ascitic fluid leak at the puncture site (rectified with single suture)
    - Consider placing an ostomy bag instead of gauze if fluid leak persists; this allows quantification of the fluid leak and eliminates dressing changes
- Trauma: Puncture of vasculature, organs, or hollow viscera
    - Local bleeding can usually be controlled with a figure-of-8 suture, but severe cases may require operative repair
- Infection: Cellulitis, abdominal wall abscess, peritonitis (rare)
- Hypotension with large-volume paracentesis (>5 L)
    - An uncommon, poorly documented complication
    - Colloid or albumin infusion to prevent this can be considered (mixed literature support)

SAFETY/QUALITY TIPS

- **Procedural**
    - Bedside ultrasonography may be employed to confirm presence of ascites before needle placement and may help in identifying anatomic anomalies such as bowel adhesions
    - Modify the site of paracentesis to avoid abdominal scars and visible veins. Scars are often sites where bowel is tethered by adhesions.
    - While sterility is certainly desirable, paracentesis can be, and is, safely performed in non-sterile fashion
    - Should an occlusion occur while aspirating fluid, release suction, consider repositioning the position to increase the amount of fluid near the needle, and then proceed with slow, intermittent aspiration
    - Do not continuously aspirate fluid once the peritoneum is reached. This may suction bowel toward your needle, causing an occlusion at best or a perforation at worst.
- **Cognitive**
    - Do not postpone an indicated paracentesis procedure due to thrombocytopenia or elevated INR—risk of major complication is low (2% in one series) (Grabau, CM et.al), and there is little evidence that trying to correct coagulopathy with blood products lowers this complication rate.
    - If no ascites pocket is detected on ultrasound, SBP is less likely and can be ruled out with computed tomography-guided paracentesis if needed. Complications are more likely if emergency department (ED)-based paracentesis is attempted in the absence of sonographically confirmed ascites.
    - Have a low threshold to send a cell count with differential, even if the tap is therapeutic. SBP is notoriously clinically occult.
    - Laboratory: Consider the following additional ascites fluid tests (based on clinical suspicion):
        + Bilirubin: Bowel or biliary perforation
        + Protein and glucose: SBP or gut perforation
        + Lactate dehydrogenase (LDH): SBP or malignancy
        + Amylase/triglyceride: Chylous ascites
        + Cytology: Malignancy
        + Tuberculosis smear/culture

ASCITIC FLUID INTERPRETATION

- Strongly suspect SBP if there are >250 neutrophils/μL or >500 WBCs/μL
- Low protein (higher risk to develop SBP), low glucose, and elevated LDH suggest SBP
- Correct for a hemorrhagic tap by subtracting 1 WBC for every 250 RBC/mm
- Serum-ascites albumin gradient (SAAG): Ascites can be classified based on this gradient. The SAAG is the difference between the measured serum and ascitic albumin concentrations. SAAG = [Albumin in Serum] − [Albumin in Ascitic Fluid]
- SAAG ≥1.1 correlates with conditions that increase portal pressure (transudates)

- SAAG <1.1 correlates with conditions that produce exudates
  - High gradient (≥1.1 g/dL): Transudative
    - Cirrhosis
    - Heart failure
    - Budd–Chiari syndrome (hepatic vein thrombosis)
    - Constrictive pericarditis
  - Low gradient (<1.1 g/dL): Exudative
    - Cancer (primary peritoneal carcinomatosis or metastases)
    - Tuberculosis peritonitis
    - Pancreatic ascites
    - Nephrotic syndrome
    - Serositis in connective tissue diseases

Acknowledgment

Thank you to prior author Brian Kwong and Mark Clark.

Suggested Readings

De Gottardi A, Thevenot T, Spahr L, et al. Risk of complications after abdominal paracentesis in cirrhotic patients: a prospective study. *Clin Gastro Hep*. 2009;7(8):906–909.

Grabau CM, Crago SF, Hoff LK, et al. Performance standards for therapeutic abdominal paracentesis. *Hepatology*. 2004;40:484.

Marx JA. Peritoneal procedures. In: Roberts JR, Hedges JR, eds. *Clinical Procedures in Emergency Medicine*. 4th ed. Philadelphia, PA: WB Saunders; 2004:851–856.

Orman ES, Hayashi PH, Bataller R, et al. Paracentesis is associated with reduced mortality in patients hospitalized with cirrhosis and ascites. *Clin Gastroenterol Hepatol*. 2014;12(3):496–503.

Runyon BA. Ascites and spontaneous bacterial peritonitis. In: Feldman M, Friedman L, Brandt LJ, eds. *Sleisenger and Fordtran's Gastrointestinal and Liver Diseases*. 8th ed. Elsevier, Philadelphia; 2010:1517.

29

Gastroesophageal Balloon Tamponade and the Sengstaken–Blakemore Tube

David Diller

INDICATIONS

- Unstable patients with gastroesophageal varices receiving maximal medical therapy
- Endoscopy is unavailable or unsuccessful

CONTRAINDICATIONS

- Esophageal strictures or recent gastroesophageal surgery
- Relative:
  - No active bleeding
  - Incomplete equipment
  - Source of bleeding likely gastric

- **General Basic Steps**
  - **Gather supplies**
  - **Prepare patient—intubate**
  - **Placement and gastric balloon inflation**
  - **Traction**
  - **Esophageal balloon inflation**

SUPPLIES

- Sengstaken–Blakemore (SB) tube (triple lumen tube) or Minnesota tube (quadruple lumen tube). The fourth port is for suctioning the proximal esophagus.
- Salem Sump (double-lumen nasogastric tube) and silk ties to create necessary fourth lumen (not needed if using a Minnesota tube)
- 60-mL Luer lock syringe
- 60-mL Piston syringe
- 2 Christmas tree catheter adapters
- 2 Three-way stopcocks
- 2 Heplock caps
- Surgilube
- 1 Sterile gauze bandage roll (Kerlix)
- 1 L NS (normal saline)
- Kelly clamps (padded)
- 2 wall-suction units
- Straight connector
- Manual sphygmomanometer

TECHNIQUE

- Preparation
- Secure the airway. The patient will be intubated in almost all scenarios. Raise the head of the bed to 45 degrees.

- Assemble attachments to gastric balloon and esophageal balloon ports
- Test for air leaks using 60-cc Luer lock syringe
  - Gastric balloon—Inflate 250-cc air
  - Esophageal balloon—Inflate 60-cc air
- Deflate the balloons completely
- If using an SB tube, create fourth lumen:
  - Place the distal tip of Salem Sump 2 cm proximal to the esophageal balloon and secure with silk ties **(FIGURE 29.1)**

Placement and Gastric Balloon Inflation

  - Lubricate the gastroesophageal balloon tamponade (GEBT). Insert orogastrically so that the 50-cm mark aligns with the patient's lip. Can insert nasally; however, the oral route is preferred **(FIGURE 29.2)**.
  - Confirm placement via air insufflation through gastric port and auscultation for gastric sounds
  - Connect gastric port to 60 to 120 mm Hg intermittent suction. Inflate the gastric balloon with 50 cc of air.
  - **Confirm with chest x-ray that the inflated balloon is in the stomach**
  - Inflate additional 200 cc of air into gastric balloon, for a total of 250 cc of air
  - Affix padded Kelly clamp to gastric balloon port

Traction

  - The proximal end of the GEBT needs to be secured with traction
  - Attach Kerlix distal to SB tube ports by creating a slip knot. Secure the opposing end to 1-L NS bag (or similar weight).
  - Hang Kerlix over the IV pole, allowing the 1-L NS bag to hang freely, applying traction to the SB tube

Esophageal Balloon Inflation

  - Connect sphygmomanometer to the three-way stopcock on esophageal balloon port
  - Inflate the esophageal balloon to 30 to 45 mm Hg (typically 50–70 cc air), using lowest pressure necessary

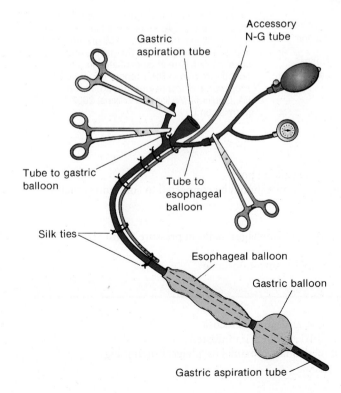

Gastric aspiration tube

Accessory N-G tube

Tube to gastric balloon

Tube to esophageal balloon

Silk ties

Esophageal balloon

Gastric balloon

Gastric aspiration tube

FIGURE 29.1 Modified Sengstaken–Blakemore tube. Also available is the Minnesota tube, which has a built-in esophageal port. (Reused with permission from Yamada T. *Textbook of Gastroenterology.* 4th ed. Vol 1. Philadelphia, PA: Lippincott Williams & Wilkins; 2003:707.)

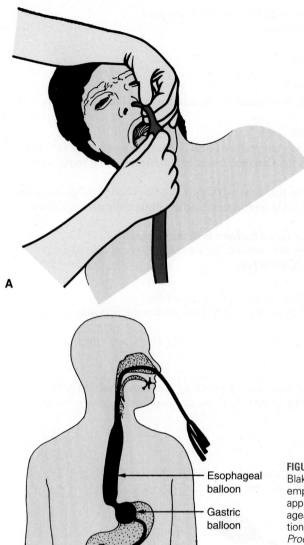

A

B

Esophageal balloon

Gastric balloon

FIGURE 29.2 The placement of an Sengstaken-Blakemore tube. **A:** To pass the tube, fold the empty balloon around itself, and give the patient appropriate analgesia. **B:** The gastric and esophageal balloons are shown inflated in proper position. (From Simon RR, Brenner BE. *Emergency Procedures & Techniques*. 4th ed. Philadelphia, PA: Lippincott Williams & Wilkins; 2002:11, with permission.)

- ✛ Affix padded Kelly clamp to esophageal balloon port
- ✛ The Salem Sump or proximal esophageal port should be connected to continuous suction to clear proximal secretions
- ⊡ **Tube Maintenance**
  - ✛ Once tamponade is achieved, decrease the esophageal balloon pressure 5 mm Hg every 3 hours until 25 mm Hg is reached
  - ✛ Maintain adequate sedation as the GEBT is uncomfortable

COMPLICATIONS

- ⊡ Esophageal rupture
- ⊡ Pressure necrosis of lips, nose, esophagus, and gastric mucosa
- ⊡ Airway obstruction via migration of GEBT, unlikely if intubated
- ⊡ Aspiration pneumonitis, especially if inadequate proximal esophageal suctioning

SAFETY/QUALITY TIPS

◻ **Procedural**
+ Ensure all equipment is readily available prior to procedure
+ Confirm placement of gastric balloon via radiography prior to inflation as full inflation of gastric balloon proximal to the stomach can rupture the esophagus. There is some evidence that this can be done with ultrasound.
+ Before traction is applied, mark the depth at the mouth. The tube will stretch as it warms to body temperature, and significant migration will be noted.

◻ **Cognitive**
+ GEBT, especially when performed by practitioners who do not do it often (i.e., most emergency clinicians), carries a significant risk of potentially disastrous esophageal trauma. Placing an SB tube is appropriate in intubated, critically ill upper gastrointestinal (GI) bleed patients who are at risk to exsanguinate despite maximal medical/endoscopic therapy.
+ Ensure adequate sedation and analgesia. Use ketamine if blood pressure is a concern.
+ Recognition that balloon tamponade is a temporizing measure to endoscopy or a rescue measure if endoscopy has failed, while other therapies (surgical, angiographic) are being arranged
+ If bleeding is persistent after full inflation of the esophageal balloon, the source of bleeding is likely gastric and not esophageal

◻ **Acknowledgment**

Thank you to prior author Mitchell Adelstein and Jennifer Kaufman.

Suggested Readings

Panacek, E. Balloon tamponade of gastroesophageal varices. In: Roberts JR, Hedges JR, eds. *Clinical Procedures in Emergency Medicine*. 5th ed. Philadelphia, PA: WB Saunders; 2010:754–759.
Yamada T. *Textbook of Gastroenterology*. Vol 1. Philadelphia, PA: Lippincott Williams & Wilkins; 2003:707.

30

Hernia Reduction

Danielle K. Matilsky

INDICATIONS

- Incarcerated hernias should have attempted manual reduction
- Techniques for reduction are applicable to both the adult and pediatric patient

CONTRAINDICATIONS

- **Strangulated Hernia**
  - Recognize signs and symptoms, including extreme tenderness, skin discoloration, erythema, peritoneal signs, evidence of bowel obstruction, free air on x-ray, fever, or shock
  - If a strangulated hernia is missed and manual reduction is attempted, necrotic bowel can be introduced into the abdomen, worsening clinical outcome

RISK/CONSENTS

- Mild pain during procedure is common, but should resolve when hernia is reduced
- Risk of incomplete reduction or unsuccessful reduction
- Medications for procedural sedation may be used and sedation risks should be addressed
- Alternative therapy usually is surgical repair of defect

LANDMARKS AND ETIOLOGY

- **Groin**
  - *Indirect inguinal hernia*—occurs superior to the inguinal ligament and passes through the inguinal ring into the inguinal canal
  - *Direct inguinal hernia*—protrusion through an acquired weakness in Hesselbach triangle formed by the rectus sheath, inferior epigastric vessels, and the inguinal ligament; does not pass through inguinal canal
  - *Femoral hernia*—peritoneal contents protrude into the femoral canal inferior to the inguinal ligament; more prevalent in females
- **Ventral**
  - *Incisional hernia*—iatrogenic due to breakdown of fascial closure after abdominal surgery
  - *Umbilical hernia*—due to failure of closure of the umbilical ring, with a high incidence occurring in children
  - *Spigelian hernia*—also known as a lateral ventral hernia, arises when peritoneum protrudes through Spigelian fascia
- **Pelvic**
  - *Perineal hernia*—often develops after pelvic surgery or in patients with chronic constipation or atrophy of pelvic floor muscles and can contain fluid, fat, or intestinal contents

TECHNIQUE

- **Preparation**
  - Provide adequate analgesia and sedation
  - Ice or cold compress applied to the hernia may assist reduction
- **Positioning**
  - Place patient in 20-degree Trendelenburg position for groin hernias, or in position such that gravity assists reduction
  - Supine positioning is adequate for reduction of umbilical, ventral, and incisional hernias
  - Allow patient to remain in position for up to 30 minutes to allow for spontaneous reduction

- **Reduction**
    - ✚ Position thumb and index finger along the lateral edges of the defect with your nondominant hand
    - ✚ Gently reduce the hernia through the external and internal rings using slow steady pressure, guiding the proximal portion first
    - ✚ Successful reduction is indicated by disappearance of the hernia mass, reduction in pain, and often a gurgling sound
    - ✚ Repeated failed attempts or significant pain should prompt surgical consultation

COMPLICATIONS

- Injury to underlying bowel due to excessive force
- Reduction of bowel into a preperitoneal location
- Development of a Richter hernia in which one side of the bowel wall remains incarcerated in the fascial defect after reduction
- *Reduction en masse*—return of strangulated bowel to the abdomen, leading to further bowel ischemia and necrosis

SAFETY/QUALITY TIPS

- **Procedural**
    - ✚ Start with adequate positioning and analgesia to increase likelihood of success
    - ✚ A period of proper positioning and ice application will increase likelihood of success
    - ✚ Consider ultrasonography to evaluate anatomy and confirm etiology of mass, especially in children or when it is not a clinically obvious hernia
- **Cognitive**
    - ✚ Recognize signs of strangulation and involve surgical services early
    - ✚ Pediatric populations have a high incidence of hernias and can be diagnostically difficult as hernias tend to spontaneously reduce and symptoms may be nonspecific, such as irritability, intermittent vomiting, or abdominal pain
    - ✚ Complications are greater with femoral hernias, advanced age, and female gender
    - ✚ Chronically incarcerated hernias may not be amenable to nonsurgical reduction, and are not usually associated with strangulation or significant pain

- **Acknowledgment**

Thank you to prior author Melissa Rockefeller and Eric Perez.

Suggested Readings

Knoop, Stack LB, Storrow AB. *Atlas of Emergency Medicine*. 2nd ed. New York, NY: McGraw-Hill; 2002:207–208.

Manthey DE. Abdominal hernia reduction. In: Roberts, JR, Hedges JR, eds. *Clinical Procedures in Emergency Medicine*. 4th ed. Philadelphia, PA: WB Saunders; 2004:860–867.

Mensching JJ, Musielewicz AJ. Abdominal wall hernias. *Emerg Med Clin North Am*. 1996;14(4):739–756.

Richard AT, Quinn TH, Fitzgibbons RJ. Abdominal wall hernias. In: Mulholland MW, Lillemoe KD, Doherty GM, et al. eds. *Greenfield's Surgery: Scientific Principles and Practice*. 4th ed. Philadelphia, PA: Lippincott Williams & Wilkins; 2006:1159–1198.

Tintanalli J, Kelen GD, Stapczynski JS. *Emergency Medicine: A Comprehensive Study Guide*. 6th ed. New York, NY: McGraw-Hill; 2004:527–230.

31

Nasogastric Tube Placement

Simran Buttar and Jennifer B. Stratton

INDICATIONS

- Aspiration of gastric fluid, air, or blood
  + Evaluation of upper gastrointestinal (GI) bleed (volume and/or presence of blood)
  + Decompression of obstructed GI tract (i.e., small bowel obstruction)
  + Prevention of aspiration and gastric dilatation (i.e., in intubated patients)
- Lavage or removal of toxins (e.g., overdose, poisonings)
- Administration of medication, oral contrast, and nutrients **(TABLE 31.1)**

CONTRAINDICATIONS

- **Absolute Contraindications**
  + Facial trauma with possible cribriform-plate fracture
    + Concern for passage into intracranial space
- **Relative Contraindications**
  + Severe coagulopathy
    + If critical, consider the orogastric route, which may cause less bleeding
  + Alkali ingestions or esophageal strictures
    + Placement may cause esophageal rupture
  + History of gastric bypass surgery/lap band placement
    + Risk for intestinal perforation

- **General Basic Steps**
  + **Position patient**
  + **Analgesia**
  + **Measure nasogastric tube (NGT)**
  + **Insertion**
  + **Confirmation of placement**
  + **Secure tube**

EQUIPMENT NEEDED

- NGT
- Viscous lidocaine
- Cetacaine spray (optional)
- Nebulizer equipment and 4% lidocaine (optional)
- A cup of water with straw
- Tapered syringe (30–60 cc)
- Suction
- Tape

TABLE 31.1. COMMON REASONS FOR NGT PLACEMENT

Bright red blood per rectum
Hematemesis/Coffee-ground emesis
Small bowel obstruction
Intubated patient

TECHNIQUE

Patient Preparation

+ Elevate the head of the patient's bed to upright position (if possible)
+ Place an emesis basin on the patient's lap
+ Select the patent nostril for tube placement
  + Have the patient occlude one nostril at a time and sniff
  + It may be necessary to switch to the opposite nostril if one side proves to be too difficult
+ In awake patients, anesthetize selected nare at least 5 minutes before attempting tube placement
  + Inject lidocaine gel (5 mL of 2% viscous lidocaine) via a 10-mL syringe. Ask the patient to sniff and swallow. The patient can orally swallow additional 5 mL of viscous lidocaine to further anesthetize the posterior pharynx.
  + Consider using benzocaine (Cetacaine) spray on the posterior pharynx
  + Consider nebulized lidocaine (2.5 mL of 4% lidocaine) via a face mask as an alternative to gels and sprays
+ Immediately after opening the NGT package, place the small (easily misplaced) "connector" in a safe place; it is frequently missing/lost when you want to connect the NGT to suction
+ Estimate tube insertion distance
  + Measure the tube from the patient's xiphoid process to the earlobe through the tip of the nose. Add 15 cm to this distance and mark on the NGT with a small amount of tape.
+ Lubricate NGT with viscous lidocaine or Surgilube

Insertion

+ Insert the tube (usual adult size 16-French or 18-French) into the selected nostril, aiming along the floor of the nose, posteriorly and caudally
+ Once in the nasopharynx, have the patient flex his head forward to aid tube placement into the esophagus
+ Pause as the tube enters the oropharynx and have the patient swallow water via straw to aid in the passage of tube, and then rapidly advance the tube into the stomach to the predetermined depth

Confirmation of Placement

+ Patient is able to speak clearly
  + If the patient has difficulty speaking or is coughing, the tube is likely in the trachea and needs to be removed
+ Aspirate gastric contents
+ Insufflation of air through a 50- or 60-mL syringe into the end of the NGT while auscultating over the stomach should reveal borborygmi (gurgling in stomach)
  + If the patient burps after insufflation, the tube is likely in the esophagus and needs to be advanced

Secure the Tube

+ Clean and dry the tube, if necessary
+ Tape the NGT at the nose entry site with emphasis of alleviating pressure of the tube on the nose
+ Secure the tube to the patient's gown for added stability
+ The air vent pigtail can be used as a cap for suction lumen when the tube is not in use

Chest X-ray Confirmation

+ It is not required to routinely confirm NGT placement with chest x-ray as the tube can be clinically confirmed via aspiration of gastric contents
+ If a chest x-ray is planned for endotracheal tube placement, consider obtaining after NGT placement
+ If the patient is unconscious, consider x-ray confirmation, especially if charcoal is to be administered through the NGT

COMPLICATIONS

- Epistaxis
- Tracheal intubation
- Esophageal/gastric perforation

- Aspiration
- Sinusitis or otitis media
- Ulceration of mucosa
- Esophageal stricture
- Necrosis or bleeding of nasal mucosa from improperly secured tube
- Intracranial insertion

SAFETY/QUALITY TIPS

- **Procedural**
  - The keys to success are adequate anesthesia and cooperation, tilting the head forward, and having the patient swallow water as tube is advanced
  - While passing the NGT, point the proximal end of the tube away from staff and self; vomiting during insertion can spray out of the proximal tube end
  - Consider using a sedative in patients who have difficulty tolerating the procedure
  - In the intubated, nonagitated, and noncombative patient, gently lifting the jaw forward or pushing the trachea to the patient's left can ease the passage of the NGT
  - An alternative method of orogastric tube (OGT) placement in an intubated patient is performing laryngoscopy and placing the tube into the esophagus under direct visualization. A bougie, with deflection pointed posteriorly rather than anteriorly, can be used as an adjunct.
  - Use intermittent suction—constant suction can lead to gastric mucosal damage
  - If the NGT has been confirmed to be in the stomach and there is minimal return during lavage, the drainage holes may be clogged, the tube may be a hold of the gastric wall, or the stomach may be empty—consider decreasing the vacuum pressure setting or you can attempt to push air into the venting lumen with a large syringe.

- **Cognitive**
  - NGT placement might require multiple attempts
    - There is a higher incidence of insertion into the pulmonary tree in this group. Alternative techniques include using Magill forceps and a gum-elastic bougie.
    - Larger-sized NGTs may be difficult to pass in narrow nasal passages, whereas smaller-sized tubes may bend too easily and curl in the patient's mouth (FIGURE 31.1)
    - If there are any concerns that the patient may bite down, do not place your fingers in the mouth
  - In patients who are unconscious or have altered mental status, consider airway protection via intubation before NGT insertion to prevent aspiration
  - In the case of hematemesis, NGT lavage is used to remove blood irritating the stomach, to determine the amount of blood, and to determine whether bleeding persists. It is not performed in order to diagnose a bleed; a negative NGT aspirate does not rule out a clinically important bleed.

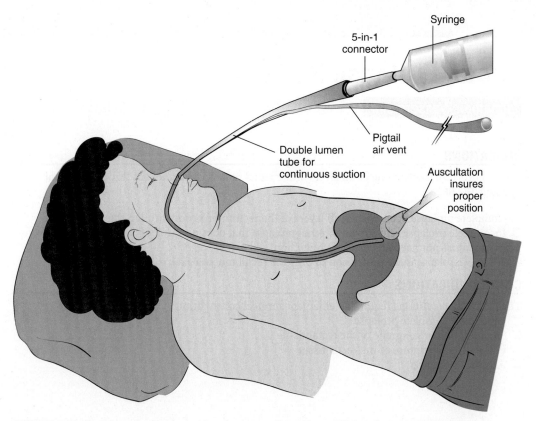

FIGURE 31.1 Confirmation of nasogastric tube placement. (From Simon HK, Lewander W. Gastric intubation. In: Henretig FM, King C, eds. *Textbook of Pediatric Emergency Procedures*. Philadelphia, PA: Williams & Wilkins; 1997:912, with permission.)

⊞ Acknowledgment

Thank you to prior author William Bagley.

Suggested Reading

Samuels LE. Nasogastric and Feeding tube placement. In: Roberts JR and Hedges JR, eds. Clinical Procedures in Emergency Medicine, 4th ed. Philadelphia. WB Saunders; 2004:809–819.

32

Rectal Prolapse Reduction

Jonathan Wassermann

INDICATIONS

A rectal prolapse is when one or all layers of the rectal mucosa protrude out through the anal opening (FIGURE 32.1).

- ⊞ Complete prolapse occurs when all layers of the rectum protrude through the anal opening
- ⊞ Incomplete prolapse refers to an internal prolapse that does not project through the anal opening and does not need an emergent reduction
- ⊞ Mucosal prolapse is the protrusion of only the rectal mucosa externally

CONTRAINDICATIONS

The following conditions require an emergent surgical consultation:
- ⊞ Irreducible complete prolapse
- ⊞ Strangulation or gangrene of the rectal tissue
- ⊞ Perforation or rupture of the rectal tissue
- ⊞ Anal incontinence

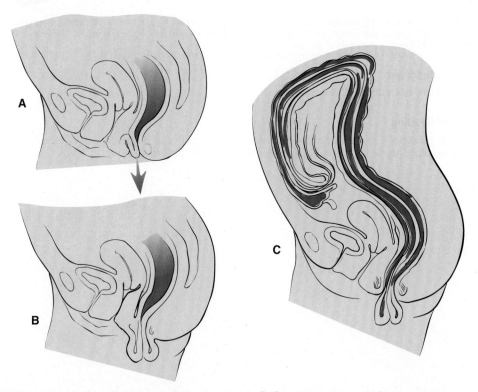

FIGURE 32.1 Anatomy of a rectal prolapse. **A:** Partial prolapse. **B:** Complete prolapse. **C:** Prolapsed intussusception. (From Schwartz G. Reducing a rectal prolapse. In: Henretig FM, King C, eds. *Textbook of Pediatric Emergency Procedures*. Philadelphia, PA: Williams & Wilkins; 1997:948, with permission.)

LANDMARKS

- A thick muscle layer palpable between the thumb and forefinger suggests a complete prolapse. This will present with the folds in a concentric ring pattern.
- In a mucosal prolapse, the mucosal folds originate from the central lumen of the protrusion and extend outward in a radial manner
- Mucosal prolapses tend to extend not beyond 4 cm from the anus, whereas complete prolapses may extend up to 15 cm from the anal verge

- **General Basic Steps**
  - **Patient preparation**
  - **Prolapse reduction**
  - **Postreduction care**

TECHNIQUE

- **Patient Preparation**
  - Place the patient in the lateral decubitus position with knees up toward the chin
  - Analgesia/sedation should be given for relaxation of sphincter muscles as well as relief of anxiety and pain
  - It is useful to have an assistant hold the buttocks apart
  - If significant edema is present, granulated sugar or salt may be applied to the prolapsed tissue to reduce the swelling. Attempt to reduce again after 15 minutes.
- **Reduction**
  - Place thumbs on either side of the lumen with the fingers grasping the exterior of the protrusion (**FIGURE 32.2**)
  - Constant, gentle circumferential pressure is applied from the thumbs at the portion closest to the lumen to guide the walls inward as the prolapse is rolled back in through the anal opening from distal to proximal
- **Postreduction Care**
  - After complete reduction, perform a digital rectal examination to evaluate for any masses that may have been the lead point causing the prolapse
  - Surgical follow-up should be arranged following a successful reduction
  - Patients should be educated regarding increased dietary fiber, adequate fluid intake, and avoidance of straining. Stool softeners should be prescribed to reduce likelihood of constipation.

COMPLICATIONS

- Failure of reduction
- Mucosal ulceration
- Necrosis of the rectal wall
- Bleeding
- Incontinence

SAFETY/QUALITY TIPS

- **Procedural**
  - Successful reduction depends on proper analgesia/sedation and constant, slow, steady pressure
- **Cognitive**
  - Rectal prolapse can be mistaken for hemorrhoids, polyps, cystocele, or carcinoma
  - If particularly painful, prolapse may be complicated by incarceration or necrosis of rectal wall
  - Rectal prolapse in children is often associated with cystic fibrosis, parasitic infection, malnutrition, and constipation

Complete rectal prolapse

Partial rectal prolapse

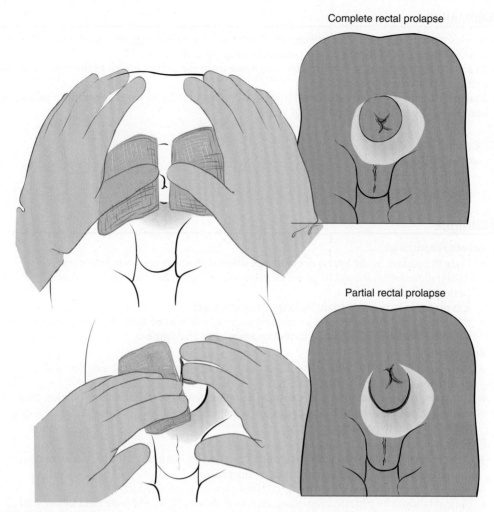

FIGURE 32.2 Rectal prolapse reduction. (From Schwartz G. Reducing a rectal prolapse. In: Henretig FM, King C, eds. *Textbook of Pediatric Emergency Procedures*. Philadelphia, PA: Williams & Wilkins; 1997:949, with permission.)

✚ Acknowledgment

Thank you to prior author Kari Scantlebury.

Suggested Readings

Coates WC. Anorectal procedures. In: Roberts JR, Custalow CB, Thomsen TW, et al. eds. *Roberts & Hedges' Clinical Procedures in Emergency Medicine*. 6th ed. Philadelphia, PA: WB Saunders; 2014:880–891.

Coburn WM III, Russell MA, Hofstetter WL. Sucrose as an aid to manual reduction of incarcerated rectal prolapse. *Ann Emerg Med*. 1997;30(3):347–349.

33

Excision of Acutely Thrombosed External Hemorrhoids

Amy B. Caggiula and Hamza Guend

INDICATIONS

- A thrombosed, painful external hemorrhoid that has been symptomatic for less than 72 hours, not improved with conservative measures
  - Decision to excise should also be based on severity of pain and clinical course. If the patient presents with improving pain, medical management is likely preferable.
  - After 72 hours, most patients have decreased pain and spontaneous resolution of symptoms

CONTRAINDICATIONS

- **Relative Contraindications**
  - Inflammatory bowel disease—high rate of fistula formation
  - Perianal infection
  - Known coagulopathy
  - Portal hypertension

LANDMARKS

- Internal hemorrhoids originate above the dentate line
  - Can prolapse and extend outside the anal canal (FIGURE 33.1)
- External hemorrhoids originate *below* the dentate line

- **General Basic Steps**
  - **Prepare patient**
  - **Anesthetize**
  - **Incise**
  - **Remove clot**
  - **Pack wound**

TECHNIQUE

- **Patient Preparation**
  - Place the patient in the prone jackknife or left lateral decubitus position
    - For prone jackknife positioning, place rolled towels beneath the patient's pelvis to elevate buttocks
    - Gently spread the buttocks and maintain the positioning with tape
  - Prepare the area with povidone–iodine solution (Betadine) using sterile gloves
  - Inject 1% lidocaine with epinephrine or 0.5% bupivacaine into the base of the thrombosed hemorrhoid
    - Avoid multiple injection sites to decrease bleeding
    - Topical lidocaine gel can be used in the anal canal to supplement local anesthesia
    - Intravenous analgesia is highly recommended
    - Alternatively, a perianal block can be performed by injecting a local anesthetic into the sphincter complex in the anterior, posterior, and lateral positions

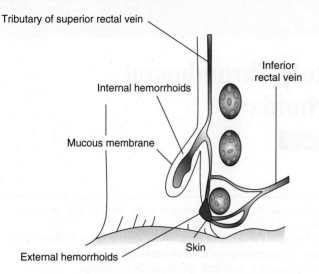

FIGURE 33.1 Varicosed tributary of the superior rectal vein forming the internal hemorrhoid. (From Snell RS. *Clinical anatomy,* 7th ed. Philadelphia: Lippincott Williams & Wilkins; 2004:427, with permission).

- **Incision**
  - Test the adequacy of the local anesthesia by grasping the hemorrhoid with forceps
  - Using a no. 15 scalpel blade, make an *elliptical incision* around the thrombosis with the long axis in the *radial* direction relative to the anus
    - Never incise in a circumferential axis
    - Control bleeding with direct pressure
  - Elevate skin edges with a forceps and excise to expose underlying thrombus
  - Remove the clot and any overlying skin using a forceps or by applying pressure
    - After the clot is removed, have an assistant spread the incision, exposing the base of the hemorrhoid to allow visualization and removal of additional clots
  - If significant bleeding occurs that is not controlled with direct pressure, hemostasis can be achieved with a suture or silver nitrate
  - Pack the wound loosely with standard cotton gauze or iodoform packing to prevent skin edges from reapproximating prematurely, and apply a pressure dressing
- **Follow-up Care**
  - Counsel the patient to apply direct pressure if bleeding occurs
  - Dressing may be removed after 12 hours, at which point the patient should begin taking sitz baths three to four times daily
  - Prescribe stool softeners and fiber supplements as needed. Avoid opiate pain medication, and instruct the patient to increase oral fluid intake.
  - Follow-up should be arranged in 2 to 4 weeks. The patient must return sooner if he or she experiences severe pain, uncontrolled bleeding, or signs of infection.

SAFETY/QUALITY TIPS

- **Procedural**
  - Incision should always be *radial* relative to the anus. A circumferential incision around the anus can result in significant anal stenosis.
  - Deep incisions can damage the external anal sphincter and result in incontinence **(FIGURE 33.2)**

✚ Cognitive

- ✚ Most hemorrhoids will resolve without intervention; symptom control with expectant management or referral is reasonable in most cases
- ✚ It is important to counsel patients on appropriate aftercare and follow-up to complications such as pain, bleeding, and infection
- ✚ Refer lesions suspicious for carcinoma to a colorectal surgeon for evaluation
- ✚ Pressure from a thrombus can cause overlying skin to necrose and ulcerate, leading to spontaneous drainage and resolution of symptoms. Excising the thrombus in these cases is usually unnecessary.
- ✚ Thrombosis of external hemorrhoids may recur or occur synchronously with prolapse and strangulation of internal hemorrhoids. Surgical intervention to excise the underlying vein or decrease blood flow to the hemorrhoidal tissue should be considered for these patients.

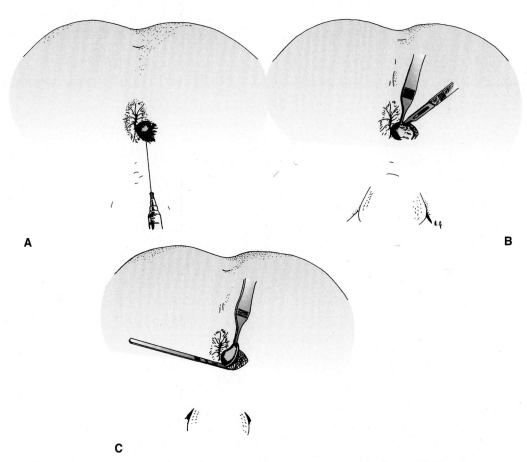

FIGURE 33.2 Anesthetize an external thrombosed hemorrhoid with 1% lidocaine with epinephrine **(A)** with a no. 15 or no. 11 blade; excise the hemorrhoid in an elliptical fashion at its base **(B)**. Be certain also to excise a wedge of skin and the subcutaneous tissue that contain additional clots, as shown above **(C)**. (From Simon RR, Brenner BE. *Emergency Procedures & Techniques*. 4th ed. Philadelphia, PA: Lippincott Williams & Wilkins; 2002:28, with permission.)

⊡ **Acknowledgment**

Thank you to prior author Laura Withers and Mitchell Bernstein.

Suggested Readings

Bharathi RS, Chakladar A, Dabas AK, et al. Evidence based switch to perianal block for ano-rectal surgeries. *Intl J Surg.* 2010;8:29–31.

Reichman EF. Chapter 68. External Hemorrhoid Management. In: Reichman EF, ed. *Emergency Medicine Procedures*, 2nd ed. New York NY: McGraw Hill; 2013.

Singer M. Hemorrhoids. In: Beck DE, Roberts PL, Saclarides TJ, et al. eds. *The ASCRS Textbook of Colon and Rectal Surgery.* 2nd ed. New York, NY: Springer; 2011:175–202.

Strear CM, Coates WC. Anorectal procedures. In: Roberts JR, Hedges JR, eds. *Clinical Procedures in Emergency Medicine.* 4th ed. Philadelphia, PA: WB Saunders; 2004:871–874.

34

Bedside Gallbladder Ultrasonography

Lara Zucconi Vanyo and Kaushal H. Shah

INDICATIONS

- Clinical suspicion of cholecystitis or biliary colic:
  - Abdominal pain, particularly right upper quadrant (RUQ), epigastric
  - Right flank pain
  - Right shoulder pain
  - Nausea/vomiting
  - Sepsis without source

CONTRAINDICATIONS

- None: No contrast or radiation

RISKS/CONSENT ISSUES

- Allergy to the ultrasonography gel

LANDMARKS

- RUQ of abdomen at expected location of gallbladder (GB)

TECHNIQUE

- Using a standard 3.5- to 5.0-MHz probe, scan the RUQ of the abdomen in the longitudinal plane under the costal margin using the liver as an acoustic window (FIGURE 34.1)
- If the GB is not readily identified:
  - Ask the patient to take slow deep breaths because the GB moves significantly with respiration
  - Have the patient move to the left lateral decubitus position
  - Place the probe in the intercostal space to avoid bowel gas and rib shadows
- Once the GB is found, confirm by identifying associated structures:
  - Echogenic gallstones in the lumen casting echolucent shadows (FIGURE 34.2)
  - Main lobar fissure of the liver points toward the GB neck and also connects the portal vein
  - Common bile duct (CBD) usually runs between the GB and the portal vein (FIGURE 34.3)
- Identify signs of cholecystitis (TABLE 34.1)

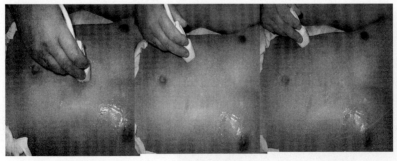

First   Second   Third

FIGURE 34.1 Biliary ultrasonography: To locate the gallbladder, do a costal margin sweep first.

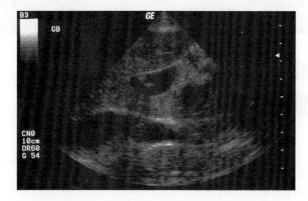

FIGURE 34.2 Echogenic gallstones casting acoustic shadows. (Courtesy of Kaushal Shah, MD.)

SAFETY/QUALITY TIPS

⊞ **Procedural**
+ Always visualize the GB in more than one plane (e.g., longitudinal and transverse) to completely view the structure
+ Eliciting pain by pressing on the ribs rather than the GB may give a false-positive sonographic Murphy sign
+ Patients who have not eaten recently will often have a dilated, more easily identifiable GB
+ The *halo sign* occurs when echolucent pericholecystic fluid surrounds the entire GB owing to inflammation; it is a very specific sign for cholecystitis
+ The *WES sign* is present when the GB is contracted around a gallstone and ultrasonography demonstrates only the anterior GB **W**all, the **E**chogenicity of the stone, and a **S**hadow

⊞ **Cognitive**
+ FIGURE 34.4 shows the recommended clinical approach to bedside ultrasonography of the GB
+ Early cholecystitis can be sonographically subtle; if point-of-care ultrasound is negative or equivocal but clinical concern is high, pursue consultative ultrasonography or computed tomography
+ Limited, goal-directed ultrasonography is within the capacity of the emergency physician (EP). The EP is not expected to identify subtle abnormalities in the hepatobiliary system.
+ GB wall thickening is a nonspecific finding because it can occur with other disease states such as congestive heart failure (CHF), liver disease, and renal disease
+ Gallstones and a positive sonographic Murphy sign have a sensitivity >90% in the hands of EPs in multiple studies

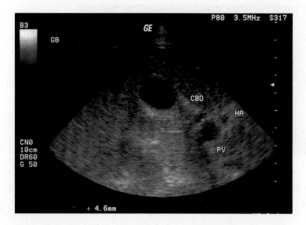

FIGURE 34.3 "Mickey Mouse" sign comprises the common bile duct (*CBD*), portal vein (*PV*), and hepatic artery (*HA*). (Courtesy of Kaushal Shah, MD.)

TABLE 34.1. SONOGRAPHIC SIGNS OF CHOLECYSTITIS

Presence of gallstones
Sonographic Murphy sign: Tenderness with probe pressure directly on the sonographically identified GB
Anterior GB wall thickness >3 mm
Pericholecystic fluid
Common bile duct >6 mm (more consistent with choledocholithiasis)

GB, gallbladder.

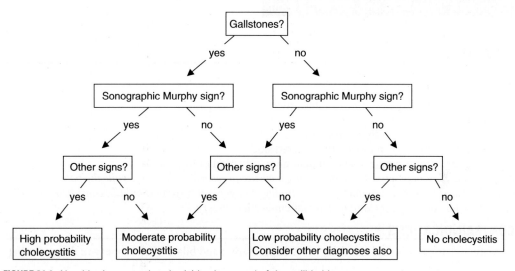

FIGURE 34.4 Algorithmic approach to bedside ultrasound of the gallbladder.

Suggested Readings

Blaivas M, Harwood RA, Lambert MJ. Decreasing length of stay with emergency ultrasound examination of the gallbladder. *Acad Emerg Med.* 1999;6(10):1020–1023.

Kendall JL, Shimp RJ. Performance and interpretation of focused right upper quadrant ultrasound by emergency physicians. *J Emerg Med.* 2001;21(1):7–13.

Ma OJ, Mateer JR. *Emergency Ultrasound.* New York, NY: McGraw-Hill; 2003.

Rosen CL, Brown DF, Chang Y, et al. Ultrasonography by emergency physicians in patients with suspected cholecystitis. *Am J Emerg Med.* 2001;19(1):32–36.

Shah K, Wolfe R. Hepatobiliary ultrasound. *Emerg Med Clin North Am.* 2004;22(3):661–673.

35

Manual Testicular Detorsion

Julie K. A. Kasarjian and Clinton J. Coil

INDICATIONS

- Testicular torsion

Signs and symptoms include:
- Acute scrotal pain/swelling or intermittent testicular pain
- Testicular tenderness
- High-riding testis with horizontal lie
- Absent cremasteric reflex on the affected side
- Negative Prehn sign (no relief of pain upon elevation of the testis)

Manual detorsion may serve as a temporizing measure to reperfuse the testis while the patient is awaiting definitive surgical management. A urologist or general surgeon should be consulted immediately when torsion is suspected to prepare for emergency surgery.

CONTRAINDICATIONS

- Manual detorsion should not delay scrotal exploration and bilateral orchiopexy in the operating room (OR)
- Spermatic cord anesthesia should be used only after discussing with the consulting urologist because it may blunt the subjective end point of detorsion efforts (relief of pain)

RISKS/CONSENT ISSUES

- Pain (sedation and local anesthesia may be used)
- Local bleeding and/or infection if spermatic cord anesthesia is administered
- Manual detorsion does not replace the absolute need for surgical scrotal exploration/orchiopexy

LANDMARKS

- If considering spermatic cord anesthesia/block, identify the spermatic cord at the external inguinal ring. Alternatively, if severe edema is present, palpate cord at pubic tubercle over pubis.

- **General Basic Steps**
  - **Patient preparation**
  - **Local anesthesia (optional)**
  - **Detorsion**
  - **Confirmation**

TECHNIQUE

- **Patient Preparation**
  - Place the patient in reclining, supine, or lithotomy position
  - Consider light procedural sedation

⬓ **Local Anesthesia (optional)**
  ✦ Ensure that the consulting urologist or general surgeon does not object to providing local anesthesia
⬓ **Spermatic Cord Block**
  ✦ Sterilize the skin overlying the spermatic cord
  ✦ Insert small (30-gauge) needle directly into the spermatic cord **(FIGURE 35.1)**
  ✦ Aspirate for blood to ensure the needle is not intravascular
  ✦ Slowly inject 10 mL of 1% plain lidocaine (maximum 3 mg/kg)
⬓ **Detorsion**
  ✦ The most common direction for torsion to occur is lateral to medial
  ✦ The initial attempt at detorsion should therefore be medial to lateral **(FIGURES 35.2 and 35.3)**. Imagine you are "opening a book."
  ✦ Multiple rotations of the testicle may be necessary for complete detorsion; the degree of torsion may be guided by the patient's pain relief
  ✦ One-third of cases are torsed in the opposite direction. If initial detorsion efforts appear ineffective/painful, attempt to detorse laterally to medially.
⬓ **Confirmation**
  ✦ Relief of pain
  ✦ Restoration of anatomy
  ✦ Eventual return of cremasteric reflex
  ✦ Color Doppler ultrasonogram shows return or improvement of flow

COMPLICATIONS

⬓ Unsuccessful manual detorsion
⬓ Patient unable to tolerate procedure (consider procedural sedation)
⬓ Testicular loss due to prolonged ischemia

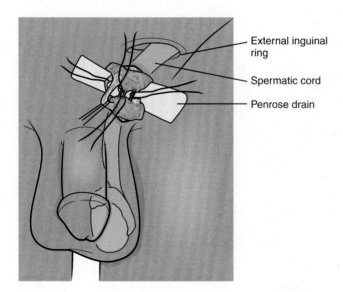

External inguinal ring

Spermatic cord

Penrose drain

FIGURE 35.1 Injecting lidocaine at the superficial inguinal ring to achieve a spermatic cord block.

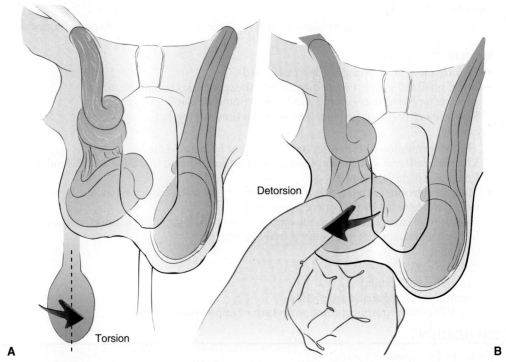

A

Torsion

B

Detorsion

FIGURE 35.2 Manual detorsion. **A:** Torsion of the testis with two inward twists has resulted in a new high-lying position. **B:** The testis is grasped with the fingers and rotated outwardly with two full 360-degree twists. (From Cronan KM, Zderic SA. Manual detorsion of the testes. In: Henretig FM, King C, eds. *Textbook of Pediatric Emergency Procedures*. Philadelphia, PA: Williams & Wilkins; 1997:1005, with permission.)

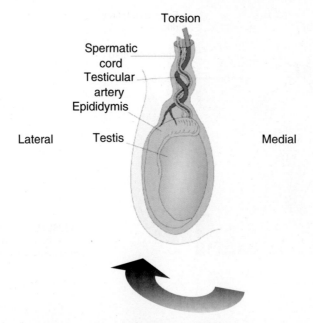

Torsion

Spermatic cord

Testicular artery

Epididymis

Lateral

Testis

Medial

FIGURE 35.3 Right spermatic cord torsion. Manual detorsion using 180 degrees or more of medial-to-lateral ("opening a book") rotation, lifting slightly upward to release the cremasteric muscle (caudal to cranial). To detorse left testis, use similar, medial-to-lateral, rotation. (From Matfin G, Editor: Porth CM. Disorders of the male genitourinary system. In: *Pathophysiology: Concepts of Altered Health States*. Philadelphia, PA: Lippincott Williams & Wilkins; 2004. Accessed August 18, 2006, at http://connection.lww.com/Products/porth7e/Imagebank.asp.)

SAFETY/QUALITY TIPS

◻ **Procedural**

➕ Most patients with testicular torsion will not allow manipulation of the testicle without some combination of anesthesia, analgesia, and sedation

➕ Rotation in wrong direction is not uncommon; gentle rotation in the opposite direction is indicated if the initial maneuver does not help or seems to make things worse

➕ Use of Doppler ultrasound prior to and after the procedure is valuable to assess the procedure's necessity and efficacy

◻ **Cognitive**

➕ Torsion is a testicle-threatening emergency; do not delay diagnosis and definitive (operative) treatment. Manual detorsion is a temporizing measure and not a substitute for emergent surgery.

➕ Although torsion can occur at any age, the most common presentation is either during the first year of life or at puberty

➕ Some patients with torsion will give a potentially misleading history of minor trauma

➕ Ultrasonography may assist in the diagnosis, but results can be misleading, and should therefore not substitute for definitive diagnosis through operative exploration

➕ The most common misdiagnosis is epididymitis, which generally presents with epididymal tenderness, an intact cremasteric reflex on the affected side, positive Prehn sign (relief of pain upon elevation of the testis), and positive urinalysis and/or history of sexually transmitted diseases. Any concern for torsion should prompt an appropriate evaluation.

Suggested Readings

Ban KM, Easter JS. Selected urologic problems. In: Marx JA, Hockberger RS, Walls RM, eds. *Rosen's Emergency Medicine: Concepts and Clinical Practice*. 8th ed. Philadelphia, PA: Saunders; 2014:1326–1354.

Davis JE, Silverman MA. Urologic procedures. In: Roberts JR, Custalow CB, Thomsen TW, et al. eds. *Roberts & Hedges' Clinical Procedures in Emergency Medicine*. 6th ed. Philadelphia, PA: Saunders; 2014: 1113–1154.

36

Phimosis Reduction

Ari M. Lipsky

INDICATIONS

- Relief of urinary retention

CONTRAINDICATIONS

- No true emergency exists
- Successful, blind insertion of Foley catheter
    + Physiologic (i.e., normal) phimosis especially in younger boys (<3 years old)
    + Preferred treatment may be medical (local skin care, topical steroids) or surgical but non–emergent (dilation or circumcision by a urologist)
    + It is uncommon that phimosis needs to be treated emergently in the emergency department (ED); inability to reduce the prepuce is not in itself an indication for emergent surgical intervention
- Coagulopathy (relative contraindication)

RISKS/CONSENT ISSUES

- Pain (local anesthesia will be given)
- Local bleeding
- Infection (sterile technique will be used)
- Scarring at the site of incision/dilation (though definitive treatment will likely include circumcision, removing the scarred tissue)
- Damage to glans penis and urethral meatus

> - General Basic Steps
>   + Patient preparation
>   + Anesthesia
>   + Dilation or dorsal slit
>   + Dressing

SUPPLIES

- Povidone–iodine or chlorhexidine
- 1% Lidocaine without epinephrine
- 5-mL syringe
- 27-gauge needle
- Sterile field supplies
- Sterile gloves
- Straight hemostat
- Straight scissors
- Topical antibiotic ointment
- Gauze
- Paper tape

TECHNIQUE

- Patient Preparation
    + Position: Supine with legs slightly abducted
    + Clean penis and surrounding region with antiseptic solution

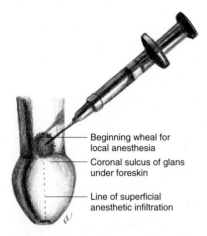

- Beginning wheal for local anesthesia
- Coronal sulcus of glans under foreskin
- Line of superficial anesthetic infiltration

FIGURE 36.1 Local anesthesia.(Courtesy of Kim Kiser.)

+ Sterile drape revealing only the genital region
+ Consider light procedural sedation as well

■ **Anesthesia**

Use 1% lidocaine without epinephrine. The options for anesthesia include:
+ **Local:** Beginning proximally at the coronal sulcus, infiltrate lidocaine into the dorsum of the foreskin, at midline, proceeding distally to the tip of the foreskin **(FIGURE 36.1)**
+ **Dorsal nerve block:** Provides anesthesia only to the dorsum of the penis **(FIGURE 36.2)**
  + Using a 27-gauge needle, inject lidocaine subcutaneously at the base of the dorsum of the penis just inferior to the pubic symphysis
  + Begin on one side of the base of the penis and inject 3 to 5 mL and then withdraw the needle back to the surface of the skin (without coming out of the skin) and direct the needle to the opposite side and again inject 3 to 5 mL
+ **Penile ring block:** Provides anesthesia to the entire distal penis **(FIGURE 36.3)**
  + Perform the dorsal nerve block as above
  + Using the same technique as above, ventrally infiltrate lidocaine, thereby producing a ring of subcutaneous lidocaine at the base of the penis

■ **Dilation Only**

The phimotic constriction can often be relieved temporarily with dilation alone, allowing for prompt outpatient referral to a urologist for definitive treatment.
+ With a hemostat, test and ensure adequate anesthesia. A penile ring block will likely be the most effective type of anesthesia for this procedure.

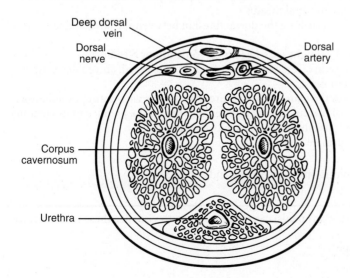

Deep dorsal vein
Dorsal nerve
Dorsal artery
Corpus cavernosum
Urethra

FIGURE 36.2 Dorsal nerve block. (Courtesy of Kim Kiser.)

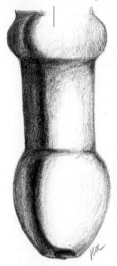

Wheal from subcutaneous
anesthetic at base of penis

FIGURE 36.3 Penile ring block.
(Courtesy of Kim Kiser.)

+ Pull the foreskin distally (away from the glans) to ensure that the glans and urethral meatus
  are not damaged
+ Slowly advance a hemostat through the foreskin opening and gradually dilate by opening the
  instrument
+ Expect some bleeding, and do not be afraid if you cut/tear the foreskin somewhat
+ Ensure that the patient can urinate easily
+ Consider placing a Foley catheter until a urologist can see the patient

▢ **Dorsal Slit**
  + With a hemostat, test and ensure adequate anesthesia (whether a penile block or local
    anesthesia is used)
  + Insert a closed straight hemostat dorsally between the glans penis and foreskin all the way to
    the coronal sulcus (take care not to injure the urethral meatus)
  + Carefully separate any adhesions that may be present by opening the instrument
  + Insert one jaw of the open hemostat to the coronal sulcus, along the path taken previously
    (i.e., between the glans and overlying foreskin)
  + Ensure that there is tenting of the foreskin caused by the inner jaw of the hemostat to ensure
    that the inner jaw is not in the urethral meatus
  + Close the hemostat, effectively crushing the dorsal foreskin between the jaws, and leave in
    place for 3 to 5 minutes
  + Cut the crushed foreskin with straight scissors (expect some minor bleeding)
    + If the inner and outer foreskin layers separate and continue to bleed, absorbable sutures
      may be used to obtain hemostasis
  + Retract the foreskin and clean the glans penis and urethral meatus with antiseptic solution
  + Inspect the glans and urethral meatus for any injuries, and return the prepuce to its anatomic
    location (to avoid iatrogenic paraphimosis, especially if sutured)
  + Ensure that the patient can urinate easily

▢ **Dressing**
  + Dress the wound with antibiotic ointment, gauze, and paper tape

COMPLICATIONS

▢ Injury to the urethral meatus or glans penis; care must be taken to visualize these two structures
  throughout the procedure
▢ Bleeding from cut/dilated tissue
▢ Infection

SAFETY/QUALITY TIPS

🔲 **Procedural**

+ Adequate anesthesia is a key aspect of this procedure; infiltrate lidocaine generously and allow sufficient time for it to work

+ Lidocaine containing epinephrine should not be used because of the potential for vasoconstriction and penile necrosis (FIGURE 36.4)

🔲 **Cognitive**

+ Most phimoses can be managed as an outpatient; performing a phimotic dilation or dorsal slit is indicated only if urinary obstruction exists and cannot be relieved by a Foley catheter

+ Do not be concerned about dilating/cutting the foreskin, as it will likely be removed with subsequent circumcision

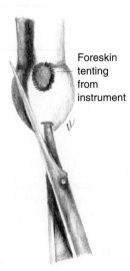

Foreskin tenting from instrument

FIGURE 36.4 Dorsal slit. (Courtesy of Kim Kiser.)

🔲 **Acknowledgment**

Thank you to prior author Richard G. Newell and Dan Chavira.

Suggested Readings

Ban KM, Easter JS. Selected urologic problems. In: Marx JA, Hockberger RS, Walls RM, eds. *Rosen's Emergency Medicine: Concepts and Clinical Practice*. 8th ed. Philadelphia, PA: Saunders; 2014:1326–1354.

Davis JE, Silverman MA. Urologic procedures. In: Roberts JR, Custalow CB, Thomsen TW, et al. eds. *Roberts & Hedges' Clinical Procedures in Emergency Medicine*. 6th ed. Philadelphia, PA: Saunders; 2014:1113–1154.

Ghory HZ. Phimosis and paraphimosis. http://emedicine.medscape.com/article/777539. Accessed April 7, 2014.

37

Paraphimosis Reduction

Ari M. Lipsky

INDICATION

- Paraphimosis (foreskin trapped proximal to coronal sulcus) is a urologic emergency, and reduction is always indicated when the condition is present

CONTRAINDICATIONS

- None

RISKS/CONSENT ISSUES

- Pain (local anesthesia will be given)
- Local bleeding
- Infection (sterile technique will be used)
- Scarring at site of incision/dilation (though definitive treatment will likely include circumcision, removing the scarred tissue)
- Damage to glans penis and urethral meatus

- **General Basic Steps**

If manual reduction fails to restore normal anatomy, proceed to assisted manual reduction; if that fails as well, proceed to phimotic ring incision. A urologist should be contacted if manual reduction fails, and will need to be actively involved if emergency circumcision is required because of reduction failure.

- **Patient preparation**
- **Anesthesia**
- **Manual reduction**
- **Assisted manual reduction** (FIGURE 37.1)
- **Phimotic ring incision**

TECHNIQUE

- **Patient Preparation**
    - Position: Supine with legs slightly abducted
    - Consider light procedural sedation as well
- **Anesthesia**
    - A topical anesthetic may be all that is necessary
        - Apply viscous lidocaine or eutectic mixture of local anesthetics (EMLA) to the inner layer of the foreskin
        - Also serves as a lubricant
    - If further anesthesia is necessary, progress from local, to dorsal nerve block, and, finally, to penile ring block
        - See chapter 36 for details and pictures of penile anesthesia
        - When providing local anesthesia with lidocaine (without epinephrine), be sure to infiltrate into the constricting ring as well
- **Manual Reduction**
    - Using your hands or an elastic bandage, manually compress the glans and foreskin for 3 to 5 minutes to remove as much edema as possible

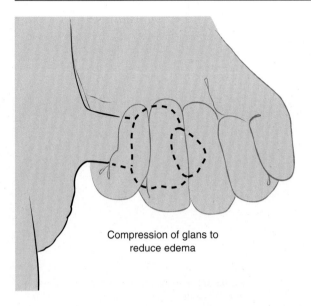

Compression of glans to
reduce edema

FIGURE 37.1 Technique for compression of glans to reduce edema and allow for manual reduction of paraphimosis. (From Green M, Strange GR. Paraphimosis reduction. In: Henretig FM, King C, eds. *Textbook of Pediatric Emergency Procedures*. Philadelphia, PA: Williams & Wilkins; 1997:1008, with permission.)

+ Place both thumbs on the glans penis and apply slow, steady pressure while using your other fingers just proximal to the phimotic ring to pull the foreskin over the glans penis **(FIGURE 37.2)**
+ Successful reduction occurs when the phimotic foreskin is reduced back to normal position over the glans
+ If unsuccessful, proceed to assisted manual reduction methods

☐ **Assisted Manual Reduction**
+ Start with less invasive techniques and proceed to more invasive as needed
+ Iced-glove method
  + Place a mixture of crushed ice and cold water in a glove and tie closed the cuffed end
  + Invert the thumb of the glove by pushing it into the glove/ice water mixture, producing a condom-like apparatus surrounded by ice water
  + Place as much of the penis as possible into the thumb of the glove, which will provide compression and vasoconstriction (both decreasing edema)
  + Allow to sit for 10 minutes
  + Attempt manual reduction as outlined earlier
  + If unsuccessful, proceed to the Babcock clamp method
+ Additional techniques described for reducing foreskin edema before reduction include the application of sugar (or a dextrose solution) to the foreskin; making multiple puncture wounds; injecting hyaluronidase; and aspiration. Manual reduction is then reattempted. The utility of these methods is unclear.

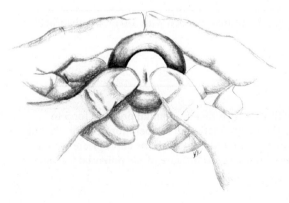

FIGURE 37.2 Manual reduction of paraphimosis. With the thumbs on the glans penis and the fingertips on the tight band of foreskin, the glans is pushed as the foreskin is pulled over the glans. Courtesy of Kim Kiser.

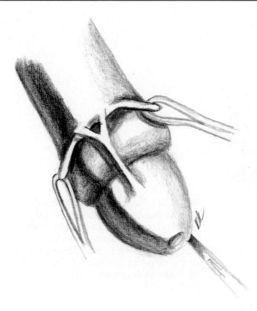

FIGURE 37.3 Babcock clamp method. (Courtesy of Kim Kiser.)

+ Babcock clamp method (**FIGURE 37.3**)
    + Ensure adequate anesthesia (e.g., penile ring block as described in chapter 36)
    + Use six Babcock clamps (no serrated edges) to evenly and circumferentially grasp the phimotic ring
    + Apply slow, steady, distal traction on the Babcock clamps while using your thumbs to apply proximal pressure to the glans
    + If reduction is unsuccessful, proceed to phimotic ring incision
▢ **Phimotic Ring Incision**
    + Ideally performed by a urologist in the operating room, it may be performed by an emergency physician comfortable with this procedure, if instructed to do so by the consulting urologist
    + Ensure adequate anesthesia and sedation
    + Place sterile drapes to reveal only the genital region
    + Clean penis and surrounding region with antiseptic solution
    + Using straight scissors or a no. 15 blade, incise the dorsal skin, subcutaneous tissue, and the constricting ring
    + When the phimotic ring is incised, it will spring open, revealing a diamond-shaped defect
    + Reduce the foreskin over the glans penis and complete the dorsal slit by extending the incision as needed (see chapter 36 for dorsal slit technique)
    + The incision may be repaired with nonabsorbable sutures (e.g., 4-0 nylon)

COMPLICATIONS

▢ Laceration or tear to the skin of the penile shaft (suture if needed with 3-0 or 4-0 absorbable material)
▢ Bleeding and/or infection if tissue incised

SAFETY/QUALITY TIPS

▢ **Procedural**
    + Most paraphimoses can be reduced with very firm, steady, manual pressure for 5 to 10 minutes; however, this requires the right combination of cooperation, anesthesia, analgesia, and sedation. Do not withhold procedural sedation from the appropriate patient.
    + Lidocaine containing epinephrine should not be used because of the potential for vasoconstriction and penile necrosis

⊡ **Cognitive**

+ Paraphimosis is a urologic emergency; the patient cannot be released from care until the paraphimosis is reduced
+ A urologist should be consulted early, especially if initial attempts at manual reduction fail
+ An important iatrogenic cause of paraphimosis is neglecting to replace the foreskin after retraction for procedures (e.g., Foley catheter insertion) or examination

⊡ **Acknowledgment**

Thank you to prior author Richard Newell and Dan Chavira.

Suggested Readings

Ban KM, Easter JS. Selected urologic problems. In: Marx JA, Hockberger RS, Walls RM, eds. *Rosen's Emergency Medicine: Concepts and Clinical Practice*. 8th ed. Philadelphia, PA: Saunders; 2014:1326–1354.

Davis JE, Silverman MA. Urologic procedures. In: Roberts JR, Custalow CB, Thomsen TW, et al. eds. *Roberts & Hedges' Clinical Procedures in Emergency Medicine*. 6th ed. Philadelphia, PA: Saunders; 2014:1113–1154.

Ghory HZ. Phimosis and paraphimosis. http://emedicine.medscape.com/article/777539. Accessed April 7, 2014.

38

Suprapubic Catheterization

Neil Patel and Amy H. Kaji

INDICATIONS

- Urethral trauma (e.g., partial or full transection)
- Urethral stricture
- Chronic urethral infection
- Urinary retention in which a urethral catheter cannot be passed (e.g., prostate obstruction, gynecologic malignancy or other pelvic mass, neurogenic bladder)
- Patients requiring a long-term indwelling urethral catheter
- Phimosis

CONTRAINDICATIONS

- An empty or nonpalpable urinary bladder
- History of previous lower abdominal surgery
- Lower abdominal wound or cellulitis
- Previous pelvic radiation with resultant scarring
- Presence of a femoral–femoral bypass graft in the suprapubic subcutaneous tissue
- Significant uncorrected coagulopathy
- Known bladder cancer

- **General Basic Steps**
  - **Patient preparation**
  - **Urinary bladder localization**
  - **Needle insertion**
  - **Foley catheter insertion**
  - **Securing the catheter**

LANDMARKS

- In the adult, the urinary bladder is a pelvic organ located immediately posterior to and extending slightly above the symphysis pubis (FIGURE 38.1)
- In the child, the urinary bladder is still an abdominal organ, located in the midline, slightly superior to the symphysis pubis

SUPPLIES

- Povidone–iodine antiseptic solution
- Sterile gloves and drapes
- Suprapubic catheterization kit (e.g., Cook cystostomy kit), which typically includes:
  - Local anesthetic (1% lidocaine), 10-mL syringe, 25-gauge needle
  - 22-gauge, 1.5-inch (for children) or 3-inch (for adults) spinal needle
  - 4- × 4-cm gauze pads
  - J-tip guidewire
  - Scalpel (no. 11 blade)
  - Dilator
  - Introducer sheath

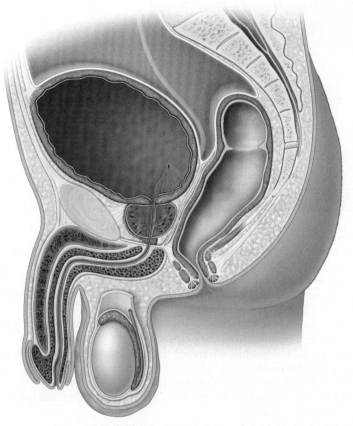

FIGURE 38.1 Relationship of bladder to symphysis pubis. (From Moore KL, Dalley AF, Agur AMR. *Clinically Oriented Anatomy.* 7th ed. Baltimore, MD: Lippincott Williams & Wilkins; 2013:374, with permission.)

- Foley catheter (size should be 1 French smaller than the diameter of the introducer sheath)
- Sterile, closed system urinary drainage bag
- Sterile dressing

TECHNIQUE

- **Patient Preparation**
  - Place the patient in the supine position with the abdomen and pubic region exposed
  - Place small children in the frog-legged supine position; a parent or guardian may hold and help calm the child in his or her lap
  - Sterilize, prepare, and drape the lower abdomen and pubic region with povidone–iodine solution
  - Shave the hair in the suprapubic region beforehand, if necessary
  - Observe sterile technique throughout the remainder of the procedure
- **Urinary Bladder Localization**
  - Palpate the bladder 1 to 2 cm above the symphysis pubis in the midline
  - To facilitate bladder localization, ensure that the patient is well hydrated and has not recently voided
  - If available, use bedside ultrasonography to identify the bladder, which appears as an anechoic mass in the lower abdomen when full **(FIGURE 38.2)**
  - If the bladder cannot be located or appears to be empty, delay the procedure until the bladder is distended

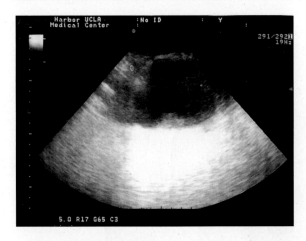

FIGURE 38.2 Transverse sonogram of urinary bladder. (Courtesy of Dr. Patel and Dr. Kaji.)

⊡ **Needle Insertion**

+ Identify the needle insertion point at the midline by measuring 1 to 2 cm cephalad to the superior aspect of the symphysis pubis
+ Using a 25-gauge needle and 1% lidocaine, raise a small wheal at the needle insertion site
+ Attach a 22-gauge spinal needle of appropriate length (1.5 inch for children and 3 inch for adults) to a 10-or 20-mL syringe containing 1% lidocaine
+ Enter the insertion point at a 20- to 30-degree angle *caudad* from the perpendicular in adults, and 20 to 30 degrees *cephalad* from the perpendicular in small children
+ Inject 5 mL of 1% lidocaine while advancing the needle toward the bladder, intermittently pausing to aspirate for urine
+ Once urine is aspirated, the needle should be advanced no further
+ If no urine is aspirated, withdraw the needle to just below the skin and redirect either 10 degrees cephalad or caudad

⊡ **Foley Catheter Insertion Using Seldinger Technique (FIGURE 38.3)**

+ Keeping the spinal needle in place, unscrew the syringe and advance a J-tipped guidewire through the needle into the bladder
+ Remove the needle over the guidewire, leaving the guidewire in place

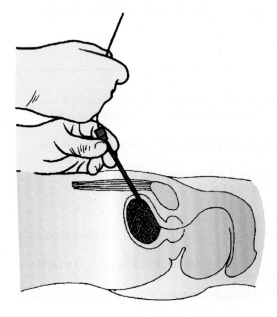

FIGURE 38.3 Technique of suprapubic catheterization with a small-gauge intracath. (From Simon RR, Brenner BF. *Emergency Procedures and Techniques.* 4th ed. Philadelphia, PA: Lippincott Williams & Wilkins; 2002:434, with permission.)

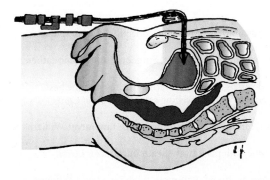

FIGURE 38.4 Trocar taped over 4- × 4-cm gauze pads after insertion. (From Simon RR, Brenner BF. *Emergency Procedures and Techniques*. 4th ed. Philadelphia, PA: Lippincott Williams & Wilkins; 2002:434, with permission.)

+ Use a no. 11 blade to make a stab incision adjacent to the guidewire
+ Advance a dilator and introducer sheath into the bladder over the guidewire
+ Remove the dilator and guidewire, leaving only the sheath in place
+ Advance a Foley catheter through the introducer sheath
    + The size of the Foley catheter should be 1 French smaller than the diameter of the introducer
+ Inflate the Foley balloon with 10 mL of normal saline or sterile water and attach the catheter to a reservoir bag
+ Remove the peel-away introducer sheath. Pull back on the Foley catheter until resistance is met, which indicates that the balloon is against the inner wall of the bladder.
- **Securing the Catheter (FIGURE 38.4)**
    + Place sterile dressing around the catheter insertion site and affix the tube to the lateral aspect of the patient's abdomen or thigh with cloth tape to prevent kinking of the tube

COMPLICATIONS

- Hematuria (usually transient)
- Hematoma
- Infection (intra-abdominal, bladder, or skin)
- Bowel perforation
- Leakage around the catheter site
- Bladder stones

SAFETY/QUALITY TIPS

- **Procedural**
    + Whenever possible, use ultrasonography to guide aspiration or catheter placement
    + To avoid bowel injury, consider placing the patient in the Trendelenburg position
    + Use adequate local anesthesia. For the pediatric age group, procedural sedation may be warranted, or the use of nitrous oxide may be helpful.
- **Cognitive**
    + Avoid procedure if the bladder cannot be easily palpated or visualized with ultrasound
    + A patient with a greatly distended bladder, in whom a conventional urethral catheter cannot be placed, requires cystostomy performed expeditiously. If a urology consultant is not immediately available, the procedure should be attempted by the emergency clinician.
    + If a formal suprapubic catheterization kit is not available, a single-lumen central venous catheter kit may be substituted as a temporizing measure

Suggested Readings

Gochman RF, Karasic RB, Heller MB. Use of portable ultrasound to assist urine collection by suprapubic aspiration. *Ann Emerg Med.* 1991;20:631–635.

Harrison SC, Lawrence WT, Moreley R, et al. British Association of Urological Surgeons' suprapubic catheter practice guidelines. *BJU Int.* 2011;107(1):77–85.

Katsumi HK, Kalisvaart JF, Ronningen LD, et al. Urethral versus suprapubic catheter: choosing the best bladder management for male spinal cord injury patients with indwelling catheters. *Spinal Cord.* 2010;48(4):325–329.

Moore KL, Dalley AF, Agur AMR. *Clinically Oriented Anatomy.* 7th ed. Baltimore, MD: Lippincott Williams & Wilkins; 2013:374.

O'Brien WM. Percutaneous placement of a suprapubic tube with peel-away sheath introducer. *J Urol.* 1991;145:1015–1016.

Simon RR, Brenner BF. *Emergency Procedures and Techniques.* 4th ed. Baltimore, MD: Lippincott Williams & Wilkins; 2002:432–434.

39

Priapism: Intracavernous Aspiration

Timothy Horeczko and Ari M. Lipsky

INDICATIONS

- To alleviate compartment syndrome in ischemic low-flow (veno-occlusive) priapism
- May be caused by:
  + Trauma (genital, pelvic, perineal)
  + Thromboembolism (sickle cell disease, leukemia)
  + Medications (cyclic guanosine monophosphate [cGMP] inhibitors, neuroleptics, erectile-dysfunction treatment, cocaine/marijuana/ecstasy, and others)
  + Neoplasm (primary or metastatic)
  + Neurologic disorders (spinal cord injury, spinal stenosis)
  + Infection (recent infection with *Mycoplasma pneumoniae*, malaria)

CONTRAINDICATIONS

- **Absolute Contraindications**
  + Nonischemic high-flow (arterial) priapism
    + Use history, physical, and selected laboratory tests to help distinguish low- from high-flow priapism. Note especially that high-flow priapism is usually not painful.
    + See "Technique" section for further methods of differentiation
  + Priapism relieved noninvasively
    + Medical treatment of underlying etiology
    + Maneuvers (e.g., ice packs to groin, "steal phenomenon")
- **Relative Contraindications**
  + Coagulopathy

RISKS/CONSENT ISSUES

- Major risk of priapism with or without treatment is long-term impotence. This should be explained clearly to the patient and documented.
- Procedure may cause pain (anesthesia will be given)
- Needle puncture may cause local bleeding and scarring
- Potential for infection (sterile technique will be used)
- If phenylephrine is injected, untoward cardiac effects may be seen (the patient must be monitored)

> **General Basic Steps**
>
> If aspiration does not result in detumescence, continue with the subsequent steps. If, after completing the steps below, detumescence is not achieved or maintained, emergent urologic evaluation is required.
> + **Anesthesia (penile nerve block)**
> + **Verify priapism is ischemic/low-flow (penile blood gas)**
> + **Aspiration**
> + **Irrigation**
> + **Injection/aspiration cycles**
> + **Dressing**

LANDMARKS

- Needle aspiration/irrigation of one of the paired cavernosa is performed dorsolaterally on the shaft of the penis, at either the 3- or 9 o'clock position. This technique avoids the corpus spongiosum and urethra ventrally and the neurovascular bundle and penile vein dorsally.

SUPPLIES

- ☐ Povidone–iodine or chlorhexidine
- ☐ 1% Lidocaine without epinephrine
- ☐ 27-gauge needle (for penile block)
- ☐ Sterile field supplies
- ☐ Sterile gloves
- ☐ Scalp vein ("butterfly") needle
    - ✦ Prepubescent boys: 21 to 23 gauge
    - ✦ Adolescents and adults: 19 gauge
- ☐ Three-way stopcock
- ☐ 10-mL empty syringe
- ☐ 10-mL syringe with normal saline
- ☐ 10-mL syringe with phenylephrine solution (see text below)
- ☐ 4- × 4-cm gauze
- ☐ Kerlix™ (bandage roll) gauze or Coban™ (self-adhesive bandage roll) gauze

TECHNIQUE

- ☐ **Anesthesia**
    - ✦ Perform a penile ring block: Clean the base of the penis with povidone–iodine or chlorhexidine (preferred) solution. Use 1% lidocaine and a 27-gauge needle to perform a ring block around the entire base of the penile shaft (see chapter 36 for details).
    - ✦ Consider systemic analgesia as well
- ☐ **Verification**
    - ✦ Perform a penile blood gas: Clean the shaft of the penis as above. If the ring block is incomplete, infiltrate 1 mL of 1% lidocaine with a tuberculin syringe for supplemental local anesthesia. Use a scalp vein ("butterfly") needle attached to the syringe to puncture perpendicularly at the 3- or 9 o'clock position on the penile shaft to draw blood gas **(FIGURE 39.1)**.
        - ✦ Note the color of aspirated blood. As a guideline, low-flow priapism is more consistent with the following: pH <7.0 to 7.25, Po_2 <30 mm Hg, and Pco_2 >60 mm Hg. A high-flow lesion will more closely reflect normal arterial values.

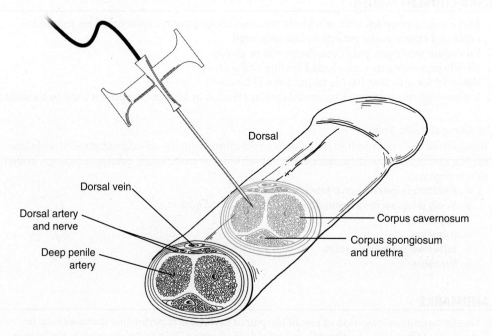

FIGURE 39.1 Cross section of penis and placement of needle. (Courtesy of Tim Horeczko.)

- A penile Doppler ultrasonography may be considered, if available, to aid in distinguishing high- from low-flow priapism
- *Penile aspiration is indicated only for low-flow priapism* **(FIGURE 39.2)**

◻ **Aspiration**
  - **Patient Preparation**
    - Establish IV access and place the patient on oxygen and monitor
    - Consider procedural sedation for patients unable to tolerate procedure
    - Prepare sterile field; swab copiously with antiseptic solution from glans to the base of the penis
    - Perform penile nerve block as described above if not previously done
  - **Penile Aspiration**
    - Palpate either of the paired, engorged corpora cavernosa at 3- or 9 o'clock position (avoiding the dorsal penile vein at 12 o'clock position)
    - Attach an appropriate-size scalp ("butterfly") needle and a 10-mL empty syringe to a three-way stopcock
    - Place the needle into one corpus cavernosum perpendicularly at 3- or 9 o'clock position midshaft, aspirating on insertion (Figure 39.1). Advance the needle only enough to ensure blood return.

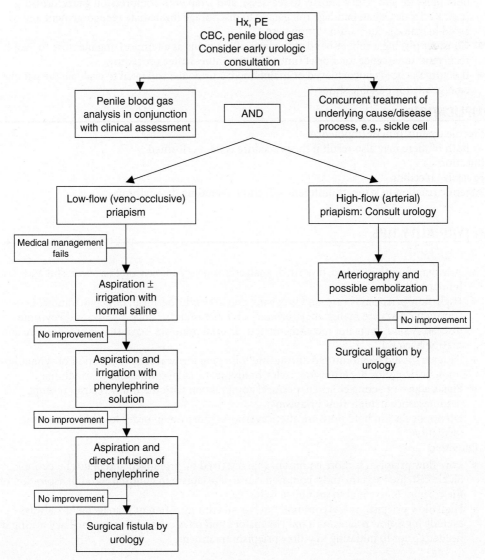

FIGURE 39.2 Priapism algorithm. Hx, history; PE, physical examination; CBC, complete blood count.

+ It is necessary to aspirate only from one corpus cavernosum as there is communication between the two corpora. (This also applies to subsequent irrigation and injection, if needed.)

◻ **Irrigation**
+ If there is inadequate return of blood or lack of initial detumescence with aspiration, irrigate with a small amount (1 mL) of 0.9% saline to flush the clot and allow for further aspiration
+ Aspirate blood while compressing the shaft until the penis detumesces, taking care not to dislodge the needle or cause laceration

◻ **Injection/Aspiration Cycles**
+ If there is minimal response to direct aspiration and irrigation, inject dilute phenylephrine solution into the corpus cavernosum. To prepare the solution, mix 0.1 mg phenylephrine in 4.9 mL of 0.9% saline (to yield 200 µg/mL). In prepubescent boys, infuse 0.5 mL of this solution (100 µg), and in adolescents and adults, infuse 1 mL (200 µg) at a time. *Repeat this every 5 to 10 minutes until (a) detumescence; (b) an hour of injection/aspiration cycles; or (c) a maximum dose of 1,500 µg, whichever comes first.*

◻ **Dressing**
+ After the procedure, remove the needle, hold pressure for 5 minutes (may have the patient hold pressure and return shortly to reassess), and wrap with compression gauze/dressing (e.g., Kerlix or Coban bandage roll gauze) to discourage immediate reengorgement and to avoid hematoma formation
+ Consider placing a rubber band at the base of the penis as a temporizing measure to avoid recurrent tumescence for a brief time (15–20 minutes) after procedure
+ If detumescence is not achieved or maintained, a urologist will need to evaluate the patient emergently for possible shunt

COMPLICATIONS

◻ Erectile dysfunction or impotence
+ Both of these may also result if the procedure is *not* performed
◻ Infection
◻ Excessive bleeding
◻ Systemic reaction to sympathomimetic injection, including dysrhythmia

SAFETY/QUALITY TIPS

◻ **Procedural**
+ Adequate anesthesia (and, if needed, analgesia/sedation) is central to a successful and humane procedure
+ High-flow priapism is rare, and is usually due to penile, perineal, or pelvic trauma. Less common causes are malignancy (primary and metastatic), Fabry disease, and Peyronie disease. Aspiration is not recommended in arterial priapism because it is not effective and may be harmful.
+ Patients should be monitored during and following intracavernous injection of sympathomimetic drugs for hypertension, reflex bradycardia, tachycardia, and dysrhythmia
+ **Piesis sign**—in young children, perineal compression with the thumb causes prompt detumescence in high-flow priapism
+ Do not neglect to hold pressure after cavernosal puncture in order to avoid hematoma formation

◻ **Cognitive**
+ Low-flow priapism is more common, characterized by prolonged and painful erection. Sickle cell disease is the most common cause of priapism in children. Prompt aspiration of the corpora is essential to minimize ischemia.
+ High-flow priapism is less common but has an entirely different management—always exclude high-flow priapism (if only by history and physical, or by using ancillary testing if needed) prior to initiating low-flow priapism treatment

Suggested Readings

Bassett J, Rajfer J. Diagnostic and therapeutic options for the management of ischemic and nonischemic priapism. *Rev Urol.* 2010;12(1):56–63.

Donaldson JF, Rees RW, Steinbrecher HA. Priapism in children: a comprehensive review and clinical guideline. *J Pediatr Urol.* 2014;10:11–25.

Kovac JR, Mak SK, Garcia MM, et al. A pathophysiology-based approach to the management of early priapism. *Asian J Androl.* 2013;15:20–26.

Montague DK, Jarow J, Broderick GA, et al; for the American Urological Association. Guideline to the management of priapism (2003). Reviewed and validity confirmed, 2010. https://www.auanet.org/education/guidelines/priapism.cfm. Accessed February 25, 2014.

Shrewsberry A, Weiss A, Ritenour WM. Recent advances in the medical and surgical treatment of priapism. *Curr Urol Rep.* 2010;11:405–413.

40

Bedside Renal Ultrasonography: Limited, Goal-Directed

Robert P. Favelukes

INDICATIONS

- Confirmation of the diagnosis of obstructive uropathy in patients suspected of ureteral colic
  - + Abdominal or flank pain
  - + Hematuria
  - + Groin pain
- Acute urinary retention
- Known or suspected acute renal failure
- Laboratory evidence of renal failure
- Oliguria or anuria
- Painless hematuria or proteinuria
- Suspected renal abscess
- Infected urine with fever and abdominal or flank pain
- Suspected or known abdominal trauma

CONTRAINDICATIONS

- None

RISKS/CONSENT ISSUES

- Allergy to the ultrasonography gel

LANDMARKS

- The right kidney is usually located inferior and posterior to the liver
- The left kidney is located inferior to the spleen
- The bladder should be imaged in the suprapubic region

TECHNIQUE

- A 3.5-MHz probe is commonly suitable for most adults, although a 5.0-MHz probe can be used in patients with a thinner body habitus and in children
- **The Right Kidney**
  - + With the patient supine, start at the midaxillary line at the level of the lower ribs holding the probe in the longitudinal axis or slightly oblique and scan laterally until the sagittal view of the hepatorenal space (Morison pouch) and the right kidney are visible
  - + Rotate the probe 90 degrees to obtain a transverse image of the kidney. Move the probe superiorly and inferiorly to locate the renal hilum and visualize the full extent of the parenchyma (FIGURE 40.1).
- **The Left Kidney**
  - + The left kidney is most easily located by placing the probe hand against the bed while scanning the left flank at the posterior axillary line at the level of the lower ribs
  - + Rotate the probe 90 degrees to obtain a transverse view of the left kidney
- **The Bladder**
  - + The bladder is best imaged when it is moderately filled at the time of examination
  - + Place the probe suprapubically in the transverse plane. Angle the probe toward the patient's feet. Color Doppler techniques can be used over the trigone area to verify the presence of ureteral flow jets indicating urine flow into the bladder.
  - + Rotate the probe 90 degrees to obtain a sagittal view

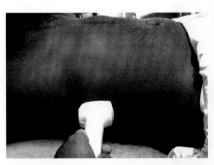 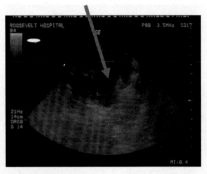

FIGURE 40.1 Renal ultrasonography (photo courtesy of Dr. Charles Martinez).

SONOGRAPHIC SIGNS OF OBSTRUCTIVE UROPATHY

- Hydronephrosis: Large, echo-free areas seen within the echogenic renal sinus **(FIGURE 40.2)**
- Hydroureter: Echo-free tubular structure arising from the renal sinus
- Stones: Ureteral stones are rarely visualized. These will appear as echogenic structures with posterior acoustic shadowing **(FIGURE 40.3)**.
- Absence of ureteral flow jets

OTHER COMMON AND EMERGENT ABNORMALITIES

- Renal abscesses: Typically solitary, round hypoechoic masses
- Renal masses: May be isoechoic, hypoechoic, or hyperechoic in their appearance
- Renal cysts: Anechoic, smooth surface, round or oval, typically eccentrically placed

SAFETY/QUALITY TIPS

- **Procedural**
  + Always visualize the kidney and bladder in two planes (e.g., sagittal and transverse)
  + Always scan both kidneys. If hydronephrosis is seen bilaterally, suspect a urinary outlet obstruction, particularly if there is a distended bladder **(FIGURE 40.4)** and oliguria.
  + Prominent renal pyramids and renal cysts can mimic hydronephrosis
  + The afferent and efferent vessels of the kidney can sometimes be mistaken for a dilated ureter; color Doppler can differentiate mild hydronephrosis from blood vessels
- **Cognitive**
  + Limited, goal-directed ultrasonography of the kidneys, looking for hydronephrosis as evidence of ureteral obstruction, is within the scope of the emergency physician
  + Many patients with ample evidence of kidney stone (concordant history and physical with hematuria and unilateral hydronephrosis) can be managed without computed tomography
  + The sensitivity of detecting clinically relevant abnormalities due to nephro/urolithiasis is 92%
  + Hydronephrosis is a nonspecific finding because it can occur with other states, such as abdominal aortic aneurysm (AAA), pregnancy, or intra-abdominal masses compressing the ureters and urinary outlet obstruction **(FIGURE 40.5)**
  + Presence of hydronephrosis may be masked by dehydration
  + In the absence of trauma, a perinephric fluid collection may represent calyceal rupture and extravasation of urine resulting from high-grade obstruction
  + Always scan the aorta to rule out an AAA in the patient with flank/abdominal pain with risk factors of AAA

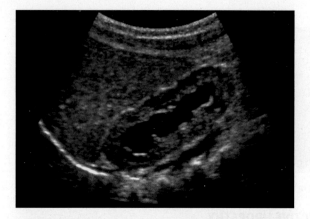

FIGURE 40.2 Hydronephrosis.

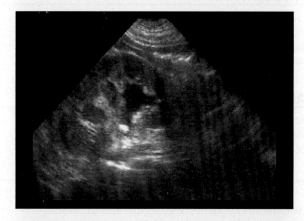

FIGURE 40.3 Echogenic stone casting acoustic shadow.

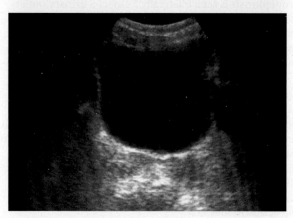

FIGURE 40.4 Bladder filled with urine.

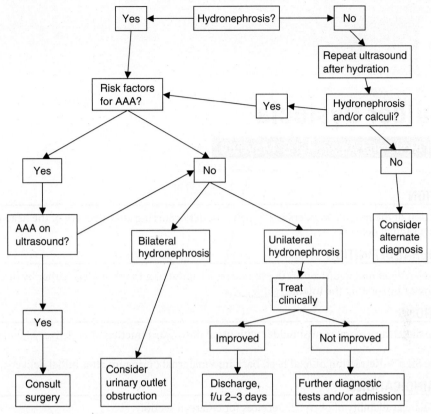

FIGURE 40.5 Hydronephrosis algorithm. AAA, abdominal aortic aneurysm.

Acknowledgment

Thank you to prior author Diana Valcich and Marina Del Rios.

Suggested Readings

Brown DF, Rosen CL, Wolfe RE. Renal ultrasonography. *Emerg Med Clin North Am.* 1997;15(4):877–893.
Ma OJ, Mateer JR. *Emergency Ultrasound.* New York, NY: McGraw-Hill; 2003.

41

Shoulder Dystocia

Olabiyi Akala and Alexander S. Maybury

DEFINITION

🞦 Impaction of the infant shoulders in the pelvic outlet occurring after delivery of the head during a vertex vaginal delivery

PROCEDURAL DEFINITION

🞦 Maneuvers intended to disimpact the shoulders by adducting the shoulders, either by direct pressure or by rotating the infant's trunk

INDICATIONS

🞦 Failure of delivery of anterior shoulder with usual downward traction after delivery of infant head

🞦 "Turtle Sign"—Retraction of fetal head back into maternal perineum after initial delivery

CONTRAINDICATIONS

🞦 Immediate availability of obstetric services for cesarean section

CONSENT

🞦 None. Considered an obstetrical emergency since fetal demise can occur if the procedure is indicated and not performed.

🞦 **General Basic Steps**
  + **Recognize shoulder dystocia**
  + **Call for help immediately (including emergency department personnel and appropriate consulting services)**
  + **Prepare patient**
    + **IV, oxygen, and maternal and fetal monitor must be available**
    + **Call for assistance and obstetric, anesthesia, and pediatric backup**
    + **Drain bladder if distended**
    + **Avoid maternal pushing while attempts are made to reposition fetus**
    + **Avoid excessive head and neck traction or uterine fundal pressure**
  + **Apply maneuvers to facilitate delivery (may need to attempt multiple maneuvers)**

TECHNIQUES

🞦 **Mazzanti Maneuver (FIGURE 41.1)**
  + Adduct shoulders by applying downward or oblique suprapubic pressure to dislodge anterior shoulder from pubic symphysis
  + *Avoid* applying fundal pressure, which may cause further fetal injury

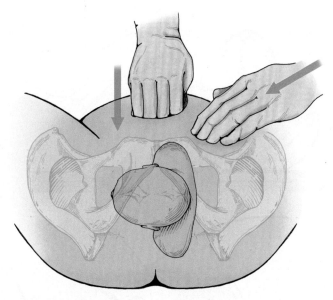

FIGURE 41.1 Mazzanti maneuver.

- **McRoberts Maneuver (FIGURE 41.2)**
  - Hyperflex maternal hips to a knee-to-chest position
  - This flattens the lumbar spine and rotates the pelvis toward the head, which frees the impacted anterior shoulder
- **Woods Screw Maneuver (FIGURE 41.3)**
  - Rotate the fetus 180 degrees by applying pressure to the clavicular surface of the posterior shoulder in an attempt to dislodge anterior shoulder
  - Do not twist the head and neck
- **Rubin Maneuver (FIGURE 41.4)**
  - Place one hand behind the posterior shoulder and adduct shoulder while rotating it anteriorly
- **Gaskin Maneuver**
  - Mother is repositioned on her hands and knees (on "all fours") and gentle downward traction is applied to posterior shoulder or upward traction applied to the anterior shoulder
- **Delivery of the Posterior Arm (FIGURE 41.5)**
  - Locate the posterior arm in the vagina
  - Apply pressure to the antecubital fossa to flex the elbow and bring the forearm across chest
  - Locate the forearm and hand and pull through the vagina to deliver the posterior shoulder
- **Clavicular Fracture**
  - Fracture the clavicle intentionally to decrease bisacromial diameter by pulling the anterior clavicle outward away from the lung to avoid causing a pneumothorax
- **Zavanelli Maneuver (FIGURE 41.6)**
  - Reverse the cardinal movements of labor and take the patient to the operating room (OR) for cesarean section
  - Relax the uterus with terbutaline (0.25 mg SC (subcutaneously)) or nitroglycerin (50–200 µg/min IV)
  - Rotate fetal head to occiput anterior position
  - Flex fetal neck and apply gentle cephalad pressure to fetal head to replace the fetus back into the pelvis
  - Prepare for cesarean section

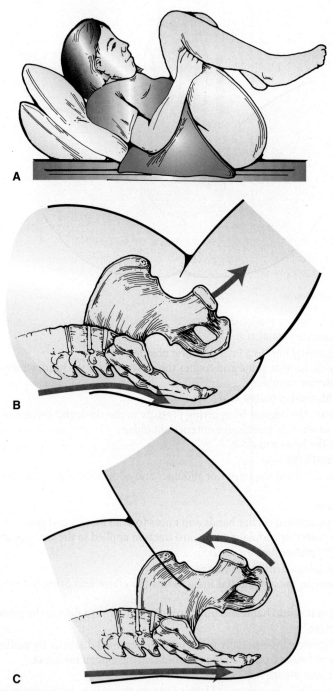

FIGURE 41.2 McRoberts maneuver.

✚ Symphysiotomy (FIGURES 41.7 and 41.8)

- ✚ Use as last resort, if all other techniques fail and cesarean delivery is unavailable
- ✚ Sterilize the skin over the pubic symphysis area with povidone–iodine solution
- ✚ Infiltrate skin and fibrocartilaginous area with local anesthetic

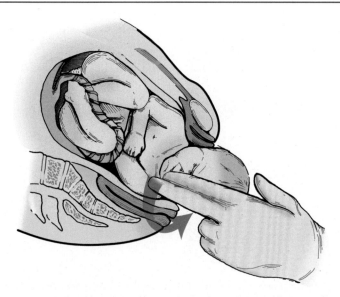

FIGURE 41.3 Woods screw maneuver.

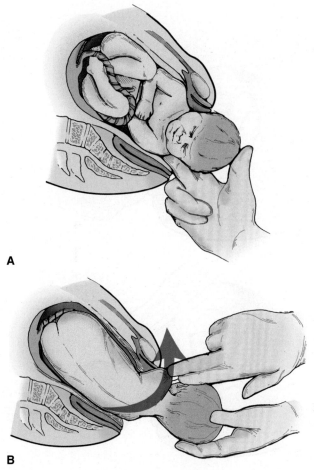

A

B

FIGURE 41.4 Rubin maneuver.

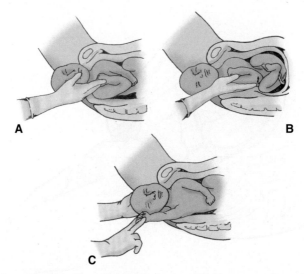

FIGURE 41.5 Delivery of posterior arm. (From Simon RR, Brenner BE. *Emergency Procedures and Techniques.* 4th ed. Philadelphia, PA: Lippincott Williams & Wilkins; 2002:214, with permission.)

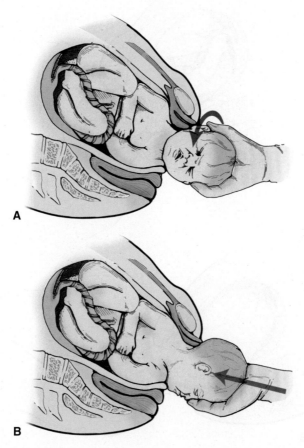

FIGURE 41.6 Zavanelli maneuver.

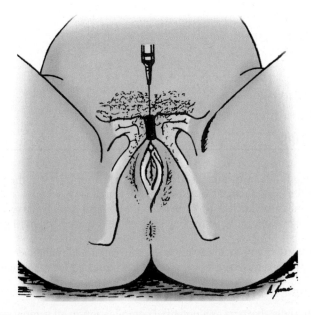

FIGURE 41.7 Infiltration of anesthetic solution over the symphysis pubis. (From Simon RR, Brenner BE. *Emergency Procedures and Techniques*. 4th ed. Philadelphia, PA: Lippincott Williams & Wilkins; 2002:220, with permission.)

+ Displace urethra laterally
+ Incise skin and fibrocartilage of pubic symphysis

COMPLICATIONS

⊞ **Fetal**
+ Brachial plexus injury due to excessive head and neck traction
+ Fractures of humerus and clavicle

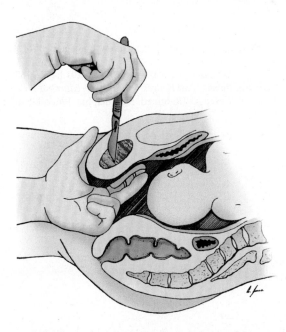

FIGURE 41.8 Make an incision into the symphysis pubis with a no. 10 blade. (From Simon RR, Brenner BE. *Emergency Procedures and Techniques*. 4th ed. Philadelphia, PA: Lippincott Williams & Wilkins; 2002:221, with permission.)

- ✦ Pneumothorax
- ✦ Hypoxic brain injury
- ✦ Fetal death
- ▢ **Maternal**
  - ✦ Hemorrhage
  - ✦ Severe perineal lacerations
  - ✦ Uterine atony

SAFETY/QUALITY TIPS

- ▢ **Procedural**
  - ✦ Avoid applying fundal pressure, which may cause further injury to the fetus
  - ✦ Never rotate the head and neck or use excessive traction
  - ✦ Noninvasive measures such as McRoberts and Mazzanti maneuvers are most often used and effective; however, multiple maneuvers may be required depending on the severity of the dystocia
  - ✦ Consider episiotomy to provide space to execute rotational maneuvers or posterior arm delivery; however, routine episiotomy is *not* indicated for management of shoulder dystocia
- ▢ **Cognitive**
  - ✦ Recognize shoulder dystocia as a potential complication in all vaginal deliveries; have an approach to shoulder dystocia in mind or ready access to a reference to guide you
  - ✦ Consult obstetrics emergently to assist with delivery and prepare for possible cesarean section
  - ✦ Be aware of how much time has elapsed since delivery of the head; fetal morbidity and mortality are significantly increased with dystocia after 7 minutes
  - ✦ After the procedure, document the maneuvers used during delivery, the time of delivery of head, shoulder, and infant, and any associated fetal or maternal injuries

▢ **Acknowledgment**

Thank you to prior author Shadi Kiriaki and Ted Korszun.

Suggested Readings

del Portal DA, Horn AE, Vilke GA, et al. Emergency department management of shoulder dystocia. *J Emerg Med.* 2014;46(3):378–382.

Grobman W. Shoulder dystocia. *Obstet and Gynecol Clin North Am.* 2013;40:59–67.

Roberts JR. Emergency Childbirth. *Roberts and Hedges' Clinical Procedures in Emergency Medicine.* Roberts JR, Custalow CB, Thomsen TW, Hedges JR. 6th ed. Philadelphia, PA: WB Saunders; 2014: chapter 56, 1155–1179.

42

Vaginal Breech Delivery

Fereshteh Sani

DEFINITION

- Presentation of the infant buttocks or feet before the head
- Considered a high-risk delivery even among seasoned obstetricians

PRESENTATION TYPES

- Frank breech—fetus with bilateral hip flexion and knees extended with feet opposite the head
- Footling (incomplete) breech—one or both hips or knees extended and presenting before buttocks
- Complete breech—bilateral hip and knee flexion with feet opposite the trunk (FIGURE 42.1)

INDICATIONS

- Imminent vaginal delivery without obstetrical backup *and* buttocks or feet of the fetus appear at the vulva

CONTRAINDICATIONS

- Placenta previa
- Spontaneous arrest of labor
- Immediate availability of obstetric services

CONSENT

- Obtain informed consent if possible and time permits

RISKS

- Peripartum fetal and maternal morbidity or mortality
- Maternal bleeding and pain
- Breech position may result from underlying fetal or uterine abnormalities

- **General Basic Steps**
  + **Examine for presenting part**
  + **Place the mother in lithotomy position**
  + **Allow natural delivery of baby as much as possible; assist without excessive traction**
  + **Flex baby's head to assist with delivery**

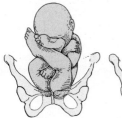
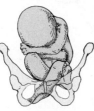
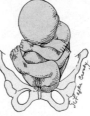

Frank breech   Footling (incomplete) breech   Complete breech

FIGURE 42.1 Fetal attitude in frank, incomplete, and complete breech presentations. (From Cruikshank DP. Breech, other malpresentations, and umbilical cord complications. In: Scott JR, Gibbs RS, Karlan BY, et al, eds. *Danforth's Obstetrics and Gynecology.* 9th ed. Philadelphia, PA: Lippincott Williams & Wilkins; 2003:382, with permission.)

TECHNIQUES

⊕ Examine the vagina to determine the presenting part

⊕ Use ultrasonography or Leopold maneuver to determine fetal lie

⊕ Consult obstetrics *emergently*

⊕ Prepare for possible cesarean section

⊕ Place the mother in the lithotomy position with a wedge under her buttocks

⊕ Consider episiotomy once the fetal anus has appeared at the vulva

⊕ Allow maternal effort to spontaneously deliver the fetal buttocks, flexed knees, and lower limbs

⊕ Avoid excessive premature traction of the fetus, which can cause undesirable positioning of the head, resulting in head and nuchal arm entrapment

⊕ If knees are extended, the physician may flex each knee (Pinard maneuver—see **FIGURE 42.2**) to facilitate delivery

⊕ Grasp the infant's bony pelvis during vaginal delivery

⊕ Rotate the fetus in the anteroposterior plane to deliver each shoulder

⊕ Shoulder delivery may be expedited by flexing the fetal elbow or adducting the extended elbow by placing a finger in the antecubital fossa

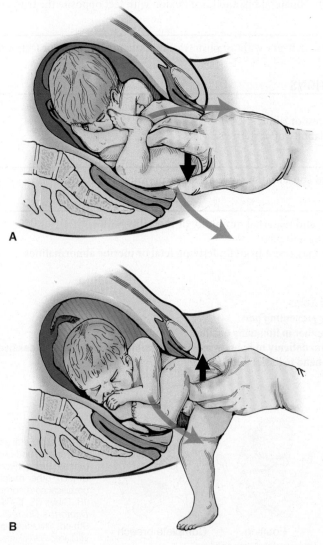

FIGURE 42.2 Pinard maneuver.

- When delivering the head, attempt to flex the neck by holding the chin and applying suprapubic pressure **(FIGURE 42.3)** or use the Mauriceau maneuver
  - The index and middle fingers are placed over the infant's maxillary bones (not in the infant's mouth) to help keep the head flexed. This should allow the mother to expel the fetus.
- Use forceps if needed
- Consider symphysiotomy as a last resort

COMPLICATIONS

- **Fetal**
  - Prolapsed cord
  - Shoulder dystocia
  - Head entrapment
  - Fetal ischemia due to excessive traction on the cord
    - This may be prevented by checking cord pulsations and forming a small loop of the cord
  - Neurologic injuries due to excessive traction or neck hyperextension during delivery
  - Visceral injuries due to excessive pressure on the abdomen during delivery

SAFETY/QUALITY TIPS

- **Procedural**
  - Avoid excessive traction on the presenting part
  - Avoid grasping the fetal abdomen instead of the bony pelvis
  - Avoid hyperextension of the neck when delivering the head
  - For head entrapment, attempt to facilitate delivery by administering terbutaline (0.25 mg SC (subcutaneously)) or nitroglycerin (50 to 200 μg/min IV) to achieve uterine relaxation
- **Cognitive**
  - Emergency breech deliveries are very high risk for both mother and baby. Make every effort to obtain obstetrics and pediatrics support.
  - The status of the fetus, mother, and fetal station determine the pace of delivery. If the baby is doing well (use ultrasound to assess heart rate if proper fetal monitoring is not available), do not rush delivery or rupture the membranes. Bring an obstetrician to bedside or, after a phone discussion with the obstetrician, move the patient to labor and delivery.

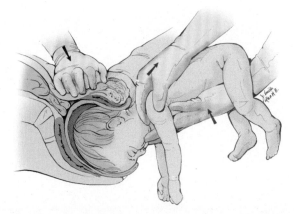

FIGURE 42.3 Breech delivery of fetal head performed by flexing the head while applying suprapubic pressure. (From Benrubi GI. *Handbook of Obstetric and Gynecologic Emergencies.* 3rd ed. Philadelphia, PA: Lippincott Williams & Wilkins; 2005:187.)

⊡ Acknowledgment

Thank you to prior author Lekha Ajit Shah and Resa Lewiss.

Suggested Readings

Benrubi GI. *Handbook of Obstetric and Gynecologic Emergencies*. 3rd ed. Philadelphia, PA: Lippincott Williams
   & Wilkins; 2005.

Reichman EF. Chapter 134. Breech Delivery. In: Reichman EF, ed. *Emergency Medicine Procedures*. 2nd ed.
   New York, NY: McGraw-Hill; 2013.

Roberts JR, Hedges JR. *Clinical Procedures in Emergency Medicine*. 4th ed. Philadelphia, PA: WB Saunders;
   2004:1128–1132.

Scott JR, Gibbs RS, Karlan BY, et al. *Danforth's Obstetrics and Gynecology*. 9th ed. Philadelphia, PA: Lippincott
   Williams & Wilkins; 2003.

Simon RR, Brenner BE. *Emergency Procedures and Techniques*. 4th ed. Philadelphia, PA: Lippincott Williams
   & Wilkins; 2002:215–221.

VanRooyen MJ, Scott JA. Emergency delivery. In: Tintinalli JE, Stapczynski J, Ma O, et al, eds. *Tintinalli's
   Emergency Medicine: A Comprehensive Study Guide*. New York, NY: McGraw-Hill; 2011.

43

Episiotomy

Jessica Hetherington Lopez

INDICATIONS

- To prevent severe spontaneous third- and fourth-degree perineal lacerations
- To increase the diameter of the soft-tissue pelvic outlet to relieve shoulder dystocia
- To facilitate delivery of fetus having nonreassuring fetal heart-rate tracings
- To facilitate delivery in malpresentations, including breech and occiput posterior presentations

CONTRAINDICATIONS

- Not recommended for routine delivery, especially in the primiparous patient

LANDMARKS (FIGURE 43.1)

- **General Basic Steps**
  - **Organize supplies**
  - **Local anesthesia**
  - **Incision**
  - **Closure**

TECHNIQUE

- **Supplies**
  - A 3-0 or 2-0 absorbable suture (polyglactin preferred or chromic catgut) on atraumatic needle
  - Needle holder
  - Tissue scissors or scalpel
  - Suture scissors
  - Gauze
  - Local anesthesia and injection materials

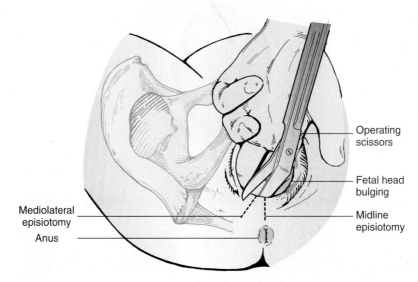

FIGURE 43.1 Episiotomy landmarks.

☐ **Initiation of Procedure**

+ For vertex presentations, episiotomy is started when the fetal head begins to stretch the perineum and when 3 to 4 cm diameter of the caput is visible during a contraction (prior to crowning)
+ For breech presentations, episiotomy is started just before extraction of the fetus
+ Inject 1% or 2% lidocaine locally in the perineum where episiotomy is planned (may also perform pudendal nerve block) (**FIGURE 43.2**)

☐ **Median or Midline Technique**

+ Most commonly performed
+ Just prior to crowning, two fingers are placed inside the vaginal introitus to expose the mucosa, posterior fourchette, and the perineal body
+ Tissue scissors are used to make a vertical incision beginning at the fourchette and extending caudally in the midline. The goal is to release the constriction caused by the perineal body.
+ Incision should be directed internally to minimize the amount of perineal skin incised
+ Incision includes the vaginal mucosa, perineal body, and the junction of the perineal body with the bulbocavernosus muscle in the perineum

☐ **Mediolateral Technique**

+ As the head crowns, two fingers are placed inside the vaginal introitus to expose the mucosa, posterior fourchette, and the perineal body
+ Tissue scissors are used to make a 3- to 5-cm incision directed downward and outward toward the lateral margin of the anal sphincter in a 45-degree angle. This incision may be either to the left or the right.
+ Incision includes the vaginal mucosa, transverse perineal and bulbocavernosus muscles, and the perineal skin

☐ **Repair: Layer Closure**

+ A 2-0 or 3-0 absorbable suture is used
+ Close the vaginal mucosa using a continuous suture from just above the apex of the incision to the mucocutaneous junction
+ Burying the closing knot minimizes the amount of scar tissue and prevents pain and dyspareunia

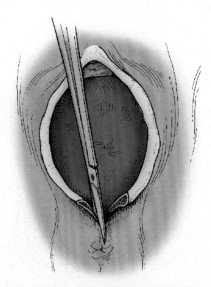

FIGURE 43.2 Midline episiotomy. As the fetal head distends, with the perineum under adequate anesthesia, a cut is made through the perineal body and the tissues of the vagina and the rectovaginal septum for the episiotomy. (From Rouse DJ, St John E. Normal labor, delivery, newborn care, and puerperium. In: Scott JR, Gibbs RS, Karlan BY, et al. eds. *Danforth's Obstetrics and Gynecology*. 9th ed. Philadelphia, PA: Lippincott Williams & Wilkins; 2003:44, with permission.)

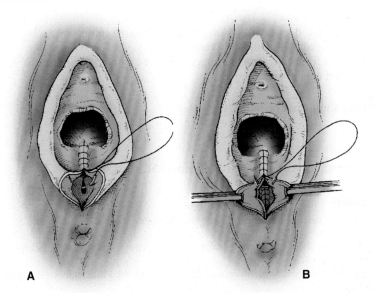

A   **B**

FIGURE 43.3 A: The episiotomy is repaired by reapproximating the vaginal mucosa in a running manner with a delayed absorbable suture. **B:** The submucosal tissue of the vagina and the subcutaneous tissue, and the fascia of the perineal body are then closed (From Rouse DJ, St John E. Normal labor, delivery, newborn care, and puerperium. In: Scott JR, Gibbs RS, Karlan BY, et al, eds. *Danforth's Obstetrics and Gynecology.* 9th ed. Philadelphia, PA: Lippincott Williams & Wilkins; 2003:44, with permission.)

- Large actively bleeding vessels may require ligation with separate absorbable sutures
- The perineal musculature is reapproximated using three to four interrupted sutures
- Closure of the superficial layers is done with several interrupted sutures through the skin and subcutaneous fascia that are loosely tied. The skin can also be closed using a running subcuticular suture.
- Finally, examine the rectum and anal sphincters with the index finger in the rectum and the thumb on the sphincter, using a pill-rolling motion to assess integrity (**FIGURE 43.3**)

COMPLICATIONS

- Hemorrhage (more common with mediolateral technique due to increased musculature incised)
- Hematoma formation
- Postpartum episiotomy pain
- Infection (cellulitis, abscess, and [rarely] necrotizing fasciitis)
- Third- and fourth-degree lacerations causing damage to the anal sphincter and rectum, respectively
- Rectovaginal fistula formation
- Incontinence
- Dyspareunia
- Sexual dysfunction
- Wound dehiscence
- Perineal laceration in subsequent deliveries

SAFETY/QUALITY TIPS

- **Procedural**
  - Start episiotomy after the head has thinned out the perineum and the fetus is expected within the next three to four contractions
  - If a scalpel is used, place a tongue blade between the infant's head and the maternal perineum before making incision to avoid trauma to the infant
  - Perform a thorough examination of the wound to evaluate for injuries to the anal sphincters and rectum

- Third- and fourth-degree lacerations involving the anal sphincters and rectal mucosa should be repaired in the operating room
- Begin perineal repair after the placenta is delivered and after full inspection and repair of the cervix and upper vaginal canal

▣ Cognitive

- Episiotomy should not be routinely performed

▣ Acknowledgment

Thank you to prior author Annie Akkara and Jennifer Stratton.

Suggested Readings

Roberts JR, Hedges JR. *Clinical Procedures in Emergency Medicine*. 4th ed. Philadelphia, PA: WB Saunders; 2004:1132–1135.

Scott JR, Gibbs RS, Karlan BY, et al. *Danforth's Obstetrics and Gynecology*. 9th ed. Philadelphia, PA: Lippincott Williams & Wilkins; 2003.

Simon RR, Brenner BE. *Emergency Procedures and Techniques*. 4th ed. Philadelphia, PA: Lippincott Williams & Wilkins; 2002:215.

44

Bedside Obstetric/Gynecologic Ultrasonography

Tsion Firew

INDICATIONS

- ⊕ Is an intrauterine pregnancy (IUP) (defined as yolk sac or fetal pole) present?
- ⊕ Abdominal or pelvic pain
- ⊕ Suspected ectopic pregnancy or risk factors for ectopic pregnancy
- ⊕ Vaginal bleeding
- ⊕ Unexplained syncope, or hypotension
- ⊕ Pelvic mass

CONTRAINDICATIONS

- ⊕ Absolute: None
- ⊕ Relative (transvaginal approach): Recent major pelvic surgery

CONSENT

- ⊕ Get verbal or written consent for the procedure, except in extremis situations

RISKS

- ⊕ No documented harmful effects on the fetus or the mother due to ultrasound exposure

LANDMARKS

- ⊕ **Transabdominal**
  - ✦ Have the patient lie supine
  - ✦ The bladder should be full in order to have an adequate acoustic window
  - ✦ Use a standard curved 3.5- to 5.0-MHz probe to scan the lower abdomen
  - ✦ Place the probe on the anterior abdominal wall, at the level of the symphysis pubis
  - ✦ For advanced gestations, place the probe more proximally
- ⊕ **Transvaginal**
  - ✦ Insert the probe into the vaginal canal
  - ✦ The uterus is midline, posterior to the bladder and anterior to the rectum **(FIGURE 44.1)**
  - ✦ The right and left ovaries are lateral to the uterus and anteromedial to the right and left iliac vessels
  - ✦ Anteroflexed uterus 90% and retroflexed in 10%

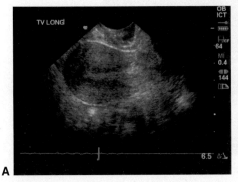 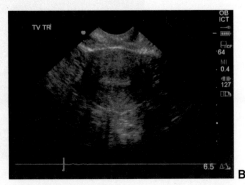

FIGURE 44.1 Transvaginal views of the uterus. A: Sagittal view. B: Transverse view.

SAFETY/QUALITY TIPS

◘ **Procedural**

✦ Transabdominal ultrasound is easier with a full bladder, and transvaginal ultrasound is easier with an empty bladder

✦ Transabdominal ultrasound should be performed prior to transvaginal ultrasound on all patients. Free fluid that may not be seen transvaginally may be appreciated transabdominally, and if an IUP can be confirmed transabdominally, a transvaginal procedure is not required.

✦ Start with bird's-eye views of the uterus, then zoom in

✦ Certain types of ectopic pregnancies can appear intrauterine. Measure the myometrial mantle; it should be >8 mm.

✦ Interpreting ultrasound of the adnexa is difficult. If an IUP is not seen, be cautious about attempting to distinguish among adnexal masses.

◘ **Cognitive**

✦ All pregnant patients without confirmed IUP, who have bleeding, pain, syncope, or hypotension should have an ultrasound performed on the index visit, either at the point of care or by consultation, regardless of their beta-human chorionic gonadotropin (β-hCG) level

✦ Inform patients that point-of-care ultrasound is not used to detect fetal anomalies or to assess fetal health; rather, the role of sonography in the emergency department is to determine where the pregnancy is, so that the pregnancy can be confirmed to be not dangerous to the mother

✦ Patients undergoing fertility treatment are at increased chance of an IUP and concurrent ectopic pregnancy (heterotopic pregnancy). Obstetric consultation is generally indicated in these circumstances.

✦ The sonographic criterion for IUP is an intrauterine sac with either a yolk sac or fetal pole. Intrauterine sacs without these contents could represent *pseudogestational sacs*, seen in ectopic pregnancy.

✦ If no IUP is confirmed, no evidence of ectopic pregnancy is found, and the patient is otherwise not at high risk for ectopic pregnancy, the patient should return to medical care (ideally in the office of an obstetrician) in 24 to 48 hours for a repeat β-hCG and ultrasound

✦ Women of childbearing age with a history of recent last menstrual period, sterilization, tubal ligation, reportedly sexually inactive, or using birth control may all be pregnant, and are at risk for ectopic pregnancy. Have a very low threshold to perform urine or serum pregnancy testing.

✦ The risk of ectopic pregnancy cannot be stratified by β-hCG. Correct interpretation of β-hCG levels must be done together with clinical and sonographic findings (**FIGURES 44.2** and **44.3**) shows the suggested approach).

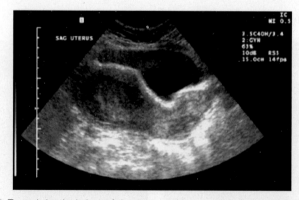

FIGURE 44.2 Transabdominal view of the uterus with a possible intrauterine pregnancy.

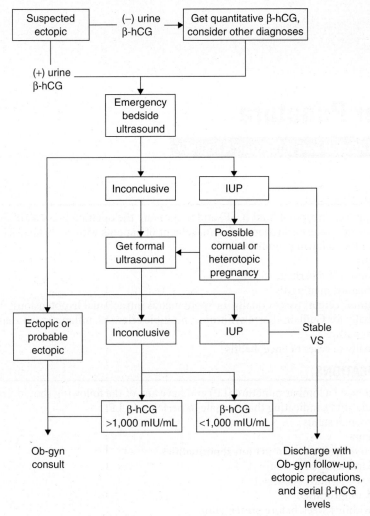

FIGURE 44.3 Emergency obstetric ultrasonography algorithm. β-hCG, beta human chorionic gonadotropin; IUP, intrauterine pregnancy; VS, vital signs.

Suggested Readings

Burgher SW, Tandy TK, Dawdy MR. Transvaginal ultrasonography by emergency physicians decreases patient time in the emergency department. *Acad Emerg Med.* 1998;5(8):802–807.

Dawson M, Mallin M. Introduction to bedside ultrasound: Vol 1. *Emergency Ultrasound Solutions.* 2013: 128–141.

45

Lumbar Puncture

Nicole M. Dubosh and Jonathan A. Edlow

INDICATIONS

- Used to obtain cerebrospinal fluid (CSF) and to measure the opening pressure of the subarachnoid space to aid in the evaluation and management of patients with acute headache or other symptoms of the following conditions:
  - Meningitis
  - Subarachnoid hemorrhage (SAH)
  - Carcinomatous meningitis
  - Pseudotumor cerebri (occasionally for spontaneous intracranial hypotension)
  - Occasionally for Guillain–Barré syndrome, multiple sclerosis, inflammatory demyelinating polyneuropathy
  - Occasionally in cases of encephalitis

CONTRAINDICATIONS

- Patients who need a lumbar puncture (LP) and have any of the following should first have a brain imaging study, indicating that it is safe to perform an LP:
  - Altered mental status
  - Papilledema
  - New focal neurologic examination abnormalities
  - Elevated intracranial pressure (ICP)
  - Age 60 years or older (relative)
  - Immunocompromised
  - Seizure within 1 week before presentation
    - Exception, pseudotumor cerebri (where by definition, the ICP is elevated)
- Suspicion of spinal cord mass, or epidural hematoma/abscess
- Skin or soft-tissue infection overlying lumbar spine
- Anatomic abnormalities: For example, patients with lumbar hardware from prior spinal surgery
- Coagulopathic patients

RISKS/CONSENT ISSUES

- Post-LP headache occurs in approximately 15% to 20% of patients. Using an atraumatic or non-cutting spinal needle decreases the incidence of this, and multiple therapies exist to treat this specific type of headache.
- The procedure can cause local pain. Local anesthesia will be given.
- Needle puncture can cause local bleeding, which is usually minimal
- Potential for introducing infection exists; however, this is extremely rare. Sterile technique will be utilized.
- Theoretical risk of damage to neural tissue exists. Such occurrences are also very rare, most often temporary, and affect spinal nerve roots, not the cord itself.

LANDMARKS

The transverse axis connecting iliac crests passes through L4 vertebral body, allowing for identification of the L4-5 and L3-4 interspaces (FIGURE 45.1)

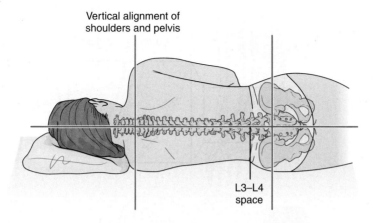

Vertical alignment of
shoulders and pelvis

L3–L4
space

FIGURE 45.1 Anatomical landmarks.

TECHNIQUE

🔲 **Patient Preparation**
  ✚ Explain the procedure to the patient and obtain patient consent
  ✚ Position the patient in either lateral decubitus or sitting position (the sitting position may be easier to use but precludes accurate ICP measurement)
🔲 **Lateral Decubitus Position**
  ✚ Have the patient lie on one side, with knees to chest and head/shoulders curled toward knees as much as possible. Placing a pillow under the head helps reduce twisting of the shoulders.
  ✚ Ensure that the lumbar spine lies parallel to the edge of the bed. (In an infant/child, or a poorly cooperative adult, it will be necessary to have an assistant hold the patient securely in the optimal position.) The top shoulder and hip should be directly above their bottom counterparts.
  ✚ A cooperative patient can be asked to curve his/her lower back, out like an "angry cat," to optimally open the spinous processes
🔲 **Sitting Position**
  ✚ Have the patient sit on the side of the bed with the bed positioned below patient's midthigh and with the feet of the patient touching floor, if possible
  ✚ Ask the patient to curve the torso forward over a bedside table positioned in front of him/her; table height should be level with patient's upper abdomen. A pillow may be placed on the table for patient's comfort.
  ✚ After positioning, but before prepping, mark the target for needle insertion with firm pressure from the Luer-lock (hub) end of a needle sheath (or some other blunt device such as a pen) firmly against the skin (which will leave a mark for several minutes and provides a visual target)
  ✚ Prepare a wide area with povidone–iodine or chlorhexidine gluconate solution
    ✦ Ensure the sterile field includes L4-5 and L3-4 interspaces. (Should first attempt at L4- 5 be unsuccessful, the L3-4 interspace will be readily accessible.)
    ✦ Use sterile drapes to frame workspace
  ✚ Reassess landmarks. It is crucial that the midline be defined.
    ✦ Sometimes, in overweight patients, feeling the spinous processes in the thoracic spine (where they are easier to palpate) and marching down will help the clinician ensure that they are in the midline
    ✦ Ultrasonography has been shown to reduce the failure rate, number of attempts, and traumatic punctures and can be used as an adjunct

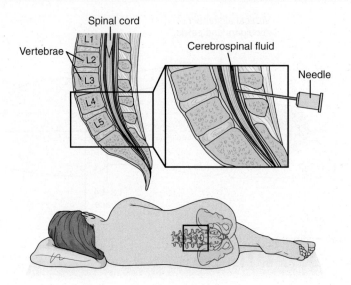

FIGURE 45.2 Needle insertion point.

Insertion

- Analgesia: Produce local anesthesia using 1% lidocaine
    - Inject the subcutaneous area with a small-bore (27-gauge) needle, and then, using a larger-bore needle (22-gauge) infiltrate the prespinous soft tissues down to the supraspinous ligament. Massaging the area afterward with your thumb will distribute the wheal and allow for reassessment of bony landmarks.
- Accessing subarachnoid space:
    - Place the nondominant thumb on L4 spinous process
    - Using the dominant hand, insert a 20- or 22-gauge atraumatic spinal needle through the skin just caudal to your thumb. Take care to orient the bevel parallel to the long axis of the spinal column, as this will minimize trauma to the longitudinally arranged dural fibers (**FIGURE 45.2**).
    - Continue advancing the needle with stylet in place until you meet resistance from the supraspinous ligament. Advance through the ligament and you will often feel a reduction in resistance (sometimes described as a slight "pop").
    - Remove the stylet. Watch the barrel of needle to look out for return of CSF as you advance very slowly. If there is no flow of CSF, rotate the needle 90 degrees (this will displace a nerve root that has floated up against the bevel).
- Measuring opening pressure:
    - Upon visualizing return of CSF, affix a three-way stopcock to the needle hub, with chamber open to the vertically-oriented manometer
    - With patient in lateral decubitus position, traditional doctrine mandates that you should have him/her slowly straighten legs and neck at this time (to make the pressure measurement accurate, though this probably only changes the number by a small amount)
    - Opening pressure is determined when CSF column ceases to climb, which usually takes approximately 1 to 2 minutes. Normal opening pressure is 6 to 20 cm H_2O in the lateral decubitus position.
    - Only recently has opening pressure been evaluated in the sitting position, with one study finding a 13-cm H_2O increase with patient sitting upright
- Collecting CSF: You may either remove the manometer or turn the stopcock to allow for CSF to bypass the manometer (**FIGURE 45.3**)
    - Collect 1 to 2 mL of CSF in each of four numbered tubes
    - If the opening pressure was elevated, it is best to measure a closing pressure; this is particularly important in cases of likely pseudotumor cerebri

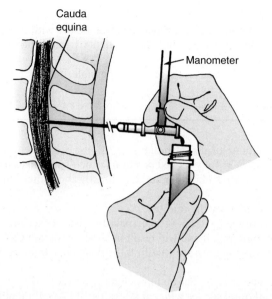

FIGURE 45.3 Turn stopcock to allow cerebrospinal fluid to drain into collecting tubes. (From Simon RR, Brenner BE. *Emergency Procedures and Techniques*. 4th ed. Philadelphia, PA: Lippincott Williams & Wilkins; 2002:199, with permission.)

+ Removing the needle: Replace the stylet completely into needle hub. Inform patient the needle is being removed. Remove the needle and place gauze over LP site for few seconds; then place a plastic adhesive dressing (e.g., Band-Aid).

☐ **Analyzing CSF:** Tightly screw the caps on the tubes of CSF to prevent loss en route to the laboratory. Most often, the following analyses are performed:
+ Tube no. 1: Cell count and differential
+ Tube no. 2: Gram stain and culture
+ Tube no. 3: Protein and glucose
+ Tube no. 4: Repeat cell count and differential

Additional analysis may be performed on tube no. 4 if appropriate volume of CSF is included. Specific requests should be made, such as Lyme serology, HSV PCR (herpes simplex virus polymerase chain reaction), India ink preparation for Cryptococcus, cytologic evaluation for malignancy, or others, as indicated by your differential diagnosis.

COMPLICATIONS

☐ **Post-LP Headache**
+ Occurs in 15% to 20% of patients
+ Therapies include hydration, caffeine, analgesics, and blood patch. Factors that correlate with increased incidence of post-LP headache include insertion of the needle perpendicular to the long axis of the cord, use of a cutting needle (vs atraumatic), and use of a larger-gauge needle. Young, thin female patients also have a higher risk of post-LP headache.

☐ **Traumatic Tap**
+ Usually (but not always) caused by passing needle further than necessary, thereby disrupting the venous plexus at anterior aspect of canal

☐ **Cerebral Herniation**
+ Occurs in the setting of elevated ICP before tap
+ History, funduscopic examination, and/or computed tomography may be used to assess ICP before LP (see "Contraindications" section). Despite the severity of this complication, it is extremely rare.

◻ **Spinal Root Herniation**
 ✛ Extremely rare; risk is minimized by replacing stylet before withdrawal of needle
 ✛ Low back pain, seen in approximately 15% of patients, treated with analgesics
 ✛ Serious bleeding is very rare
 ✛ Infection of any involved tissues is theoretically possible, but risk is minimized by sterile technique

SAFETY/QUALITY TIPS

◻ **Procedural**
 ✛ Use adequate amount of local anesthesia
 ✛ Failure to place patient in fully tucked position (which maximizes interspace opening) or failure to have the upper shoulder and hip directly above their lower counterparts will decrease success rate
 ✛ Take special care to identify the midline
 ✛ Attempting to insert needle in L5-S1 interspace because of excessive concern for "going too high" is a common pitfall and will result in failure to obtain CSF
 ✛ Failing to obtain opening pressure will limit the diagnostic information obtained from the procedure
 ✛ Do not forget to replace stylet before removing the needle
 ✛ The interspace and dural sac are wider at L3-4 than at L4-5. If LP fails at L4-5, you may be more successful at L3-4 interspace.
 ✛ In infants, the anatomical distances are remarkably smaller and the sensation of traversing different tissue densities is more subtle. Some practitioners will remove the stylet immediately after penetrating the skin and advance slowly, watching for CSF.
 ✛ Since you generally want as few red blood cells (RBCs) as possible in the final tube, when there is concern for a traumatic tap, remove extra CSF from earlier tubes, to clear the RBCs

◻ **Cognitive**
 ✛ Interpreting CSF data:
  ✛ White blood cell (WBC) count
   ▪ 0 to 5 WBCs is normal; higher values suggest an infectious process
  ✛ RBC count
   ▪ 0 to 5 RBCs is normal in an atraumatic tap
   ▪ If traumatic, expect a marked diminution of RBCs from tube no. 1 to tube no. 4. If there is no clearing on successive tubes, RBCs are highly suggestive of SAH. There is no specific RBC threshold below which SAH can be completely excluded; the best approach is to consider the RBC count from the last tube not in comparison to an earlier tube but in isolation.
  ✛ Xanthochromia
   ▪ Pink or yellow tinge is present in the supernatant of "older" lysed RBCs, suggestive of SAH
  ✛ Glucose
   ▪ Normal CSF glucose is two-thirds of the serum glucose, and is usually 50 to 80 mg/dL
   ▪ Low CSF glucose is often seen in bacterial meningitis
  ✛ Protein
   ▪ Normal CSF protein is 15 to 45 mg/dL
   ▪ Elevated protein level is nonspecific, but is seen in bacterial and aseptic meningitis, tuberculosis (TB) meningitis, Guillain–Barré syndrome, neoplastic disease, and multiple myeloma, among other pathologic processes
 ✛ Because there is approximately 150 mL of CSF in the body at any one time and 20 mL is made during any hour, one can take a large volume if needed either for diagnostic purposes or, in the case of pseudotumor, therapeutic purposes
 ✛ Remember to factor in timing from onset of symptoms to the LP being done. For example, xanthochromia may be absent in an SAH 4 to 12 hours old (becomes increasingly common with time from onset of SAH), or the number of cells in bacterial meningitis could be low in the first hours.

Acknowledgment

Thank you to prior author Amy S. Hurwitz.

Suggested Readings

Abbrescia KL, Brabson TA, Dalsey WC, et al. The effect of lower-extremity position on cerebrospinal fluid pressures. *Acad Emerg Med*. 2001;8:8–12.

Arendt K, Demaerschalk BM, Wingerchuck DM, et al. Atraumatic lumbar puncture needles: after all these years, are we still missing the point? *Neurologist*. 2009;15:17–20.

Edlow JA, Caplan LR. Avoiding pitfalls in the diagnosis of subarachnoid hemorrhage. *N Eng J Med*. 2000;342:29.

Evans RW. Complications of lumbar puncture. *Neurol Clin*. 1998;16:83–105.

Flaatten H, Thorsen T, Askeland B, et al. Puncture technique and postural puncture headache. A randomized, double-blind study comparing transverse and parallel puncture. *Acta Anaesthesiol Scand*. 1998;42(10):1209–1214.

Hasbun R, Abrahams J, Jekel J, et al. Computed tomography of the head before lumbar puncture in adults with suspected meningitis. *N Engl J Med*. 2001;345:1727–1733.

O'Malley GF, Byers S, Dominici P. Cerebrospinal fluid opening pressure is constant and reproducible between the sitting and recumbent positions. *Acad Emerg Med*. 2006;13:S136.

Shah KH, Edlow JA. Distinguishing traumatic lumbar puncture from true subarachnoid hemorrhage. *J Emerg Med*. 2002;23:67–74.

Shaikh F1, Brzezinski J, Alexander S, et al. Ultrasound imaging for lumbar punctures and epidural catheterisations: systematic review and meta-analysis. *BMJ*. 2013;346:f1720.

Straus SE, Thorpe KE, Holroyd-Leduc J. How do I perform a lumbar puncture and analyze the results to diagnose bacterial meningitis? *JAMA*. 2006;296:2012–2022.

46

Epley Maneuver

Nicole M. Dubosh and Jonathan A. Edlow

INDICATIONS

- Used to treat posterior canal benign paroxysmal positional vertigo (BPPV) that has been confirmed through a positive Hallpike test (upbeat, ipsilateral, and torsional nystagmus in the head-hanging position)
- This is also known as the *canalith repositioning maneuver* and the "modified" Epley maneuver (the originally described maneuver used premedication and had fewer steps)

CONTRAINDICATIONS

- Unstable heart disease
- Ongoing cerebrovascular ischemia
- Severe neck disease
- High-grade carotid stenosis

RISKS/CONSENT ISSUES

- There have been no reported serious adverse events such as neck fracture or carotid artery dissection
- Warn the patient that he will likely become symptomatic during the various head maneuvers, but that this will be transient
- Rarely the patient may vomit. In general, premedication is not needed.

LANDMARKS

The Epley maneuver is a four- to five-step maneuver that moves the otoliths in the plane of the posterior semicircular canal back into the utricle (**FIGURE 46.1**).

TECHNIQUE

- Patient is sitting upright in the gurney and positioned far enough back such that when he lies down, his head will overhang the edge of the gurney
- Turn the patient's head 45 degrees to the side that was positive during the Hallpike test, which was performed to confirm the diagnosis of posterior canal BPPV
- Lower the guardrail of the gurney on the opposite side to which you have turned the patient's head. Warn the patient that you are going to lower him and that he will become symptomatic.
- Place the patient in the head-hanging position, supporting the patient's head with your hands. This does not need to be done rapidly but should be done over several seconds. This step is identical to performing the Hallpike test.
- Keep the patient in the head-hanging position until the nystagmus and symptoms resolve, or at least for 30 seconds
- Turn the patient's head 90 degrees to the other side. Again, hold this position for 30 seconds or until the nystagmus and vertigo resolve.
- Tell the patient to roll onto his side and turn his head so that he is looking at the floor. Try to keep the head in the dependent position throughout. Hold this position for at least 30 seconds or until the vertigo resolves.

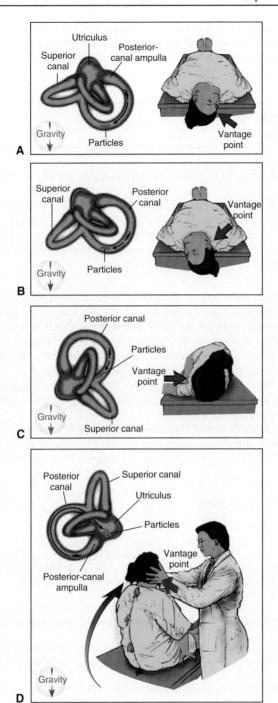

FIGURE 46.1 Bedside maneuver for the treatment of a patient with benign paroxysmal positional vertigo affecting the right ear. (From Furman JM, Cass SP. Benign paroxysmal positional vertigo. *N Engl J Med.* 1999;341:1590–1596, with permission.)

▢ Sit the patient up with his legs extended over the side of the gurney (you previously lowered the guard rails on this side to allow for this) and tilt his head forward slightly

   ✦ You can tell the patient to put his hands on your shoulder in order to assist you in lifting him up to the sitting position

COMPLICATIONS

▢ Rarely, the patient may vomit

SAFETY AND QUALITY TIPS

▢ **Procedural**

   ✦ Be sure to sit the patient far enough back in the gurney so that the head is overhanging the edge of the gurney

   ✦ Warn the patient that he will become symptomatic and to try to keep his eyes open

   ✦ Some patients with a history strongly suggesting BPPV (which is usually of the posterior semicircular canal) will have horizontal canal BPPV; the diagnostic test (supine head roll test) and the therapeutic canal repositioning maneuver (Lempert BBQ roll) are different from the test/maneuver for posterior canal BPPV

▢ **Cognitive**

   ✦ The amount of time recommended to keep the patient in the upright position after performing the Epley maneuver has changed drastically over the years. Currently, it is felt that 20 minutes is enough time for the otoliths to reattach themselves to a membrane within the utricle. After approximately 20 minutes, repeat the Hallpike test and if it is still positive, repeat the Epley maneuver. If the diagnosis is correct, the Dix–Hallpike should convert to negative. Several repetitions of the Epley may be needed.

   ✦ If the Dix–Hallpike does not convert to negative, reconsider the diagnosis

   ✦ Postural restrictions are not necessary for management of posterior canal BPPV following successful completion of the maneuver

   ✦ The Dix–Hallpike maneuver can be tricky to perform and interpret. Do not ignore signs of central vertigo syndromes because the Dix–Hallpike maneuver is "positive."

▢ **Acknowledgment**

Thank you to prior author Andrew Chang.

Suggested Readings

De Stefano A, Dispenza F, Citraro L, et al. Are postural restrictions necessary for management of posterior canal benign paroxysmal positional vertigo? *Ann Otol Rhinol Laryngol*. 2011;120(7):460–464.

Epley JM. The canalith repositioning procedure: for treatment of benign paroxysmal positional vertigo. *Otolaryngol Head Neck Sur*. 1992;107:399–404.

Fife TD, Iverson DJ, Lemper T, et al. Practice parameter: therapies for BPPV (an evidence-based review). Report of the Quality Standards Subcommittee of the American Academy of Neurology. *Neurology*. 2008;70:2067–2074.

Furman JM, Cass SP. Benign paroxysmal positional vertigo. *N Engl J Med*. 1999;341:1590–1596.

Huebner AC, Lytle SR, Doettl SM, et al. Treatment of objective and subjective BPPV. *J Am Acad Audiol*. 2013;24:600–606.

Kim JS, Oh SY, Lee SH, et al. Randomized clinical trial for apogeotropic horizontal canal BPPV. *Neurology*. 2012;78:1–8.

47

Hallpike Test (Dix–Hallpike, Nylan–Barany)

Nicole M. Dubosh and Jonathan A. Edlow

INDICATIONS

- Used to confirm the diagnosis of benign paroxysmal positional vertigo (BPPV) of the posterior semicircular canal

CONTRAINDICATIONS

- Unstable heart disease
- Ongoing cerebrovascular ischemia
- Severe cervical degenerative arthritis
- High-grade carotid stenosis

RISKS/CONSENT ISSUES

- There have been no reported serious adverse events such as neck fracture or carotid artery dissection
- Warn the patient that he will become symptomatic during the procedure, but that this will be transient. Inform the patient that this response is actually very useful.
- Rarely the patient may vomit. In general, premedication is not needed.

LANDMARKS

The Hallpike test diagnoses the inappropriate presence of otoliths in the posterior semicircular canal. This canal is oriented 45 degrees from the vertical axis (FIGURE 47.1).

TECHNIQUE

- The patient is sitting upright in the gurney and positioned far enough back such that when he lies down, his head will overhang the edge of the gurney
- Warn the patient that you are going to lower him and that he may become symptomatic. Instruct the patient to keep his eyes open as it is important for you to document both the presence and direction of nystagmus.
- Turn the patient's head 45 degrees to one side before tipping him backwards. This will orient the posterior canal into the same plane as the upcoming movement into the head-hanging position.
- Have the patient lie in the head-hanging position, supporting the patient's head with your hands. This does not need to be done overly rapidly (should be done over several seconds).
- If otoliths are present, there is usually a few seconds, delay (but not longer than approximately 10 seconds)
- The patient will develop reproduction of his symptoms and, usually, nystagmus. This indicates a positive test. Many patients will reflexively close their eyes and you may need to open their eyelids.
- Carefully observe the direction of the nystagmus
  + Direction of nystagmus is defined as the direction of the fast phase
  + Classic nystagmus in this situation is upbeat (toward the forehead) and ipsilateral (toward the involved side), as well as torsional/rotatory
  + Downbeat or vertical nystagmus can indicate a central cause of vertigo and requires further evaluation
- Help the patient back to the sitting up position

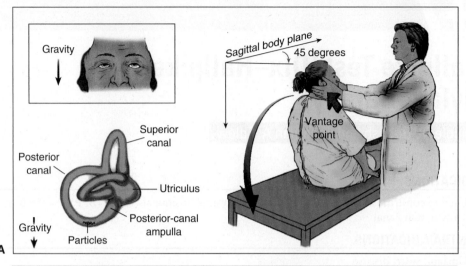

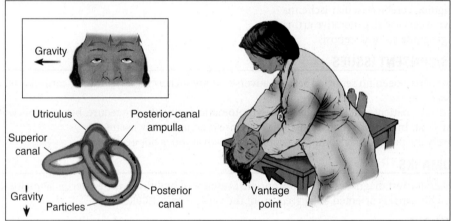

FIGURE 47.1 The Dix–Hallpike test of a patient with benign paroxysmal positional vertigo affecting the right ear. (From Furman JM, Cass SP. Benign paroxysmal positional vertigo. *N Engl J Med*. 1999;341:1590–1596, with permission.)

- ✛ Most patients will become dizzy from orthostasis, and it is important to distinguish this from positional vertigo
- ✛ If a patient had a positive result on Hallpike test, the eyes usually reverse direction when the patient sits up
- ⊡ Test both sides; apart from the rare situation in which otoliths are present bilaterally, this test should be positive on one side and negative on the other

COMPLICATIONS

⊡ The patient may occasionally vomit

SAFETY/QUALITY TIPS

⊡ **Procedural**
- ✛ Be sure to sit the patient far enough back in the gurney so that the head is overhanging the edge of the gurney
- ✛ Always start with the patient's head turned 45 degrees to one side and then lay him in the head-hanging position. Although it is possible to get a positive test result by laying the patient down and then turning his head 45 degrees to one side, this alternative way is not

as provocative in moving the otoliths and is more likely to result in a false-negative test result.
+ Warn the patient that he will become symptomatic and to keep his eyes open

☐ **Cognitive**
+ It is critical to know that most patients with dizziness from central reasons (e.g., a cerebellar tumor or a multiple sclerosis plaque) will have worse dizziness when they move their head. Therefore, the Dix–Hallpike test will be falsely positive in patients with other causes of dizziness that are ongoing. Patients with BPPV are asymptomatic at rest.
+ Observe the direction of the nystagmus and recognize that downbeating or vertical nystagmus can indicate a central cause of vertigo and warrants further evaluation
+ Recognize that patients with horizontal canal BPPV (approximately 10%–15% of cases) will have a negative Dix–Hallpike on both sides (see below). In addition, patients whose otoliths are fixed on the cupola of the posterior canal (not free floating) will not have latency of the nystagmus and the nystagmus lasts longer and does not fatigue.
+ Unless there is bilateral posterior semicircular canal BPV, only one side will test positive during the Hallpike test
+ It is important to note which side is positive during the Hallpike test as this will be the starting position for the Epley maneuver, which is used to treat BPPV of the posterior semicircular canal
+ Some patients with a history strongly suggesting BPPV (which is usually of the posterior semicircular canal) will have horizontal canal BPPV; the diagnostic test (supine head roll test) and the therapeutic canal repositioning maneuver (Lempert BBQ roll) are different from the test/maneuver for posterior canal BPPV

☐ **Acknowledgment**

Thank you to prior author Andrew Chang.

Suggested Readings

Fife TD, Iverson DJ, Lemper T, et al. Practice parameter: therapies for BPPV (an evidence-based review). Report of the Quality Standards Subcommittee of the American Academy of Neurology. *Neurology.* 2008;70:2067–2074.

Furman JM, Cass SP. Benign paroxysmal positional vertigo. *N Engl J Med.* 1999;341:1590–1596.

Lee SH, Kim JS. Benign paroxysmal positional vertigo. *J Clin Neurol.* 2010;6:51–63.

48

Occipital Nerve Block

Nissa J. Ali and Jonathan A. Edlow

INTRODUCTION

- Occipital neuralgia is neuropathic pain that is classically described as a persistent dull pain at the base of the skull with intermittent, sudden shocklike pain or paresthesias radiating from the back of the head over the scalp to behind the eyes. The pain follows the distribution of the greater occipital nerve (GON) and the lesser occipital nerve (LON).[1]
- Thought to be from irritation or trauma to the GON and LON. Possible causes include muscle entrapment of the nerves, inflammation or repetitive microtrauma from hyperextension of the neck (i.e., computer monitors with a focal point too high).
- Usually unilateral
- Tenderness over the nerve is associated with a positive response to occipital nerve block (ONB) injections[2]
- Indicated only if a history and physical examination do not suggest potential intracranial processes

INDICATIONS

- ONBs are traditionally used for the treatment of headache associated with occipital neuralgia[3]
- Although not typically used as treatment in emergency medicine, studies have found ONBs to be effective in the treatment of migraine,[4] cluster,[5] and cervicogenic[6] headaches

CONTRAINDICATIONS

- Allergy to analgesic compounds or steroids
- Lack of a clear-cut diagnosis
- Suspected intracranial process or focal neurologic deficits on examination

LANDMARKS

- The GON arises from the C2 nerve root and becomes superficial medial to the palpated occipital artery at the level of the superior nuchal line. It runs laterally to the external occipital protuberance and medially to the mastoid process.
- The occipital artery can be palpated one-third of the way from the inion to the mastoid process
- The LON arises from the cervical plexus. It becomes superficial at the inferior nuchal line.
- The GON perforates the semispinalis capitis and trapezius muscles. One study found that the GON emerges from the semispinalis approximately 3.0 cm inferior to the occipital protuberance and 1.5 cm lateral to midline.[7]

SUPPLIES

- Antiseptic solution
- Local anesthetic (i.e., 1% lidocaine, 4 mL, and 0.25% bupivacaine, 4 mL)
- Injectable steroids (i.e., methylprednisolone, betamethasone, or triamcinolone)
- 25- or 27-gauge 1.5-inch needle, 12-mL sterile syringe

TECHNIQUE

❏ Preparation

+ In a 12-mL sterile syringe, draw up a total of 8 mL of local anesthetic and 80 mg of methyl-prednisolone for a first time block or 40 mg of methylprednisolone for a repeat block
  + Commonly used anesthetic agents include a mixture of 4 mL of a quick-acting local anesthetic for immediate results, such as 1% lidocaine, with 4 mL of a longer-acting local anesthetic, such as 0.25% bupivacaine
  + Injectable steroids include methylprednisolone, triamcinolone, or betamethasone (**FIGURE 48.1**)
+ Place the patient in a sitting position, leaning forward, with the forehead resting on a padded bedside table with the neck in a flexed position
+ Prepare the skin/hair with an antiseptic solution
+ Anesthetize the superficial skin of the injection site with a small wheal of lidocaine

❏ Distal Injection Technique

+ This classic technique injects the GON at the level of the superior nuchal line, a region with no muscle. This is the suggested approach.
+ Palpate the occipital artery one-third of the way from the inion to the mastoid process. Using a 25- or 27-gauge 1.5-inch needle, aim just medial to the occipital artery at the level of the superior nuchal line.
+ Advance the needle perpendicularly until the needle touches the skull or until a paresthesia is elicited (the patient should be warned of this prior to starting). Withdraw the needle approximately 2 to 4 mm and redirect superiorly.
+ After gentle aspiration to confirm that the needle is not in a vessel, 5 mL of the solution should be injected in a fanlike distribution. (Note: The solution should inject easily; resistance to injection is a sign of inappropriate needle positioning.)
+ Further block of the LON and several superficial branches of the GON can be achieved by directing the needle laterally and slightly inferior with injection of an additional 4 mL of solution, after gentle aspiration
+ Massage/compress the injected area to distribute the anesthetic and to minimize hematoma formation

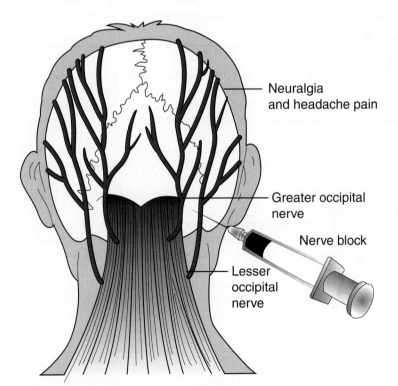

Figure 48.1 Block of the greater occipital nerve.

◻ **Proximal Injection Technique**
  ✦ This alternative technique injects the location where the GON exits the muscle. Proximal injections also cause paraspinal muscle infiltration with anesthetics, which may lead to additional benefits from trigger-point injections.[8]
  ✦ Follow the preparation steps as listed above
  ✦ The most commonly referenced proximal injection area is located 3 cm inferior to the occipital protuberance and 1.5 cm laterally to midline. After gentle aspiration, infiltrate the muscle in this area with the solution in a fanlike distribution.
  ✦ Massage/compress the injected area
◻ **Maximal Occipital Scalp Tenderness Technique**
  ✦ This alternative technique is based on the hypothesis that the point of maximal tenderness will encompass the GON. Although it may or may not encompass the nerve, the approach has demonstrated positive results.[9]
  ✦ Follow the preparation steps as listed above
  ✦ Palpate the area of maximal occipital scalp tenderness for the injection point, which should correlate to the expected GON superficial location
  ✦ After gentle aspiration, infiltrate the subcutaneous tissue with the solution in a fanlike distribution
  ✦ Massage/compress the injected area

COMPLICATIONS

◻ ONB complications are rare and almost never serious
◻ Risk of inadvertent injection of local anesthetic into the occipital artery or one of its branches with secondary arrhythmias. Given the small dose of local anesthetic recommended, this is mostly a theoretical risk.
◻ Risk of inadvertent needle placement into the foramen magnum with subsequent total spine anesthesia
◻ Postblock ecchymosis, hematoma formation, or tenderness
◻ Case reports have described rare alopecia and cutaneous atrophy with local steroid injections[3,9]
◻ Transient dizziness/lightheadedness or nausea directly following the injection
◻ Bleeding, infection, or adverse reaction to the anesthetic/steroid may occur

SAFETY/QUALITY TIPS

Procedural
  ✦ Care must be taken to use the appropriate landmarks and technique, as noted above, to avoid inadvertent needle placement in the foramen magnum
  ✦ Ultrasound guidance has been used to assist in accurately locating the GON[10]
  ✦ Although anticoagulation is not an absolute contraindication, use of a small-diameter needle is recommended
  ✦ Postinjection manual compression and/or ice packs over the injection site for 20 minutes after administration of the block are suggested to help minimize hematoma formation
Cognitive
  ✦ Failure of a ONB to relieve headache is most commonly due to a cause other than occipital neuralgia
  ✦ Patients who fail to respond to the block should be reevaluated for other diagnoses
  ✦ Positive response to the block does not conclusively demonstrate occipital neuralgia or other benign causes of headache as the etiology. Keep dangerous conditions in mind.

✚ Acknowledgment

Thank you to prior author Jay Smith.

References

Ashkenazi A, Levin M. Three common neuralgias. How to manage trigeminal, occipital, and postherpetic pain. *Postgrad Med.* 2004;116(3):16–32,48.

Afridi SK, Shields KG, Bhola R, et al. Greater occipital nerve injection in primary headache syndromes—prolonged effects from a single injection. *Pain.* 2006;122(1–2):126–129.

Ward JB. Greater occipital nerve block. *Semin Neurol.* 2003;23(1):59–62.

Weibelt S, Andress-Rothrock D, King W, et al. Suboccipital nerve blocks for suppression of chronic migraine: safety, efficacy and predictors of outcome. *Headache.* 2010;50:1041–1044.

Lambru G, Bakar NA, Stahlhut L, et al. Greater occipital nerve blocks in chronic cluster headache: a prospective open-label study. *Eur J Neurol.* 2014;21(2):338–343.

Gabrhelik T, Michalek P, Adamus M. Pulsed radiofrequency therapy versus greater occipital nerve block in the management of refractory cervicogenic headache—a pilot study. *Praque Med Rep.* 2011;112(4):279–287.

Mosser SW, Guyuron B, Janis JE, et al. The anatomy of the greater occipital nerve: implications for the etiology of migraine headaches. *Plast Reconstructr Surg.* 2004;113(2):693–697.

Young WB. Blocking the greater occipital nerve: utility in headache management. *Curr Pain Headache Rep.* 2010;14:404–408.

Shields KG, Levy MJ, Goadsby PJ. Alopecia and cutaneous atrophy after greater occipital nerve infiltration with corticosteroid. *Neurology.* 2004;63(11):2193–2194.

Shim JH, Ko SY, Bang MR, et al. Ultrasound-guided greater occipital nerve block for patients with occipital headache and short term follow up. *Korean J Anesthesiol.* 2011;61(1):50–54.

49

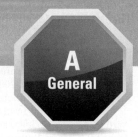

A
General

Methylene Blue Injection/ Open Joint Evaluation

Felipe Teran

INDICATIONS

- When there is clinical suspicion of communication between a traumatic wound and joint space
- When intra-articular air within the joint space is seen on radiographs

CONTRAINDICATIONS

- Evidence of overlying cellulitis on the site of arthrocentesis
- Patients taking serotonergic psychiatric drugs (risk of serotonin syndrome) and those having glucose-6-phosphate dehydrogenase deficiency (risk of anemia and methemoglobinemia) **(FIGURE 49.1)**

RISKS/CONSENT ISSUES

- Risk of iatrogenic septic arthritis
- Risk of iatrogenic hemarthrosis
- Allergic reaction to local anesthetic
- Pain during and after procedure

LANDMARKS

- In most cases approach is via the extensor surface of joints (avoids vessels and nerves)
- Specific landmarks should be utilized depending on the joint
- If available, ultrasound can be used to facilitate arthrocentesis

TECHNIQUE

- **Prepare the Methylene Blue Injection**
  - Methylene blue usually comes in 1-mL ampoules. There are no exact dilutional guidelines; we recommend diluting 1 mL of methylene blue with 29 mL normal saline in a 30-mL syringe.
  - Attach an 18- or 20-gauge needle to the syringe
- **Prepare the Joint Before Injection**
  - Prepare the skin using either a povidone–iodine solution or a chlorhexidine solution and a large sterile drape
  - Using a small-gauge needle, deposit a small wheal of either 1% or 2% lidocaine for local anesthesia
- **Inject the Joint**
  - Enter the joint space using standard arthrocentesis technique
  - Inject the methylene blue solution into the affected joint space until the joint is fully distended or methylene blue exudes from the wound
- The amount of solution necessary to fully distend the joint is mostly dependent on the joint in question
- The shoulder can hold ~30 mL and the knee can hold approximately 60 mL

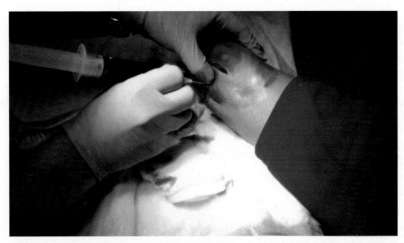

Figure 49.1 Arthrocentesis with injection of methylene blue dilution to assess traumatic arthrotomy in a patient with a deep laceration over the elbow. (Courtesy of Felipe Teran, MD.)

- Studies support injecting up to the maximum tolerated volume of the joint or until fluid begins to extravasate through the wound
- A positive test is considered if any extravasation of fluid is seen from the wound

COMPLICATIONS

- Septic arthritis
- Bleeding
- Allergic reaction
- Damage to the articular surface during arthrocentesis

SAFETY/QUALITY TIPS

- **Procedural**
  + Arthrocentesis is a painful procedure. Provide adequate analgesia and local anesthesia.
  + Ultrasound guidance may be used to avoid damage to neurovascular structures
  + Flexion and extension of the joint can increase the chance of fluid extravasating through a violated joint capsule
  + Avoid extravasation of methylene blue into soft tissues; this can cause local skin necrosis
  + Remember to dilute the methylene blue adequately to avoid thrombophlebitis
  + Although controversy exists regarding the ideal volume, injection of insufficient methylene blue solution may lead to a false-negative test. We recommend injecting the maximum tolerated volume to optimize sensitivity of the test.
- **Cognitive**
  + Maintain a high clinical suspicion for possible open joint injuries. If traumatic arthrotomy is slightly suspected, the patient should be surgically explored.
  + A theoretical limitation is the presence of an intra-articular fracture. It is possible that the injected solution could extravasate through the fracture site into the surrounding soft tissue instead of the arthrotomy site. Consider x-ray if fracture seems clinically likely.
  + If traumatic arthrotomy is confirmed, definitive treatment includes broad-spectrum antibiotics and urgent (within 6 hours) surgical exploration and irrigation of the joint and soft tissues to prevent joint destruction
  + Antibiotic regimen depends on the Gustilo classification for open fractures:
    + **Type I** (open fractures with a skin wound <1 cm)
      - Cefazolin (1 g IV) is adequate for coverage. Clindamycin (900 mg IV) can be used for patients with allergies to penicillin or cephalosporins.

+ **Type II** (open fractures with a skin wound >1 cm)
  - An aminoglycoside (i.e., gentamicin 600 mg) should be added to the type I regimen
+ **Type III** (open fractures with extensive soft-tissue damage/loss, segmental fractures, amputation)
  - An aminoglycoside (i.e., gentamicin 600 mg) should be added to the type I regimen
+ If vascular injury or anaerobic contamination of joint is suspected (i.e., farm injury), penicillin (20 million units IV) should be added

☐ Acknowledgment

Thank you to prior author Jennifer Teng and Kaushal Shah.

Suggested Readings

Bond MC, Perron AD, Abraham MK. *Orthopedic Emergencies: Expert Management for the Emergency Physician.* New York, NY: Cambridge University Press; 2013.

Keese GR, Boody AR, Wongworawat MD, et al. The accuracy of the saline load test in the diagnosis of traumatic knee arthrotomies. *J Orthop Trauma.* 2007;21(7):442–443.

Metzger P, Carney J, Kuhn K, et al. Sensitivity of the saline load test with or without methylene blue dye in the diagnosis of artificial traumatic knee arthrotomies. *J Orthop Trauma.* 2012;26(6):347–349.

Roberts JR, Custalow CB, Thomsen TW, et al. *Roberts & Hedges' Clinical Procedures in Emergency Medicine.* 6th ed. Philadelphia, PA: Elsevier Saunders; 2014.

50

Colles Fracture Reduction with Hematoma Block

Rebecca T. Brafman

INDICATIONS

- A Colles fracture is a transverse fracture through the distal 2 to 3 cm of the radial metaphysis where the distal fragment is dorsally displaced and angulated. The most common mechanism is a fall on an outstretched hand.
- Closed reduction is indicated if distal fragment has a dorsal tilt >10 degrees, an intra-articular fracture is present and has a >1 mm step-off, or there is >2 mm radial shortening
- General goals are to reduce displaced fragments and maintain reduction during healing

CONTRAINDICATIONS

- Hematoma block contraindicated if:
  + History of allergy to local anesthetics
  + Overlying skin infection or dirty skin
- Reduction contraindicated if open fracture exists

PROCEDURAL RISKS/CONSENT ISSUES

- Pain (site of needle insertion)
- Bleeding (local at needle puncture site)
- Infection (theoretical risk of iatrogenic infection)

- **General Basic Steps**
  + **Obtain radiographs**
  + **Hematoma block**
  + **Reduction**
  + **Splinting**
  + **Postreduction steps**

LANDMARKS: RADIOGRAPHIC

- Standard radiographs should include a posteroanterior (PA) and a lateral projection
- Clearly describe fractures as pediatric or adult, extra-articular or intra-articular, comminuted or noncomminuted, angulated or not angulated
- In adults, several measurements are used to determine the extent of deformity
  + Radial height (PA view): Two parallel lines drawn perpendicularly to the long axis of the radius, one through the tip of the radial styloid and the other at the articular surface of the radius
    + **Normal radial height is 9.9 to 17.3 mm**
  + Radial inclination (PA view): A line drawn through the articular surface of the radius, perpendicular to its long axis. A line is then drawn tangent from the tip of the radial styloid.
    + **Normal radial inclination is 15 to 25 degrees**
  + Volar tilt (lateral view): A line drawn perpendicularly to the long axis of the radius. A line is then drawn tangent to it along the articular surface from the dorsal to palmar surface of the radius.
    + **Normal volar tilt is 10 to 25 degrees**

SUPPLIES

- Povidone–iodine or chlorhexidine solution
- 25-gauge needle and 10- to 20-mL syringe for hematoma block
- Local anesthesia: 1% lidocaine without epinephrine or bupivacaine 0.5%
- Reduction materials: Gauze bandage roll for finger trap, traction weights (8–10 lb)
- Splinting materials: Web roll, plaster, elastic compression bandage

TECHNIQUE

- **Clinical Assessment**
  - Inspection: Identify the skeletal deformity. Classic finding is the so-called dinner-fork deformity, produced by dorsal displacement of the distal fracture fragments.
  - Palpation: Note any step-off, crepitus, and the point of maximal tenderness
  - Test neurovascular status: Acute median nerve compression is common in these injuries, especially in severely displaced, high-energy fractures. Pay close attention to finger sensation.
  - Evaluate for a distal radioulnar joint (DRUJ) dislocation: Caused by a disruption of the triangular fibrocartilage complex which stabilizes the joint. Orthopedic consultation is necessary for this injury.
    - X-rays may be reported as normal; physical examination is the key to diagnosis
    - Wrist has limited range of motion, with crepitus on supination and pronation
    - Loss of the ulnar styloid contour with volar ulna dislocation and prominence of the ulnar styloid with dorsal dislocation
    - More frequently with associated ulnar styloid fracture
  - Evaluate for a Salter–Harris type I fracture in pediatric patients
    - Tenderness over the distal radial physis
    - Only radiologic finding may be displacement or absence of the pronator quadratus fat pad sign
    - Low threshold to splint and arrange orthopedic follow-up
    - Rarely results in a growth disturbance
    - Consider child abuse in patients <1 year of age with this injury **(FIGURE 50.1)**
- **Hematoma Block**
  - Prepare skin over fracture site with povidone–iodine or chlorhexidine solution
  - Insert a 25-gauge needle dorsally into the hematoma at the fracture site approximately 30 degrees to the skin. Guide the needle tip into the fracture space by sliding along the fractured surface of the distal fragment. Placement is confirmed by the aspiration of blood.
  - Slowly inject 5 to 10 mL of 1% lidocaine without epinephrine into the fracture cavity and another 5 mL into the surrounding periosteum
    - Lidocaine will provide anesthesia for approximately 1 to 2 hours
    - Bupivacaine 0.5% may also be used if available and has a significantly longer duration of action (4 to 6 hours)
  - Allow 10 to 15 minutes for the anesthesia to become effective
- **Reduction (Jones Method):** Goal is to restore the normal anatomy (radial height, radial inclination, volar tilt, and intra-articular step-off) through traction and manipulation **(FIGURE 50.2)**
  - Place patient's fingers in a finger trap device with the elbow in 90 degrees of flexion
  - Suspend 8 to 10 lb of weight from elbow (distal humerus specifically) for 5 to 10 minutes to disimpact fracture fragments
  - While in traction, apply dorsal pressure over the distal fragment with your thumbs while simultaneously applying volar pressure over the proximal segment with your fingers to continue to disimpact the fragments
  - Apply volar force to the distal fragments to realign them into anatomic position
  - Remove the traction weight
- **Splinting:** A sugar-tong splint maintains the reduction and allows for swelling without compromising circulation
  - Extends from the dorsal metacarpal–phalangeal joints around the elbow to the midpalmar crease
  - The splint should be premeasured and created with six to eight layers of thickness

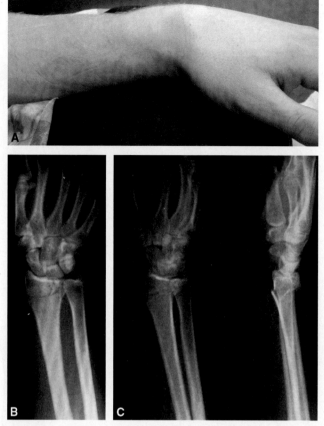

FIGURE 50.1 A: "Dinner-fork" deformity of Colles fracture. **B, C:** Colles fracture. (From Silverberg M. Colles' and Smith's fractures. In: Greenberg MI, ed. *Greenberg's Text-Atlas of Emergency Medicine*. Philadelphia, PA: Lippincott Williams & Wilkins; 2005:483, with permission.)

+ The elbow is placed in 90 degrees of flexion, the forearm in pronation, and the wrist in slight flexion and slight ulnar deviation
   + Extensive flexion, >20 degrees, can cause median nerve compression
   + The position of the forearm can be controversial (neutral vs. slight supination). Leave the decision up to the orthopedist who will be following up with the patient.
   + The metacarpal–phalangeal joints should not be immobilized to reduce the risk of potential stiffness
+ A reverse sugar-tong splint provides an equally effective alternative to the traditional sugar-tong splint, while avoiding splint buckling at the elbow. In this case, the splint fold will be located distally at the first web space of the hand, instead of at the elbow as described above (Figure 50.2).

Postreduction Steps
+ Obtain postreduction x-rays to evaluate reduction
   + The volar tilt of the radius should be restored to anatomic position, but neutral position or zero degree is considered acceptable. The radial height should be within 2 mm of the ulna.
+ Document neurovascular status after the procedure
+ Arrange follow-up
   + Orthopedic follow-up within 3 days to assess reduction, need for surgical intervention, and eventual conversion to a short arm cast
   + Repeat radiographies are recommended weekly for 2 to 3 weeks to ensure maintenance of the reduction

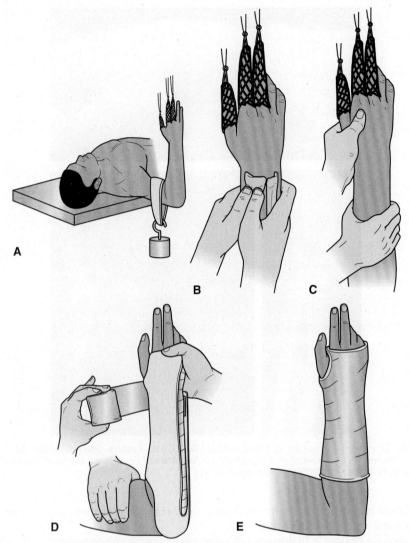

FIGURE 50.2 Colles fracture reduction. **A:** Fingers are placed in finger trap. **B:** After disimpaction of fragments with dorsal pressure, the fracture is reduced by applying a volar force to the distal segments. **C:** Adjust wrist into proper position for immobilization. (Modified from Simon RR, Brenner BE. *Emergency Procedures and Techniques.* 4th ed. Philadelphia, PA: Lippincott Williams & Wilkins; 2002:273.) **D:** Apply sugar-tong splint with wrist in neutral position. **E:** Cover with elastic bandage. (Modified from Simon RR, Brenner BE. *Emergency Procedures and Techniques.* 4th ed. Philadelphia, PA: Lippincott Williams & Wilkins; 2002:273.)

COMPLICATIONS

- ⊞ Median/ulnar nerve injury or compression
  - ✛ Resulting from the original injury or after closed reduction from traction placed on the nerve, direct pressure from a splint, or secondary to swelling
  - ✛ Carpal tunnel syndrome: Pain and paresthesias in the median nerve distribution
- ⊞ Compartment syndrome
- ⊞ Loss of fracture reduction (more common in comminuted or severely displaced fractures)
- ⊞ Nonunion or malunion—angling, shortening
- ⊞ Posttraumatic arthritis (from injury itself or reduction)
- ⊞ Tendon rupture, particularly the extensor pollicis longus
- ⊞ Reflex sympathetic dystrophy: A syndrome of paresthesias, pain, stiffness, and changes in skin temperature and color (complicates 3% of distal radius fractures)

SAFETY/QUALITY TIPS

◘ **Procedural**
  + Immediate orthopedic assessment is indicated for open fractures, inadequate reduction, or any neurovascular deficit
  + Document neurovascular function both before and after the reduction, including symptoms of carpal tunnel syndrome
    + Assess motor function with finger extension (radial nerve), thumb opposition (median nerve), and finger abduction (ulnar nerve)
  + If hematoma block is ineffective, procedural sedation is indicated to achieve proper reduction

◘ **Cognitive**
  + Prior to fracture reduction, evaluate for DRUJ dislocation and, in pediatric patients, look for Salter–Harris type 1 fractures. Have low threshold to splint if tenderness over the physis is present.
  + Consider risk factors for loss of reduction in more unstable fractures. Inadequate reduction can lead to radial shortening, limited range of motion, and chronic pain.
    + Fracture pattern: Dorsal comminution beyond the midaxial plane of the radius, intra-articular fracture, associated ulnar fracture
    + Severity of the primary displacement: Dorsal angulation >20 degrees or radial shortening >5 mm
    + Patient factors: Age >60 years, poor bone quality
  + Instruct the patient on range-of-motion exercises for fingers and shoulder to reduce stiffness

◘ **Acknowledgment**
Thank you to prior author Turandot Saul and Ami Kirit Dave.

Suggested Readings
Berquist TH. *Imaging of Orthopedic Trauma.* New York, NY: Raven Press; 1992.
Egol KE, Koval KJ, Zuckerman JD. *Handbook of Fractures.* 4th ed. New York, NY: McGraw-Hill; 2010.
Keats TE, Sistrom C. *Atlas of Radiologic Measurement.* St. Louis, MO: Mosby; 2001.
Leventhal JM. The field of child maltreatment enters its fifth decade. *Child Abuse Neglect.* 2003;27(1):1–4.

51

Extensor Tendon Repair

Robert Dalton Cox

INDICATIONS

- For repair of a partial or complete tendon injury
- Partial laceration of the extensor tendons proximal to the metacarpophalangeal (MCP) joint may or may not require repair; those at or distal to the MCP joint level must be repaired

CONTRAINDICATIONS

- Delayed closure and/or referral to a hand specialist or orthopedic surgeon may be more appropriate in the following circumstances:
  - Severe contamination or acute infection
  - Injuries due to human teeth (clenched fist injury or "fight bite")
  - Delayed presentation of injury
  - Extensive injury requiring prolonged use of tourniquet (longer than 20–30 minutes)
  - Penetration of laceration into a joint capsule
- These cases may be taken to the operating room for surgical exploration, irrigation, and intravenous (IV) antibiotics

RISKS/CONSENT ISSUES

- Pain
- Bleeding
- Infection (theoretical risk of iatrogenic infection)
- Risk of injuring other structures—tendons, vessels, nerves
- Laceration may need to be extended to allow adequate exploration or access to the surgical field

- **General Basic Steps**
  - **Patient preparation (ring removal, tourniquet, irrigation)**
  - **Local anesthesia or nerve block**
  - **Thorough wound evaluation**
  - **Tendon repair**
  - **Apply appropriate splint**

LANDMARKS

The anatomic location of open extensor tendon injuries in the wrist or hand drives treatment decisions and emergency department (ED) management. The Verdan classification system divides the hand and wrist into eight zones (TABLE 51.1 and FIGURE 51.1), which helps determine if tendon repair should be attempted in the ED.

TECHNIQUE

- **Preparation**
  - Remove all rings immediately!
  - Radiographs, as indicated, should be employed to assess for associated fracture, foreign body, or joint space disruption
  - Place the patient in a comfortable position, preferably supine, with the injury site easily accessible
  - Obtain proper lighting to optimize wound exploration, which should include thorough assessment for tendon injury and foreign bodies
  - Sterile technique should be employed

TABLE 51.1. THE VERDAN CLASSIFICATION SYSTEM		
Zone	Finger	Thumb
I	DIP joint	IP joint
II	Middle phalanx	Proximal phalanx
III	PIP joint	MCP joint
IV	Proximal phalanx	Metacarpal
V	MCP joint	CMC joint
VI	Metacarpals	
VII	Carpals	
VIII	Proximal wrist and distal forearm	

DIP, distal interphalangeal; IP, interphalangeal; PIP, proximal interphalangeal; MCP, metacarpophalangeal; CMC, carpometacarpal.

✦ Adequate anesthesia should be administered once the initial neurovascular examination is complete. Lidocaine 1% to 2% with epinephrine can be used in the hand except in areas supplied by end arteries. Local infiltration or an appropriate nerve block can be used.

✦ The wound should be thoroughly irrigated and free of contamination. Debridement of grossly contaminated tissue may be necessary.

✦ Good hemostasis is critical to wound exploration and tendon repair
   ✦ Elevate the arm for 1 minute to facilitate drainage of blood before applying a tourniquet
   ✦ Inflate a blood pressure cuff to 260 to 280 mm Hg and clamp the cuff tubes to avoid air leak, or use commercial tourniquets for arm or finger
   ✦ Apply the tourniquet for no longer than 20 minutes

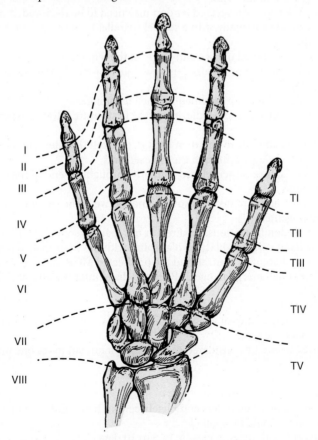

FIGURE 51.1 Extensor tendon repair landmarks.

- ▢ **Materials:** Choice of suture material depends on the location of the tendon injury
  - ✛ For repair of complete laceration injuries on the dorsum of the hand, nonabsorbable, synthetic (polyester) sutures are preferred (Ethilon)
    - ✛ Nylon sutures are acceptable, although colored nylon may be visible beneath the skin
    - ✛ Chromic and plain gut should not be used in complete tendon laceration, as they will dissolve before adequate tendon healing has occurred
    - ✛ Partial tendon injuries can be repaired with fine synthetic, absorbable sutures such as polyglactin (Vicryl)
    - ✛ Avoid silk sutures
  - ✛ Size 4-0 sutures are appropriate for most extensor tendons; 5-0 sutures may be needed for smaller tendons. Smaller, tapered needles should be used to avoid tearing the tendon.
  - ✛ Instruments: Needle holder, two skin hooks and retractors, sharp and blunt-nosed scissors, hemostats, single-toothed forceps
- ▢ **Procedure:** For open tendon injuries that will be repaired by a hand surgeon, primary skin closure and immobilization, unless otherwise noted, can be done outside of the operating room
  - ✛ Zones VII (wrist) and VIII (distal forearm)
    - ✛ Extensor tendon lacerations in these areas are complex and should generally be repaired by an orthopedic/hand surgeon
    - ✛ Management includes irrigation, local wound care with primary repair of the skin, and the application of a volar splint with the wrist at 35 to 45 degrees of extension and the MCPs at 10 to 15 degrees of flexion
    - ✛ Outpatient follow-up with a hand surgeon should be arranged within 1 to 5 days
  - ✛ Zone VI (metacarpal/dorsal hand)
    - ✛ Most extensor tendon injuries in zone VI can be repaired outside of the operating room
    - ✛ The distal end of a severed tendon is usually found by passively extending the affected digit to bring the end into view
    - ✛ The proximal portion of a severed tendon may need to be retrieved; it may be necessary to extend the wound proximally with a scalpel (parallel to the course of the tendon) to obtain adequate exposure
    - ✛ Repair technique is based on size and shape of the tendon
      - ▬ Smaller tendons may be repaired using a figure-of-8 or horizontal mattress suture **(FIGURE 51.2B)**
      - ▬ The modified Kessler or modified Bunnell techniques
        - ▬ Using a small, tapered needle, insert the first suture into the exposed, cut end of the tendon
        - ▬ Next weave the suture out, then back in through the lateral tendon margins, and then back out again through the exposed end
        - ▬ The same suture is then placed similarly through the end of the opposite half of the cut tendon
        - ▬ The suture ends are tied in a square knot between the cut ends, bringing the two halves together
    - ✛ All extensor tendon lacerations, repaired or unrepaired, should be immobilized and referred to a hand surgeon. Place a volar splint with the wrist in 45 degrees of extension, the affected MCP joint in neutral, and the unaffected MCP joints in 15 degrees of flexion. Allow the proximal interphalangeal (PIP) and distal interphalangeal (DIP) joints full range of motion.
  - ✛ Zone V (MCP joint)
    - ✛ Owing to the complexities of a tendon injury in this region, repair should be done by an orthopedic/hand surgeon
    - ✛ Open injuries should be considered secondary to a human tooth bite until proven otherwise
      - ▬ Obtain radiographs
      - ▬ Copiously irrigate the wound
      - ▬ Leave the wound open unless completely certain that it did not enter the mouth
      - ▬ A volar splint should be applied
      - ▬ IV antibiotics with delayed closure in 5 to 10 days

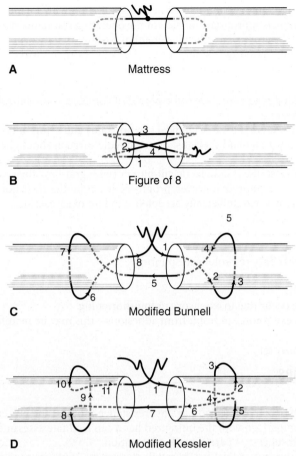

FIGURE 51.2 A: Horizontal mattress. **B:** Figure-of-8 stitch. **C:** Modified Bunnell. **D:** Modified Kessler suture technique.

+ Zone IV (proximal phalanx)
    + Management is variable and should be discussed with a hand surgeon
    + Lacerations of a single lateral slip can either be repaired or left unrepaired and splinted. Using 5-0 nonabsorbable suture material, a running suture or simple interrupted sutures with buried knots are appropriate for this area.
    + Apply splint from the forearm to the digit, leaving the DIP with full mobility. The PIP joint should be left in neutral position.
+ Zone III (PIP)
    + Wounds suspected of penetrating the joint are generally taken to the operating room for exploration and irrigation
    + Laceration of the central slip can result in long-term Boutonniere deformity (flexion of the PIP and hyperextension at the DIP due to unopposed flexion of the flexor digitorum superficialis [FDS])
    + Close the open skin laceration primarily
    + Splint the PIP in extension (leaving the DIP and MCP with full mobility)
    + Referred to a hand surgeon for repair
+ Zones I (DIP) and II (middle phalanx)
    + Laceration of the terminal extensor mechanism (TEM) in zones I or II can result in mallet finger deformity. When evaluating closed or open injuries to zone 1 or 2, hold the PIP in extension to evaluate active extension of the DIP joint. If unidentified or left untreated, a mallet finger may develop a swan-neck deformity (hyperextension at the PIP and hyperflexion at the DIP).
    + Closed injuries are splinted with the DIP joint in extension and free range of motion of the PIP joint, and referred to a hand surgeon

+ Repair of an open injury should be done in consultation with a hand specialist
+ If repair is deemed appropriate outside of the operating room, the dermatotenodesis technique can be employed—the placement of a suture that incorporates both the tendon and the overlying skin into a single suture. The sutures are removed after 10 to 12 days and the finger splinted in extension for 6 weeks.

□ **After-care**

＋ All extensor tendon repairs require some period of complete immobilization with splinting during tendon healing

＋ Patients should be advised to seek medical care for signs and symptoms of wound infection

＋ Timely follow-up with a hand specialist or orthopedic surgeon should be provided within 1 to 5 days

＋ Many clinicians prescribe prophylactic antibiotics (with gram-positive coverage) if a tendon has been lacerated or sutured; however, prophylactic antibiotics have not been proven to reduce infection rates. No universally accepted standard of care exists.[1]

COMPLICATIONS

□ Wound infection
□ Skin breakdown secondary to prolonged splinting
□ Tendon rupture
□ Tendon subluxation
□ Loss of flexion may occur due to extensor tendon shortening
□ Loss of flexion and extension can result from adhesions—this may be manifested by a weakened grip
□ Deformity or dysfunction

SAFETY/QUALITY TIPS

□ **Procedural**

＋ Assess strength of active extension against resistance (not just the presence of passive extension). Comparison with the uninjured hand can facilitate assessment; weakness or significant pain suggests a partial tendon laceration.

＋ Adequate anesthesia is critical for thorough assessment of injury, particularly strength of extension against resistance, which may be severely limited by pain

＋ Adequate hemostasis is essential to complete tendon examination. A blood pressure cuff or other tourniquet should be employed.

＋ Remember to immobilize the affected area with a splint after repair

□ **Cognitive**

＋ Wounds should be examined through a full range of motion and in the position of injury, because the site of tendon injury frequently does not lie directly beneath the site of the skin wound

＋ Remember that it sometimes may be necessary to extend a laceration in order to fully examine, cleanse, and repair tendon injuries

＋ Little data exists on the optimal management of partial extensor tendon lacerations. It is considered optional to repair a laceration if <50% of the cross-sectional area is involved.

＋ Irrigation, skin closure, splinting, and timely follow-up with a hand surgeon are considered standard for unsutured partial tendon lacerations

Reference

1. Whittaker JP. The role of antibiotic prophylaxis in clean incised hand injuries: a prospective randomized placebo controlled double blind trial. *J Hand Surg [Br]*. 2005;30(2):162–167.

□ **Acknowledgment**
Thank you to prior author Faye Maryann Lee and Gregory S. Johnston.

Suggested Reading

Sokolove PE, Barnes DK. Extensor & flexor tendon injuries in the hand, wrist and foot. In: Roberts JR, Hedges JR, eds. *Clinical Procedures in Emergency Medicine*. 4th ed. Philadelphia, PA: WB Saunders; 2004.

52

Digital Nerve Block

Gallane Dabela Abraham

INDICATIONS

- Used to provide local anesthesia to the digits for repair, reduction, or drainage
  - Lacerations
  - Nail bed injuries
  - Infections (i.e., felons, paronychias)
  - Amputations
  - Fractures or dislocations

CONTRAINDICATIONS

- **Absolute Contraindications**
  - Transthecal technique contraindicated in cases of infection, including felon, tenosynovitis, and overlying cellulitis
  - Allergy to lidocaine, bupivacaine, or other selected anesthetic
- **Relative Contraindications**
  - Complex laceration or other injury involving multiple digits that can be more easily and adequately anesthetized with a nerve block at the wrist

RISKS/CONSENT ISSUES

- Pain (site of needle insertion)
- Bleeding (local at needle puncture site)
- Infection (theoretical risk of iatrogenic infection)
- Potential for damage to neurovascular bundle
- Paresthesias
- Possible need for additional anesthetic or alternate procedures if the initial nerve block fails

- **General Basic Steps**
  - **Aseptic technique**
  - **Choose approach and deliver anesthetic**
  - **Massage area for 25 to 30 seconds**
  - **Test for adequate analgesia**

LANDMARKS

- The common digital nerves divide into two pairs of nerves corresponding to the dorsal and volar sides of the digits
- **Palmar Nerve**
  - Located at the 4- and 8 o'clock positions when looking at a cross section of the digit
  - Supplies the volar surface of the digit and the dorsal surface distal to the distal interphalangeal (DIP) joint for the middle three fingers
  - Blocking only the palmar nerves will provide adequate anesthesia on fingertip injuries distal to the DIP for the three middle fingers
- **Digital Nerve**
  - Located at the dorsal 2- and 10 o'clock positions when looking at a cross section of the digit

✛ Supplies the nail beds of the thumb, fifth digit, and dorsal aspects of all three middle fingers up to the DIP

✛ For the thumb and fifth digit, all four nerves must be blocked for fingertip and nail bed anesthesia **(FIGURE 52.1)**

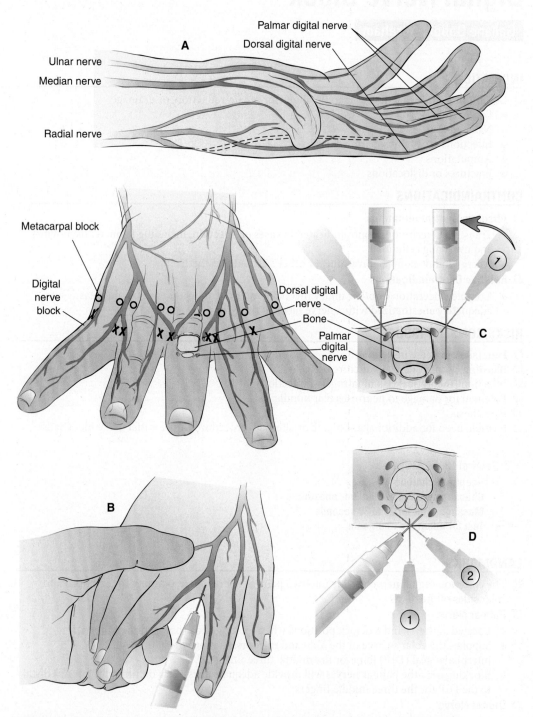

FIGURE 52.1 Dorsal technique for palmar and dorsal digital nerve block. **A:** Nerve distribution in hand. **B:** Traditional digital nerve block. **C:** Dorsal three-sided ring block. **D:** Volar three-sided ring block. (Lewis L, Stephan M. Local and regional anesthesia. In: Henretig FM, King C, eds. *Textbook of Pediatric Emergency Procedures*. Philadelphia, PA: Williams & Wilkins; 1997:481, with permission.)

TECHNIQUE: SEVEN APPROACHES

◘ **Patient Preparation**
+ Document neurovascular examination before anesthesia
+ Place patient's affected hand/foot comfortably on bedside procedure table with volar surface down (for metacarpal nerve block, traditional ring block, wing block) or volar surface up (for subcutaneous block, transthecal approach or thumb block)
+ Prepare the digit and web space by using standard aseptic technique

◘ **Equipment**
+ Lidocaine or procaine 1% to 2% (or 0.25% bupivacaine for longer, complicated procedures), 2 to 3 mL
+ An 18-gauge needle for drawing up the anesthetic
+ A 25- to 30-gauge needle for the nerve block
+ A 5-mL syringe
+ Povidone–iodine or chlorhexidine solution
+ Sterile drapes and sterile gauze
+ Gloves

◘ **Traditional Digital Block (Web-space Block or Metacarpal Nerve Block)**
+ Anesthetizes all digits except great toe
+ Prepare skin over dorsal surface of web space between metacarpal/metatarsal heads
+ Aspirate and inject subcutaneous wheal between metacarpal/metatarsal bones on dorsum of hand/foot 1 to 2 cm proximal to web space
+ Slowly advance needle through the wheal toward lateral volar surface of metacarpal/metatarsal head until slight tenting of the volar surface is appreciated
+ Aspirate and then inject 2 mL of anesthetic
+ Repeat the process on the opposite side of the finger/toe

◘ **Traditional Three-sided Ring Block**
+ Anesthetizes all digits including the dorsal, medial, and lateral nerve branches of great toe
+ Give two injections of lidocaine, one on each side of the digit
+ Locate dorsal–lateral aspect of proximal phalanx at the web space, just distal to metacarpal/phalangeal (MCP) or metatarsal/phalangeal (MTP) joint
+ Advance needle perpendicular to digit until bone is struck, aspirate and slowly inject 0.5 mL of lidocaine to anesthetize the dorsal nerve
+ Withdraw needle slightly, then redirect and advance toward volar surface and slowly inject 1 mL of lidocaine
+ Withdraw needle partially and redirect it medially over dorsal aspect of digit, aspirate and slowly inject lidocaine while withdrawing needle to anesthetize medial and dorsal aspect of digit
+ Withdraw the needle
+ Repeat procedure on medial side of digit at site of anesthetized skin
+ Massage area of infiltrated skin for 15 to 30 seconds to ensure diffusion of the anesthetic
+ Wait for 5 to 10 minutes to test for efficacy

◘ **Four-sided Ring Block**
+ Advantages: Anesthetizes volar side of digits
+ Disadvantages: May result in ischemic complications
+ Perform traditional three-sided ring block
+ Locate anesthetized volar–lateral aspect of proximal phalanx at the web space, just distal to MCP or MTP joint
+ Advance needle medially, aspirate and slowly inject 0.5 mL of lidocaine to anesthetize the volar side while withdrawing needle

◘ **Subcutaneous Block**
+ Prepare skin over volar surface at proximal skin crease
+ Pinch skin distal to proximal skin crease
+ Insert needle at midpoint of crease, aspirate and inject subcutaneous 1 to 2 mL wheal
+ Massage injected area for 15 to 30 seconds to improve diffusion process

- **Transthecal Approach**
  - Advantages: Single injection and low risk of neurovascular bundle injury
  - Disadvantage: More painful to inject through volar surface
  - Anesthetic is infused directly into the flexor tendon sheath at the proximal digital crease on volar surface
  - Fill 5-mL syringe with lidocaine
  - Insert 25-gauge needle at a 90-degree angle at the midpoint of the proximal digital crease and advance until bone is struck
  - Withdraw needle approximately 2 to 3 mm (should be in flexor tendon sheath) and redirect at a 45-degree angle to the long axis of the digit
  - Aspirate and inject 1.5 to 3 mL lidocaine while palpating tendon sheath with other hand; continue until resistance is felt
  - After removing the needle, apply pressure over the tendon proximally to facilitate distal spread
  - Wait for 2 to 3 minutes to test for efficacy of anesthesia
  - Most effective for middle three fingers (FIGURE 52.2)
- **Thumb Block**
  - All four digital nerves must be blocked for complete anesthesia of the thumb
  - Locate the flexor pollicis longus on the volar aspect of the thumb at the level of the proximal thumb flexor crease
  - The nerves lie immediately adjacent to this tendon
  - Aspirate and inject 1 to 2 mL of lidocaine along both sides of the tendon (FIGURE 52.3)
- **Wing Block**
  - Anesthetizes distal digit and nail bed
  - Prepare the distal digit by using standard aseptic technique
  - Insert 30-gauge needle perpendicular to the long axis of digit at a 45-degree angle at a point 3 mm proximal to the imaginary intersection of the lateral and proximal nail folds
  - Aspirate and inject anesthetic across the dorsum of digit parallel to proximal nail fold
  - Partially withdraw needle and redirect along lateral nail fold
  - Aspirate and inject anesthetic along the lateral nail fold
  - Repeat procedure on opposite side of digit if bilateral anesthesia is required (FIGURE 52.4)

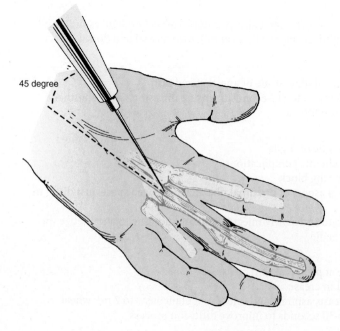

45 degree

FIGURE 52.2 Digital nerve block: Transthecal approach. The needle is directed into the proximal digital crease at a 45-degree angle to the long axis of the digit into the flexor tendon sheath where the lidocaine is deposited slowly.

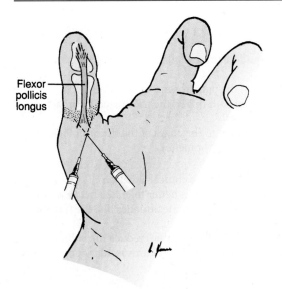

Flexor
pollicis
longus

FIGURE 52.3 Nerve block of thumb. (From Simon RR, Brenner BE. *Emergency Procedures and Techniques.* 4th ed. Philadelphia, PA: Lippincott Williams & Wilkins; 2002:136, with permission.)

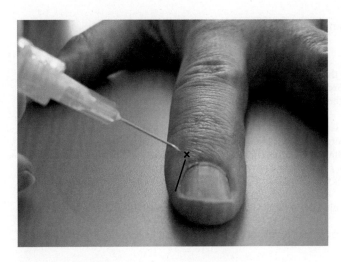

FIGURE 52.4 Wing block. 1) The needle is directed perpendicular to the long axis of digit at a 45-degree angle at a point 3 mm proximal to the imaginary intersection of the lateral and proximal nail folds. 2) Anesthetic is injected across the dorsum of digit parallel to proximal nail fold. 3) The needle is partially withdrawn and redirected along the lateral nail fold. Anesthetic is injected along the lateral nail fold.

COMPLICATIONS

- Laceration of digital nerve
- Intravascular injection may cause vasospasm and ischemia, suggested by blanching of digit
- Risk of flexor tendon injury with transthecal block
- Compartment syndrome
- Neurovascular compression and compromise due to large volume injection or four-sided ring block

SAFETY/QUALITY TIPS

- **Procedural**
  - Use adequate amounts of high concentration local anesthetic and massage the injected area for 15 to 30 seconds to improve diffusion process
  - The notion that infiltration of a digit with lidocaine that contains epinephrine will cause digital ischemia is a myth that has been debunked. There is no reason to use epinephrine

(continued)

for a regional nerve block, but it certainly can be used for direct infiltration of a finger or toe wound to promote hemostasis.
+ To achieve adequate anesthesia of the distal middle three digits, only the palmar sensory branches need to be blocked
+ Inject medially to ensure adequate anesthesia of the palmar sensory branches
+ To achieve adequate anesthesia of the thumb and fifth finger, the transthecal approach requires additional blocking of the dorsal branches
+ When blocking the thumb, extend infiltration down to the edges of the flexor pollicis longus tendon to ensure anesthesia of palmar sensory branches

☐ **Cognitive**
+ The preferred site and technique should be tailored to the clinical situation
+ Several studies have shown that the traditional ring block is better tolerated because of the thinner skin on the dorsal surface. However, single-injection techniques like the transthecal block are equally effective.
+ Higher concentrations of lidocaine or procaine (i.e., 2% lidocaine) reduce the volume required for adequate anesthesia thereby decreasing the risk of neurovascular compression and discomfort

☐ **Acknowledgment**

Thank you to prior author Tina Wu and Elizabeth M. Borock.

Suggested Readings

Dean E, Orlinsky M. Nerve blocks of the thorax and extremities. In: Roberts JR, Hedges JR, eds. *Clinical Procedures in Emergency Medicine*. 3rd ed. Philadelphia, PA: WB Saunders; 1998:484–490.

Hart RG, Fernandas FAS, Kutz JE. Transthecal digital block: an underutilized technique in the ED. *Am J Emerg Med*. 2005;23:340–342.

Hill RG Jr, Patterson JW, Parker JC, et al. Comparison of transthecal digital block and traditional digital block for anesthesia of the finger. *Ann Emerg Med*. 1995;25:604–607.

Hung VS, Bodavula VK, Dubin NH. Digital anaesthesia: comparison of the efficacy and pain associated with three digital nerve block techniques. *J Hand Surg [Br]*. 2005;30(6):581–584.

Salasche SJ. Surgery. In: Scher RK, Daniels CR, eds. *Nails: Treatment, Diagnosis, Surgery*. 2nd ed. Philadelphia, PA: WB Saunders; 1997:329.

Sarhadi NS, Shaw-Dunn J. Transthecal digital nerve block. An anatomical appraisal. *J Hand Surg*. 1998;23:490–493.

Simon RR, Brenner BE. *Emergency Procedures and Techniques*. 4th ed. Philadelphia, PA: Lippincott Williams & Wilkins; 2002:133–136.

53

Fasciotomy

Aldo Gutierrez

INDICATIONS

- For acute compartment syndrome treatment (**TABLE 53.1**)
  - Common locations for compartment syndrome include the calf, the anterior thigh, and the forearm
  - Once the diagnosis is made, early fasciotomy is advocated to reduce the risk of limb loss or dysfunction, rhabdomyolysis, lactic acidosis, and infection
  - Muscle death typically begins within 4 to 6 hours of vascular compromise; irreversible damage is usually achieved by 12 hours
  - Early consultation should be obtained with general, vascular, and/or orthopedic surgery

CONTRAINDICATIONS

- Although there are no absolute contraindications to fasciotomy in the acute setting, relative contraindications may include:
  - A nonviable extremity
  - Acute compartment syndrome associated with snake bites

RISKS/CONSENT ISSUES

- Pain
- Bleeding
- Infection
- Iatrogenic injury to nerve, muscle, and vascular structures
- Continued muscle damage, despite intervention

- **General Basic Steps**
  - **Conscious sedation and analgesia**
  - **Sterilization**
  - **Fasciotomy**
  - **Verification**

TABLE 53.1. EXTERNAL AND INTERNAL CAUSES OF COMPARTMENT SYNDROME

External causes	Internal causes
- Constrictive cast or dressing - Tight fascial closure - Prolonged limb compression during unconsciousness, paralysis, or surgery	- Edema, inflammation, or hemorrhage within a fascial compartment following trauma, *closed or open* fractures, burns, frostbite, electrocution, rhabdomyolysis, infection, or envenomation - Venous obstruction or ligation - Edema following revascularization or reperfusion - Iatrogenic extravasation of fluids from intravenous catheter or arterial line

Adapted from Moore EE. *Trauma*. 5th ed. New York, NY: McGraw Hill; 2005:903; table 41-1.

LANDMARKS

- ⬚ The forearm—there are two compartments
  - ✦ The volar compartment of the arm is accessed through a volar–ulnar incision beginning 3 cm below the medial epicondyle and running down the volar–ulnar aspect of the arm, ending 5 cm proximal to the ulnar styloid. This incision allows for soft-tissue coverage of the flexor tendons and ulnar and median nerves **(FIGURES 53.1 and 53.2)**.
  - ✦ The dorsal compartment of the arm is accessed through a dorsal incision from 2 cm below the lateral epicondyle, cutting longitudinally to the midline of the dorsum of the wrist
- ⬚ The lower leg—there are four compartments accessible by two approaches
  - ✦ Double-incision fasciotomy; two approximately 8-cm incisions are made
    - ✛ Lateral incision 1 cm anterior to the fibula
      - ▬ Begin 2 cm below the fibular head and continue two-thirds of the length of the leg—this avoids peroneal nerve where it exits the fascia
      - ▬ Make two corresponding fascial incisions; one into the anterior compartment and one into the lateral compartment **(FIGURE 53.3)**
    - ✛ Medial incision 2 cm posterior to the tibia; stay posterior incising over the gastrocnemius
      - ▬ Begin 2 cm below the tibial tuberosity and continue two-thirds the length of the leg—this course avoids the saphenous vein and nerve

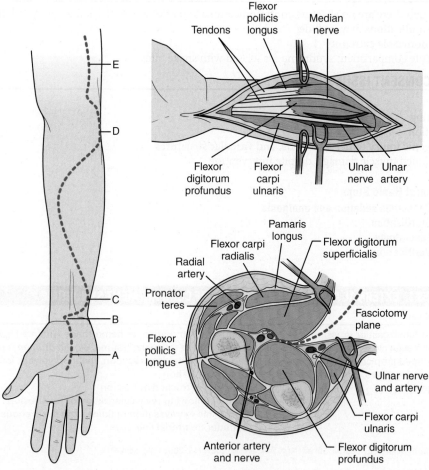

FIGURE 53.1 Volar release in the forearm. The upper illustration shows the incision that is used. The lower left picture depicts the relevant incisional anatomy. The lower right picture depicts the cross-sectional anatomy.

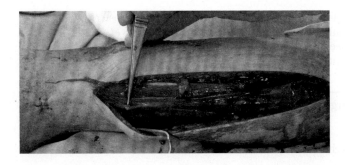

FIGURE 53.2 Fasciotomy of the forearm. (Reused with permission from Court-Brown C. *Trauma*. Philadelphia, PA: Lippincott Williams & Wilkins; 2005:501.)

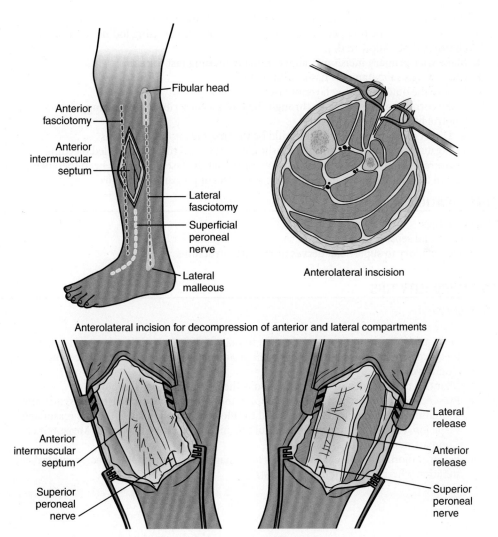

FIGURE 53.3 Anterior and lateral fasciotomy showing the superficial peroneal nerve.

- Make two corresponding fascial incisions; one into the superficial posterior compartment and other into the deep posterior compartment
+ The perifibular approach has been shown to be less efficacious, requires more exposure, may require fibulectomy, and has generally fallen out of favor

SUPPLIES

⊡ Assemble your materials: Basic surgical tray, or minimally the following:
+ No. 10 blade scalpel
+ Blunt scissors
+ Two small tissue retractors or self-retaining retractors
+ 10 to 12 surgical sponges
+ Sponge forceps
+ Three to four hemostats
+ Needle driver and absorbable sutures

TECHNIQUE

⊡ **Procedure**
+ Procedural sedation will be required for this procedure
+ The skin should be prepped and draped in a sterile manner using iodine solution or chlorhexidine. Allow to dry.
+ Make your primary incision as above, initially incising just the skin
+ Cut through subcutaneous tissue with scalpel
+ Expose the outer investing layer of fascia
+ Make corresponding incisions through the fascia as described above using scissors
+ Control bleeding as necessary
  + Direct pressure on the vessel should be the first means of hemostasis
  + Ligature or clamping of the artery should be reserved for uncontrolled bleeding
+ Measure the compartment pressures to ensure that the fasciotomy has been therapeutic and extend fascial incision as needed until compartment pressures normalize

COMPLICATIONS

⊡ Hemorrhage
⊡ Infection and sepsis
⊡ Iatrogenic injury to superficial nerves or vascular structures

SAFETY/QUALITY TIPS

⊡ **Procedural**
+ Place the extremity at level of the heart
+ Do not rely on one single measurement to make a diagnosis and make sure to perform measurements after fasciotomy has been performed to ensure successful decompression
+ Cognitive
+ Maintain a high index of suspicion, pain is the first presenting symptom
+ Presence of pulses by palpation or Doppler does not rule out compartment syndrome. The clinical examination is more useful to rule out the diagnosis; if there is reasonable suspicion, compartment pressures should be measured (see Chapter 54: Measurement of Compartment Pressures).
+ Perform thorough serial examinations to manage uncertainty. Obtain early surgical consultation where sufficient concern exists.

⊡ Acknowledgment

Thank you to prior author Gregory J. Lopez and Maurizio A. Miglietta.

Suggested Readings

Heppenstall RB. An update in compartment syndrome investigation and treatment. *Univ Penn Ortho J.* 1997;10:49–57.

Hope MJ, McQueen MM. Acute compartment syndrome in the absence of fracture. *J Orthop Trauma.* 2004;18:220.

Park S, Ahn J, Gee AO, et al. Compartment syndrome in tibial fractures. *J Orthop Trauma.* 2009;23:514.

Rizvi S, Catenacci M. Responding promptly to acute compartment syndrome. *Emerg Med.* 2008;40:12.

Ulmer T. The clinical diagnosis of compartment syndrome of the lower leg: are clinical findings predictive of the disorder? *J Orthop Trauma.* 2002;16:572.

Velhamos GC, Toutouzas KG. Vascular trauma and compartment syndromes. *Surg Clin North Am.* 2002;82:1.

54

Measurement of Compartment Pressures

Joe Pinero

INDICATIONS

- ⊕ Suspected compartment syndrome
- ⊕ Rising creatine phosphokinase (CPK) level without a source in the setting of trauma

CONTRAINDICATIONS

- ⊕ **Relative Contraindications**
  - ✚ Overlying skin cellulitis
  - ✚ Coagulopathy

RISKS/CONSENT ISSUES

- ⊕ Pain (site of needle insertion)
- ⊕ Bleeding (local at needle puncture site)
- ⊕ Infection (theoretical risk of iatrogenic infection)

- ⊕ **General Basic Steps**
  - ✚ **Sterilize field**
  - ✚ **Provide analgesia**
  - ✚ **Zero apparatus**
  - ✚ **Measure pressure in desired compartment**

LANDMARKS/RELEVANT ANATOMY

- ⊕ The forearm consists of three compartments (**FIGURE 54.1**). All compartments are entered one-third of the way from the elbow to the wrist with the arm at heart level and in supination (palm up). At this level, the posterior border of the ulna is easily palpated, just distal to the elbow.
  - ✚ The volar (palmar) compartment contains the wrist and finger flexors. The needle entry is medial to palmaris longus tendon, 1 to 2 cm deep.

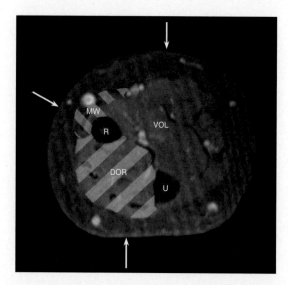

FIGURE 54.1 The three compartments of the forearm. R, radial bone; U, ulna bone; VOL, volar compartment; DOR, dorsal compartment; MW, mobile wad.

- ✦ The dorsal compartment contains the wrist and finger extensors. The needle entry is 1 to 2 cm lateral to the posterior ulna border, 1 to 2 cm deep.
  - ✦ The mobile wad contains the brachioradialis and radial flexors of the wrist. Needle insertion is 1 to 1.5 cm into the muscle, which laterally overlies the radius.
- ⊞ The buttock contains three compartments: One containing the tensor fascia lata; one containing gluteus medius and minimus; and one containing the gluteus maximus.
  - ✦ Landmarks vary from person to person
  - ✦ In all cases, the needle should be at the point of maximal tenderness
- ⊞ The thigh is composed of two compartments; the needle is easily passed into the point of maximal tenderness
  - ✦ The anterior contains the quadriceps and femoral neurovascular bundle
  - ✦ The posterior contains the hamstring group and the sciatic nerve, which gives rise to the common tibial and common fibular nerve
- ⊞ The leg contains four compartments **(FIGURE 54.2)**. All compartments are entered one-third of the way from the knee to the ankle with the leg at heart level.
  - ✦ The anterior compartment contains the tibialis anterior, responsible primarily for dorsiflexion of the foot, and the toe extensors; *this compartment is most commonly affected by compartment syndrome.* The needle entry is 1 cm lateral to the anterior border of the tibia, 1 to 3 cm deep, while the patient is supine.
  - ✦ The deep posterior compartment contains the tibialis posterior muscle (which inverts the foot) and the toe flexors. The needle entry is posterior to the medial border of the tibia, angled toward the posterior border of the fibula, 2 to 4 cm deep, with the patient supine.
  - ✦ The superficial posterior compartment contains the plantar flexors of the foot—the soleus, gastrocnemius, and plantaris muscles, as well as the sural nerve. The needle entry is either side of the midline of the calf, 2 to 4 cm deep, with the patient prone.
  - ✦ The lateral compartment is located anterolaterally and contains the foot everters as well as the fibular nerve. The needle entry is just anterior to the posterior border of the fibula, 1 to 1.5 cm deep, with the patient supine.

TECHNIQUE

- ⊞ Preparation
  - ✦ Choose the most appropriate method for compartment measurement
  - ✦ Remove possible offending factors (i.e., cast, tourniquet)
  - ✦ Identify point of maximal tenderness to palpation
  - ✦ Variety of tonometers are commercially available

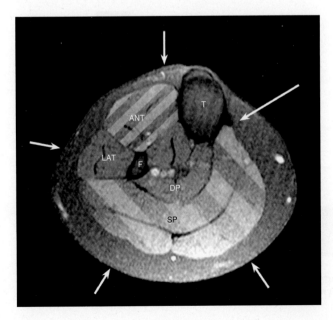

FIGURE 54.2 The four compartments of the leg. T, tibial bone; F, fibula bone; ANT, anterior compartment; LAT, lateral compartment; DP, deep posterior compartment; SP, superficial posterior compartment.

- ✦ Alternatively, measurements can be made using an arterial-line assembly
- ✦ Assemble materials
  - ✦ Arterial-line assembly, transducer, monitor, and stand
  - ✦ An 18-gauge side-port needle or slit catheter
- ✦ Set up the arterial-line transducer and apparatus as would be for inserting an arterial line
- ✦ Attach the side-port needle or slit catheter to the arterial-line assembly and flush
- ✦ Zero the apparatus at the level of the compartment
- ✦ Select your entry site and cleanse it with iodine solution or chlorhexidine. Allow to dry.
- ✦ Administer local anesthesia and/or systemic analgesia as appropriate (avoid injection of muscle or fascia as this can affect measurements)
- ✦ Insert the needle into your selected compartment, perpendicular to the skin
  - ✦ For fractures, insert at level of the fracture (± 5 cm)
  - ✦ Feel the "pop" as you enter the compartment through the deep fascia
- ✦ Verify placement by gently compressing the compartment distal to the needle
- ✦ Record the *mean* pressure (allow needle to equilibrate)
- ✦ Remove the needle from the compartment, inspect and flush as needed
- ✦ Repeat the measurement of the same compartment
- ✦ Cover puncture site with a clean, dry dressing
- ⬚ Whitesides technique (in the absence of the above) may be used
  - ✦ Assemble your materials
    - ✦ A 20-mL syringe
    - ✦ Two intravenous (IV) extension tubing sets
    - ✦ Four-way stopcock
    - ✦ Sterile saline
    - ✦ Mercury manometer (dial-style or aneroid pressure gauges are not calibrated at low pressures and should not be used)
    - ✦ An 18-gauge needle or spinal needle
  - ✦ In a sterile manner, assemble the apparatus **(FIGURE 54.3)**
    - ✦ Attach the two IV extension tubing sets to the four-way stopcock
    - ✦ Attach the 20-mL syringe to the remaining port on the four-way stopcock
    - ✦ Attach the manometer to the female-end of the apparatus
    - ✦ Attach the 18-gauge needle to the male-end of the apparatus
    - ✦ On the four-way stopcock, set the manometer's port to the "off" position. Aspirate enough sterile saline to fill half of the first section of tubing.
    - ✦ Ensure that there are no air bubbles in the column as this will affect your measurement

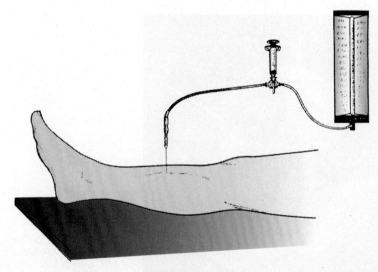

FIGURE 54.3 Schematic for a bedside compartment pressure measuring device. (From Simon RS, Brenner BE. *Emergency Procedures and Techniques.* 4th ed. Philadelphia, PA: Lippincott Williams & Wilkins; 2002:293, with permission.)

+ Prepare the site of needle insertion in sterile manner as described above
+ Insert the needle into the compartment of interest
+ Set the four-way stopcock so that all three ports are open
+ Zero the apparatus: The top of the column of saline must be at the same height as the needle
+ Slowly compress the syringe and observe the column of water in the IV tubing; the pressure at which the fluid begins to infuse is the pressure of the compartment
+ Remove the needle from the compartment
+ Cover the puncture site with a clean, dry dressing

COMPLICATIONS

☐ Infection
☐ Local bleeding or hematoma

SAFETY/QUALITY TIPS

☐ **Procedural**

+ If obtaining a measurement is difficult, check to see if there is tissue or clot occluding the needle tip. Flush with saline if necessary.
+ If your reading seems too high or too low, review your anatomy landmarks and make sure that your insertion site places you within the correct compartment and reposition the needle to assure that you are not inserted in tendon or fascia
+ Do not forget to zero the apparatus prior to obtaining your measurement
+ Whitesides technique is notoriously inaccurate and is no longer recommended
+ In one study, readings with a simple 18-gauge needle or spinal needle on an arterial-line assembly were 11.5 to 32 mm Hg above the compartment pressure, therefore their use is discouraged

☐ **Cognitive**

+ The most important error around the evaluation of compartment syndrome is delay in suspicion or diagnosis. Diminishment or loss of pulses is a late sign; the earliest sign is pain with passive flexion/extension of the involved muscles.
+ If you suspect compartment syndrome, before measurement of pressures, your first action should be to release any extrinsic compression of the limb—bivalve casts, remove restrictive or circumferential dressings and place leg level. Do not elevate the leg above the heart as this may decrease perfusion.
+ Owing to the potentially devastating complications of compartment syndrome and the low complication rate and ease of measurement, clinicians should have a low threshold for measurement of compartment pressures, especially in patients with altered mental status or who are unable to communicate
+ Compartment pressure used as an indication for fasciotomy varies from study to study
+ Beware of patient with polytrauma, crush injuries, hypotension, and/or patients on blood thinners, as these populations are at an elevated risk for developing compartment syndrome
+ Clinicians must take into account the entire clinical picture before ruling out compartment syndrome based on a recorded "low" compartment pressure or the presence of a pulse

☐ **Acknowledgment**

Thank you to prior author Gregory J. Lopez and Maurizio A. Miglietta.

Suggested Readings

Boody AR, Wongworawat MD. Accuracy in the measurement of compartment pressures: a comparison of three commonly used methods. *J Bone Joint Surg Am.* 2005;87:2415–2422.

Murdock M, Murdoch MM. Compartment syndrome: a review of the literature. *Clin Podiatr Med Surg.* 2012;29(2):301–310.

Simon RR, Brenner BE. *Emergency Procedures and Techniques.* 4th ed. Philadelphia, PA: Lippincott Williams & Wilkins; 2002:293.

Whitesides TE, Haney TC, Morimoto K, et al. Tissue pressure measurements as a determinant for the need of fasciotomy. *Clin Orthop Relat Res.* 1975;113:43–51.

55

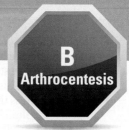

Knee Arthrocentesis

Alicia Blazejewski

INDICATIONS

- Used to evacuate abnormal fluid collections from the joint space for synovial fluid analysis
  - Septic arthritis
  - Crystal arthropathy
  - Hemarthrosis
  - Inflammatory process
- Used to diagnose occult fracture or ligamentous injury
- Used to decrease/relieve pressure in the joint to provide pain relief
- Used to inject methylene blue and test for joint capsule integrity when concerned that overlying laceration communicates with joint space
- Used to inject medication for treatment and pain relief

CONTRAINDICATIONS

- **Absolute Contraindications**
  - Abscess/cellulitis in the tissue overlying the site to be punctured (often infectious arthritis can mimic an overlying soft-tissue infection)
- **Relative Contraindications**
  - Bleeding diatheses/anticoagulant therapy
  - Prosthetic joint
  - Known bacteremia

RISKS/CONSENT ISSUES

- Potential for introducing infection (sterile technique must be utilized)
- Procedure can cause pain (local anesthesia will be given)
- Needle puncture can cause localized bleeding
- Reaccumulation of fluid may occur
- Risk of injuring articular cartilage with needle tip

- **General Basic Steps**
  - **Identify landmarks and prep area**
  - **Sterilize**
  - **Analgesia**
  - **Aspirate**

LANDMARKS

- **Parapatellar Approach**
  - Can use medial or lateral approach
  - Enter 1 cm from the edge of the patella along the superior one-third of the medial or lateral border
  - Direct the needle along the inferior surface of the patella and toward the intercondylar notch **(FIGURE 55.1)**

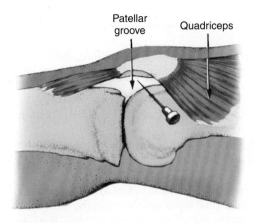

Patellar groove   Quadriceps

FIGURE 55.1 Medial parapatellar approach. (From Simon RR, Brenner BE. *Emergency Procedures and Techniques.* 4th ed. Philadelphia, PA: Lippincott Williams & Wilkins; 2002:245.)

TECHNIQUE

◻ **Equipment**
  + Chlorhexidine or povidone–iodine
  + Sterile gloves and drapes
  + Local anesthetic
  + Two syringes (one for anesthetic, one for joint fluid)
  + Tubes for fluid analysis
◻ **Patient Preparation**
  + Position the knee fully extended or passively flexed 15 degrees with a towel roll behind the popliteal region
  + Make sure the patient relaxes his/her quadriceps as this will open up the joint space
  + Confirm the landmarks and mark the needle insertion point
  + Sterilize the area with povidone–iodine solution or comparable skin antiseptic
  + Wipe the injection site with alcohol to avoid introduction of iodine into the synovium
  + Drape the area with sterile towels
◻ **Analgesia**
  + Use a small-bore (25-gauge) needle to raise a wheal of anesthetic
  + Inject lidocaine with epinephrine at the site of puncture
  + Anesthetize the subcutaneous tissue and a track toward the joint
  + Avoid entering the joint space if synovial fluid analysis is desired
◻ **Aspiration**
  + Using an 18-guage needle advance slowly toward the joint space providing negative pressure on the syringe plunger at all times
  + Angle the needle along the posterior surface of the patella toward the intercondylar notch until synovial fluid is aspirated
  + Use caution and avoid trauma to bone and articular surfaces with the needle tip
  + Free flow of fluid confirms proper needle position
  + Once the procedure is completed, withdraw the needle
  + Apply pressure over the area of insertion for 30 seconds or until bleeding stops
  + Wipe off all excess povidone–iodine solution on the skin
  + Apply clean dressing

COMPLICATIONS

◻ Iatrogenic infection
◻ Excessive pain during procedure
◻ Localized bleeding
◻ Reaccumulation of effusion
◻ Injury to articular cartilage if proper technique is not utilized

SAFETY/QUALITY TIPS

☐ Procedural

+ Send aspirated fluid for cell count with differential, Gram stain and culture, and microscopic evaluation of crystals. See Chapter 61 (Arthrocentesis Appendix: Joint Fluid Analysis) for guidance around fluid analysis.
+ If fluid aspiration is slow/inadequate, "milk" the joint space to facilitate aspiration
+ If the first syringe becomes full, use extension tubing or a clamp on the hub of the needle to avoid moving it excessively when changing syringes
+ If the needle becomes clogged with debris, gently readjust the needle, ease up on the force of aspiration, or reinject a small amount of aspirated fluid

☐ Cognitive

+ The most common cognitive error related to arthrocentesis is failure to perform; have a low threshold to collect and analyze joint fluid when septic arthritis is in the differential
+ Septic arthritis may cause skin changes similar to that of an overlying cellulitis. It is imperative that this distinction be made so that this clinical imitator is not seen as a relative contraindication to arthrocentesis, which is essential for the timely diagnosis of a septic joint.

☐ Acknowledgment

Thank you to prior author Richard F. Petrik.

Suggested Readings

Roberts JR, Custalow CB, Thomsen TW, et al. eds. *Roberts & Hedges' Clinical Procedures in Emergency Medicine.* 6th ed. Philadelphia, PA: WB Saunders; 2013.

Simon RR, Brenner BE. *Emergency Procedures and Techniques.* 4th ed. Philadelphia, PA: Williams & Wilkins; 2002.

56

Elbow Arthrocentesis

Denise Fernandez

INDICATIONS

- ⊡ Used to evacuate abnormal fluid collections from the joint space for synovial fluid analysis
  - ✦ Septic arthritis
  - ✦ Crystal arthropathy
  - ✦ Hemarthrosis
  - ✦ Inflammatory process
- ⊡ Used to diagnose occult fracture or ligamentous injury
- ⊡ Used to inject methylene blue to test for joint capsule integrity when there is an overlying laceration that potentially extends into the joint space
- ⊡ Used to decrease or relieve pressure in the joint to provide pain relief
- ⊡ Used to instill medication for treatment and pain relief

CONTRAINDICATIONS

- ⊡ **Absolute Contraindications**
  - ✦ Abscess/cellulitis overlying the procedural site (note that often infectious arthritis can mimic an overlying soft-tissue infection)
- ⊡ **Relative Contraindications**
  - ✦ Bleeding diatheses
  - ✦ Known bacteremia

RISKS/CONSENT ISSUES

- ⊡ Potential for introducing infection (sterile technique must be utilized)
- ⊡ Procedure can cause pain and discomfort (if no anesthetic allergy exists, local anesthesia will be given)
- ⊡ Needle puncture can cause localized bleeding
- ⊡ Reaccumulation of fluid may occur
- ⊡ Risk of injuring articular cartilage with needle tip

- ⊡ **General Basic Steps**
  - ✦ **Patient preparation**
  - ✦ **Sterilize area**
  - ✦ **Analgesia**
  - ✦ **Aspiration**
  - ✦ **Analyze fluid**

LANDMARKS

Arthrocentesis of the radiohumeral joint (elbow) is performed at the center of the triangle composed of the lateral epicondyle of the humerus, the olecranon, and the head of the radius (FIGURE 56.1).

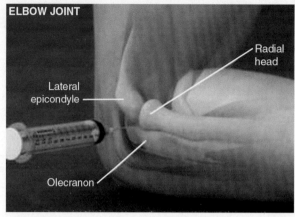

FIGURE 56.1 Landmarks for arthrocentesis of the elbow. (From Roberts RJ, Custalow CB, Thomsen TW, et al. *Roberts & Hedges' Clinical Procedures in Emergency Medicine.* 6th ed. Philadelphia, PA: WB Saunders; 2013:1088.)

TECHNIQUE

◻ **Patient Preparation**
- ✛ Position the patient supine on a stretcher and raise the head of the bed 90 degrees so that the patient is in sitting position
- ✛ Place the patient's affected arm on a procedure table
- ✛ With the elbow extended, palpate the depression between the radial head and the lateral epicondyle of the humerus. While still palpating, flex the elbow to 90 degrees and pronate the forearm. Place the palm down flat on a procedure table. If helpful, mark the insertion point or use ultrasound. If an effusion is present it should be easily palpable.
- ✛ Sterilize the area where the needle will be inserted with povidone–iodine solution or a comparable antiseptic
- ✛ Wipe the injection site with alcohol to avoid introduction of iodine into synovium
- ✛ Drape the area with sterile towels

◻ **Analgesia**
- ✛ Use a 25-gauge needle attached to a 3-mL syringe to raise a wheal of 1% lidocaine (with or without epinephrine) at the site of puncture
- ✛ Anesthetize the subcutaneous tissue and track toward the joint
- ✛ Avoid entering the joint space if synovial fluid analysis is desired for analysis

◻ **Aspiration**
- ✛ Insert a 20- or 22-gauge needle attached to a 10-mL syringe from a lateral position distal to the lateral epicondyle directing the needle medially. A lateral approach is preferred in order to avoid injury to the ulnar nerve and the superior ulnar collateral artery, which run near the medial epicondyle.
- ✛ Remember to aspirate gently as the needle is advanced
- ✛ A slight reduction in resistance is often felt as the needle passes into the joint space and synovial fluid should flow easily into the syringe
- ✛ Once the procedure is completed, withdraw the needle
- ✛ Apply pressure over the area of insertion for 30 seconds or until bleeding stops
- ✛ Wipe off all excess povidone–iodine solution of the skin
- ✛ Apply clean dressing

COMPLICATIONS

- Iatrogenic infection
- Increased pain
- Localized bleeding
- Reaccumulation of effusion
- Injury to articular cartilage if proper technique is not utilized
- Allergic reaction (to local anesthetic)

SAFETY/QUALITY TIPS

- **Procedural**
    - Use adequate local and, if necessary, systemic anesthesia/sedation to facilitate the procedure
- **Cognitive**
    - Patients presenting after joint trauma should have plain radiographs to rule out underlying fracture

- **Acknowledgment**

Thank you to prior author Joseph P. Underwood, III.

Suggested Readings

Boniface KS, Ajmera K, Cohen JS, et al. Ultrasound-guided arthrocentesis of the elbow: a posterior approach. *J Emerg Med.* 2013;45(5):698–701.

May HL, ed. *Emergency Medical Procedures.* New York, NY: Wiley; 1984.

Roberts JR, Custalow CB, Thomsen TW, et al. *Roberts & Hedges Clinical Procedures in Emergency Medicine.* 6th ed. Philadelphia, PA: WB Saunders; 2013.

Schwartz G, ed. *Principles and Practice of Emergency Medicine.* Vol 1. 4th ed. Philadelphia, PA: Lea & Febiger; 1999.

Simon RR, Brenner BE. *Emergency Procedures and Techniques.* 4th ed. Philadelphia, PA: Williams & Wilkins; 2002.

57

Ankle Arthrocentesis

Raquel F. Harrison

INDICATIONS

- ⊕ **Diagnostic**
  - ✦ Evacuate abnormal collections of fluid from the joint space for synovial fluid analysis of the following suspected conditions:
    - ✚ Septic arthritis
    - ✚ Crystal arthropathy
    - ✚ Hemarthrosis
    - ✚ Inflammatory process
  - ✦ Diagnose occult fracture or ligamentous injury
  - ✦ Inject sterile saline to test for joint capsule integrity when overlying laceration potentially extends into joint space
- ⊕ **Therapeutic**
  - ✦ Drain effusion to decrease/relieve pressure in the joint to provide pain relief
  - ✦ Instill medication for treatment and pain relief

CONTRAINDICATIONS

- ⊕ **Absolute Contraindications**
  - ✦ Abscess/cellulitis in the tissues overlying the site to be punctured (often infectious arthritis can mimic an overlying soft-tissue infection)
- ⊕ **Relative Contraindications**
  - ✦ Bleeding diatheses or anticoagulant therapy
  - ✦ Known bacteremia
  - ✦ Prosthetic joint

RISKS/CONSENT ISSUES

- ⊕ Potential for introducing infection (sterile technique must be utilized)
- ⊕ Procedure can cause pain and discomfort (local anesthesia will be given)
- ⊕ Needle puncture can cause localized bleeding
- ⊕ Reaccumulation of fluid may occur
- ⊕ Risk of injuring articular cartilage with needle tip
- ⊕ Potential for tendon and nerve damage if a medication is incorrectly instilled

> ⊕ **General Basic Steps**
> - ✚ **Position patient**
> - ✚ **Analgesia**
> - ✚ **Aspiration**
> - ✚ **Fluid analysis**

LANDMARKS

- ⊕ Two approaches are available (**FIGURE 57.1**):
  - ✦ **Medial approach** (most common):
    - ✚ Identify the malleolar sulcus which allows a portal to the tibiotalar joint space. It is a small depression that is bordered by the medial malleolus medially and the anterior tibial tendon laterally.
    - ✚ Be wary of the saphenous vein and nerve, which lie laterally to medial malleolus

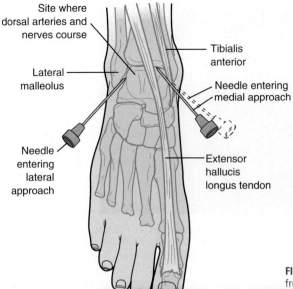

FIGURE 57.1 Arthrocentesis of the ankle. (Modified from Simon RR, Brenner BE. *Emergency Techniques and Procedures.* 4th ed. Philadelphia, PA: Lippincott Williams & Wilkins; 2002:246, with permission.)

✛ **Lateral approach:** The subtalar joint space lies approximately ½ inch proximal and medial to the distal tip of the lateral malleolus

◘ Consider the use of ultrasound to aid in identification of anatomy and the effusion pocket. The site for aspiration can be marked and then proceed with aspiration blindly. Alternatively, procedure can be done under direct visualization **(FIGURES 57.2–57.4)**.

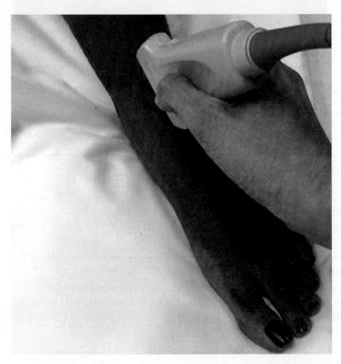

FIGURE 57.2 Placement of ultrasound probe on anterior surface of the ankle near the entry point for the medial approach. Foot should be slightly plantar-flexed. (From: Sanford SO. Arthrocentesis. In: Roberts RJ, Custalow CB, Thomsen TW, et al. eds. *Roberts and Hedges' Clinical Procedures in Emergency Medicine.* 6th ed. Philadelphia, PA: WB Saunders; 2013:1075–1094.)

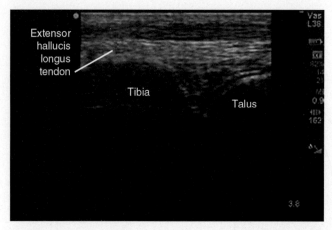

FIGURE 57.3 Ultrasound of normal ankle joint. (From: Sanford SO. Arthrocentesis. In: Roberts RJ, Custalow CB, Thomsen TW, et al. eds. *Roberts and Hedges' Clinical Procedures in Emergency Medicine.* 6th ed. Philadelphia, PA: WB Saunders; 2013:1075–1094.)

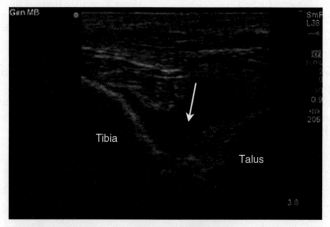

FIGURE 57.4 Ultrasound of a visualized ankle joint effusion. (From: Sanford SO. Arthrocentesis. In: Roberts RJ, Custalow CB, Thomsen TW, et al. eds. *Roberts and Hedges' Clinical Procedures in Emergency Medicine.* 6th ed. Philadelphia, PA: WB Saunders; 2013: 1075–1094.)

SUPPLIES

- Antiseptic solution, sterile gloves and drapes
- Alcohol wipes
- 1% Lidocaine
- 25- and 22-gauge needles, 10-mL syringe
- Gauze pads, bandage

TECHNIQUE

- **Patient Preparation**
  - Confirm landmarks and, if needed, mark the needle insertion point
  - Sterilize the area where the needle will be inserted with antiseptic solution
  - Wipe injection site with alcohol to avoid introduction of iodine (if used as antiseptic solution) into synovium
  - Drape the area with sterile towels

- Analgesia
  - + Use a 25-gauge needle to raise a wheal of lidocaine
  - + Inject lidocaine without epinephrine at the site of puncture
  - + Anesthetize the subcutaneous tissue and track toward the joint
  - + Avoid entering the joint space if synovial fluid analysis is desired
- Aspiration
  - + **Medial Approach**
    - + The patient should be placed in a supine position, the knee extended, and the foot slightly plantar-flexed (after identifying the landmarks with dorsiflexion)
    - + Alternatively, the patient can (if capable) sit on the side of a stretcher and hang his/her leg, placing the foot on a stool. This fixes the joint in a stable position and avoids the posterior pooling of fluid in the joint that may occur when the patient is in the supine position.
    - + Insertion: Insert a 22-gauge needle just medial to the anterior tibial tendon directing it toward the anterior edge of the medial malleolus. Take caution to avoid the saphenous nerve and vein.
    - + Advance the needle 2 to 3 cm until the joint space is entered. While advancing, gentle aspiration should be applied on the 10-mL syringe.
  - + **Lateral Approach**
    - + The patient should be placed in a supine position; the foot should be perpendicular to the leg
    - + Insertion: Insert a 22-gauge needle approximately ½ inch proximal and medial to the distal tip of the lateral malleolus directing the needle medially toward the joint space
    - + Advance the needle 2 to 3 cm until the joint space is entered. While advancing, gentle aspiration should be applied on the 10-mL syringe.
  - + Free flow of fluid confirms proper needle position
  - + Once the procedure is completed, withdraw the needle
  - + Apply pressure over the area of insertion for 30 seconds or until bleeding stops
  - + Wipe off all excess povidone–iodine/antiseptic on the skin
  - + Apply clean dressing
- Analysis of Aspirate
  - + Send aspirated fluid for cell count with differential, Gram stain and culture, and microscopic evaluation of crystals
  - + If minimal amount is collected, the fluid culture and Gram stain should be the priority

COMPLICATIONS

- Iatrogenic infection
- Increased pain
- Localized bleeding
- Reaccumulation of effusion
- Injury to articular cartilage if proper technique not utilized
- Nerve injury
- Allergic reaction to lidocaine

SAFETY/QUALITY TIPS

- Procedural
  - + Ankle arthrocentesis is very painful, and some patients will require procedural sedation
  - + Failure to advance the needle far enough into the joint space is a common mistake
- Cognitive
  - + Septic arthritis may cause skin changes similar to that of an overlying cellulitis. It is imperative that this distinction be made so that this clinical imitator is not seen as a relative contraindication to arthrocentesis, which is essential for the timely diagnosis of a septic joint.

⊡ Acknowledgment

Thank you to prior author Teresa M. Amato.

Suggested Readings

Paget SA. *Hospital for Special Surgery Manual of Rheumatology and Outpatient Orthopedic Disorders: Diagnosis and Therapy.* 5th ed. Philadelphia, PA: Lippincott Williams & Wilkins; 2006.

Sanford SO. Arthrocentesis. In: Roberts RJ, Custalow CB, Thomsen TW, et al. eds. *Roberts and Hedges' Clinical Procedures in Emergency Medicine.* 6th ed. Philadelphia, PA: WB Saunders; 2013:1075–1094.

Simon RR, Brenner BE. *Emergency Procedures and Techniques.* 3rd ed. Baltimore, MD: Williams & Wilkins; 1994.

58

Shoulder Arthrocentesis

Gina Waight

INDICATIONS

- To evacuate abnormal collections of fluid from the joint space for synovial fluid analysis, especially in the investigation of the following conditions:
  - Septic arthritis
  - Crystal arthropathy
  - Hemarthrosis
  - Inflammatory processes
- To diagnose occult fracture or ligamentous injury
- To decrease/relieve pressure in the joint for pain relief
- To assess whether an overlying laceration extends into the joint space using methylene blue
- To instill medication for treatment and pain relief

CONTRAINDICATIONS

- **Absolute Contraindications**
  - Abscess/cellulitis in the tissue overlying the puncture site
- **Relative Contraindications**
  - Known bacteremia
  - Bleeding diathesis or anticoagulant therapy
  - Prosthetic joint

- **General Basic Steps**
  - **Patient preparation**
  - **Sterile technique**
  - **Analgesia**
  - **Aspiration**

LANDMARKS

- **Anterior Approach**
  - Coracoid process and head of the humerus
- **Posterior Approach**
  - Posterolateral edge of the acromion

SUPPLIES

- Povidone–iodine or other antiseptic solution, drapes
- Lidocaine with epinephrine
- 25- and 18-gauge needles, 20-mL syringe
- Gauze pads, adhesive tape

TECHNIQUE

- **Patient Preparation**
  - The patient should sit upright with arm in slight external rotation
  - Confirm landmarks and, if needed, mark the needle insertion point
  - Sterilize the needle insertion area with povidone–iodine solution or comparable skin antiseptic

- ✦ Wipe injection site with alcohol to avoid introduction of iodine into synovium
- ✦ Drape the area with sterile towels
- ✚ **Analgesia**
  - ✦ Use a 25-gauge needle to raise a wheal of anesthetic
  - ✦ Inject lidocaine with epinephrine at the puncture site
  - ✦ Anesthetize the subcutaneous tissue and a track toward the joint
  - ✦ Avoid entering the joint space at this point if synovial fluid analysis is desired
- ✚ **Aspiration**
  - ✦ **Anterior Approach**
    - + Insert an 18-gauge needle attached to a 20-mL syringe just below and lateral to the coracoid process, medial to the head of the humerus
    - + Point the needle posterolaterally to avoid the joint capsule
    - + Gently aspirate while advancing the needle. The needle should be advanced approximately 3 cm or until fluid is aspirated (**FIGURE 58.1**).
  - ✦ **Posterior Approach**
    - + Insert an 18-gauge needle attached to a 20-mL syringe 1 cm below and 1 cm medial to the posterolateral edge of the acromion
    - + Aim the needle anteriorly toward the coracoid process
    - + Gently aspirate while advancing the needle. The needle should be advanced approximately 3 cm or until fluid is aspirated (**FIGURE 58.2**).
  - ✦ Once the required amount of fluid is obtained, withdraw the needle
  - ✦ Apply pressure over the area of insertion for 30 seconds or until bleeding stops
  - ✦ Wipe off all excess povidone–iodine on the skin
  - ✦ Apply clean dressing

COMPLICATIONS

- ✚ Iatrogenic infection
- ✚ Excessive pain during procedure
- ✚ Localized bleeding
- ✚ Reaccumulation of fluid
- ✚ Injury to articular cartilage

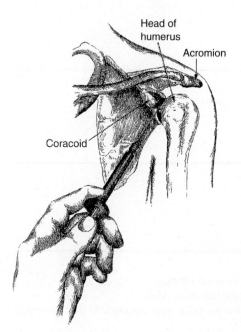

FIGURE 58.1 Anterior approach. (From Simon RR, Brenner BE. *Emergency Procedures and Techniques.* 4th ed. Philadelphia, PA: Lippincott Williams & Wilkins; 2002:242, with permission.)

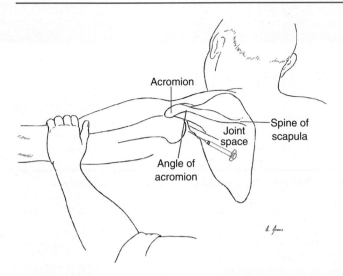

Acromion

Spine of scapula

Joint space

Angle of acromion

FIGURE 58.2 Posterior approach. (From Simon RR, Brenner BE. *Emergency Procedures and Techniques.* 4th ed. Philadelphia, PA: Lippincott Williams & Wilkins; 2002:242.)

SAFETY/QUALITY TIPS

⬚ **Procedural**
+ If unsuccessful using one approach, attempt a different approach

⬚ **Cognitive**
+ Send aspirated fluid for cell count with differential, Gram stain and culture, and microscopic evaluation of crystals
+ Septic arthritis may cause skin changes that appear similar to a cellulitis, but is not a true overlying soft-tissue infection. Arthrocentesis should not be delayed in these instances, as it is essential to the diagnosis of a septic joint.

⬚ **Acknowledgment**

Thank you to prior author Caesar R. Djavaherian.

Suggested Readings

Courtney P, Doherty M. Joint aspiration and injection. *Best Pract Res Clin Rheumatol.* 2005;19(3):345–369.

Li SF, Henderson J, Dickman E, et al. Laboratory tests in adults with monoarticular arthritis: can they rule out a septic joint? *Acad Emerg Med.* 2004;11(3):276–280.

Lossos IS, Yossepowitch O, Kandel L. Septic arthritis of the glenohumeral joint. A report of 11 cases and review of the literature. *Medicine (Baltimore).* 1998;77(3):177–187.

Schaffer TC. Joint and soft-tissue arthrocentesis. *Prim Care.* 1993;20:757–770.

Simon RR, Brenner BE. *Emergency Procedures and Techniques.* 3rd ed. Baltimore, MD: Williams & Wilkins; 1994.

59

Interphalangeal Arthrocentesis

Joel Wussow

INDICATIONS

- Evacuation of abnormal collections of fluid from the joint space for synovial fluid analysis
  + Septic arthritis
  + Crystal arthropathy
  + Hemarthrosis
  + Inflammatory process
- Diagnose occult fracture or ligamentous injury
- Decrease/relieve pressure in the joint to provide pain relief
- Inject methylene blue and test for joint capsule integrity when overlying laceration potentially extends into joint space
- Instill medication for treatment and pain relief

CONTRAINDICATIONS

- **Absolute Contraindications**
  + Abscess/cellulitis in the tissues overlying the site to be punctured (often infectious arthritis can mimic an overlying soft-tissue infection)
- **Relative Contraindications**
  + Bleeding diatheses or anticoagulant therapy
  + Prosthetic joint
  + Known bacteremia

RISKS/CONSENT ISSUES

- Potential for introducing infection (sterile technique must be utilized)
- Pain and discomfort (local anesthesia will be given)
- Needle puncture can cause localized bleeding
- Reaccumulation of fluid may occur
- Risk of injuring articular cartilage with needle tip

- **General Basic Steps**
  + **Sterilize target area and create sterile field**
  + **Confirm landmarks**
  + **Analgesia**
  + **Flex digit with distal traction**
  + **Insert needle**
  + **Aspirate**
  + **Withdraw needle**
  + **Apply pressure**

LANDMARKS

- The landmarks for aspiration of the small joints of the upper and lower extremities are similar
- The fibrous tendon sheaths, nerves, and vessels are located on the volar/plantar surface of the joint, so the dorsal approach should be used
- Approach from either side of the extensor tendons
- Remember: The undersurface of the extensor tendon is attached to the dorsal joint capsule surface

TECHNIQUE

◻ Patient Preparation

+ Confirm landmarks and, if needed, mark the needle insertion point
+ Sterilize the area with povidone–iodine solution or comparable skin antiseptic
+ Wipe injection site with alcohol to avoid introduction of iodine into synovium
+ Drape the area with sterile towels

◻ Analgesia

+ Use a 25-gauge needle to raise a wheal of anesthetic
+ Inject lidocaine without epinephrine at the site of puncture
+ Anesthetize the subcutaneous tissue and track toward the joint
+ Avoid entering the joint space if synovial fluid analysis is desired

◻ Aspiration

+ Passively flex the interphalangeal joint 20 to 30 degrees, applying distal traction
+ Assuming that the "dorsal crease line" is an imaginary line connecting the dorsal points of the interphalangeal skin creases, place the needle in the dorsal crease line as shown in **FIGURE 59.1**
+ "Lifting up" the extensor tendon with your needle, insert the needle tip under the tendon (Figure 59.1)
+ For metacarpophalangeal/metatarsophalangeal joints, passively flex the joint and apply distal traction. Note the separation between the metacarpal/metatarsal and proximal phalanx. Place the needle lateral or medial to the extensor tendon into the fossa **(FIGURE 59.2)**.
+ In the case of the first metacarpophalangeal joint, insert the needle radial to the extensor pollicis longus tendon, and medially in the case of the first metatarsophalangeal joint **(FIGURE 59.3)**
+ Free flow of fluid confirms proper needle position
+ Once the procedure is completed, withdraw the needle
+ Apply pressure over the area of insertion for 30 seconds or until bleeding stops
+ Wipe off all excess povidone–iodine on the skin
+ Apply clean dressing

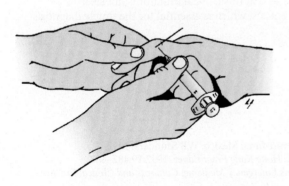

FIGURE 59.1 Insert the needle tip in the dorsal crease line at the joint. (From Simon RR, Brenner BE. *Emergency Procedures and Techniques.* 4th ed. Philadelphia, PA: Lippincott Williams & Wilkins; 2002:238. with permission.)

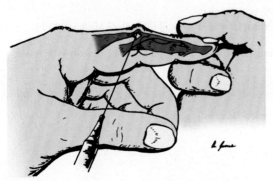

FIGURE 59.2 Distract the joint and "lift up" the extensor tendon with the needle tip. (From Simon RR, Brenner BE. *Emergency Procedures and Techniques.* 4th ed. Philadelphia, PA: Lippincott Williams and Wilkins; 2002, with permission.)

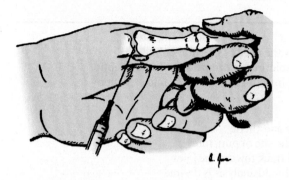

FIGURE 59.3 Arthrocentesis of the metacarpophalangeal joint of the thumb. (From Simon RR, Brenner BE. *Emergency Procedures and Techniques.* 4th ed. Philadelphia, PA: Lippincott Williams & Wilkins; 2002:238, with permission.)

COMPLICATIONS

- Iatrogenic infection
- Excessive pain during procedure
- Localized bleeding
- Reaccumulation of effusion
- Injury to articular cartilage if proper technique is not utilized

SAFETY/QUALITY TIPS

- **Procedural**
  - Sterilize the entire region—it is easy to accidentally brush up against another finger during this procedure
- **Cognitive**
  - Send aspirated fluid for cell count with differential, Gram stain and culture, and microscopic evaluation of crystals. See Chapter 61 (Arthrocentesis Appendix: Joint Fluid Analysis (FIGURE 61.2)) for a guideline of fluid analysis.
  - Septic arthritis may cause skin changes similar to that of an overlying cellulitis. It is imperative that this distinction be made so that this clinical imitator is not seen as a relative contraindication to arthrocentesis, which is essential for the timely diagnosis of a septic joint.

- **Acknowledgment**

Thank you to prior author Hina Z. Ghory.

Suggested Readings

Jastremski MS, Dumas M, Penalaver L. *Emergency Procedures.* Mexico: WB Saunders; 1992.

Lee GKW, Lau CS. Intraarticular injection of steroid. *Hong Kong Practitioner.* 1997;19:482–488.

Marx JA, Hockberger RS, Walls RM, et al. eds. *Rosen's Emergency Medicine: Concepts and Clinical Practice.* Vol 2. 5th ed. St. Louis, MO: Mosby; 2002.

May HL. *Emergency Medical Procedures.* New York, NY: Wiley; 1984.

Schwartz GR, Cayten CG, Mangelsen MA, et al. eds. *Principles and Practice of Emergency Medicine.* Vol 1. 3rd ed. Philadelphia, PA: Lea & Febiger; 1992.

Simon R, Brenner BE. *Emergency Procedures and Techniques.* 4th ed. Philadelphia, PA: Lippincott Williams & Wilkins; 2002:238.

60

Wrist (Radiocarpal) Arthrocentesis

Kenneth J. Perry

INDICATIONS

- Provide evacuation of abnormal collections of fluid from the joint space for synovial fluid analysis
  - Septic arthritis
  - Crystal arthropathy
  - Hemarthrosis
  - Inflammatory process
- Diagnose occult fracture or ligamentous injury
- Decrease/relieve pressure in the joint to provide pain relief
- Used to instill medication for treatment and pain relief
- Used to test joint integrity by injecting methylene blue when overlying laceration is present

CONTRAINDICATIONS

- **Absolute Contraindications**
  - Abscess/cellulitis in the tissues overlying the site to be punctured (infectious arthritis can often mimic an overlying soft-tissue infection)
- **Relative Contraindications**
  - Known bacteremia
  - Bleeding diatheses or anticoagulant therapy

RISKS/CONSENT ISSUES

- Potential for causing infection if not done with proper sterile technique
- Pain from the procedure (mitigate with local anesthesia)
- Bleeding from the needle
- Reaccumulation of fluid may occur
- Risk of injuring articular cartilage with needle tip

- **General Basic Steps**
  - **Patient preparation**
  - **Sterilize area**
  - **Anesthetize area**
  - **Aspiration**

LANDMARKS

- **Dorsal/Radiocarpal Approach**
  - Place the wrist in 20-degree flexion and extend the thumb
  - Palpate the dorsal radial tubercle (Lister tubercle) and the extensor pollicis longus tendon as it courses over the distal radius
  - Palpate the depression that is distal to the tubercle and on the ulnar side of the extensor carpi radialis brevis tendon
- **Ulnocarpal Approach**
  - Flex the wrist 20 degrees and palpate the depression between the ulnar styloid process and pisiform bone
  - Approach may be problematic due to multiple tendons travel through this region

TECHNIQUE

⬒ **Patient Preparation**
+ Confirm landmarks—mark the needle insertion point if needed
+ Sterilize the area where the needle will be inserted with povidone–iodine solution or comparable skin antiseptic
+ Wipe injection site with alcohol to avoid introduction of iodine solution into the synovium
+ Drape the area with sterile towels
+ Place the wrist in neutral, relaxed position
+ Apply gentle traction and ulnar deviation to the hand to open the joint space

⬒ **Analgesia**
+ Use a 25-gauge needle to infiltrate injection site with lidocaine with epinephrine
+ Anesthetize the subcutaneous tissue and a track toward the joint
+ Avoid entering the joint space if synovial fluid analysis is desired

⬒ **Aspiration**
+ Use a 22-gauge needle attached to a 5- or 10-mL syringe
+ For the radiocarpal approach, direct the needle just distal to the border of the distal radius
+ Insert the needle in the depression on the ulnar side of the extensor carpi radialis brevis tendon and between the distal radius and lunate bone **(FIGURE 60.1)**
+ For the ulnocarpal approach direct the needle between the distal border of the ulnar styloid process and the pisiformis bone **(FIGURE 60.2)**
+ Provide negative pressure on the syringe plunger as the needle is inserted in the joint cavity
+ Easy aspiration of fluid confirms proper needle position
+ Withdraw needle, apply pressure, then apply clean dressing

COMPLICATIONS

⬒ Iatrogenic infection
⬒ Increased pain
⬒ Localized bleeding
⬒ Reaccumulation of effusion
⬒ Injury to articular cartilage if proper technique is not utilized

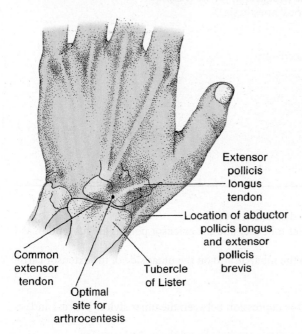

Extensor pollicis longus tendon

Location of abductor pollicis longus and extensor pollicis brevis

Common extensor tendon

Optimal site for arthrocentesis

Tubercle of Lister

FIGURE 60.1 Radiocarpal arthrocentesis. (From Simon RR, Brenner BE. *Emergency Procedures and Techniques.* 4th ed. Philadelphia, PA: Lippincott Williams & Wilkins; 2002:239, with permission.)

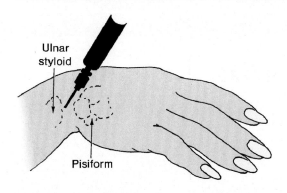

FIGURE 60.2 Ulnocarpal joint arthrocentesis. (From Simon RR, Brenner BE. *Emergency Procedures and Techniques.* 4th ed. Philadelphia, PA: Lippincott Williams & Wilkins; 2002:240, with permission.)

SAFETY/QUALITY TIPS

☐ **Procedural**
  + Procedure can be exquisitely painful; provide aggressive analgesia, sedation, or procedural sedation as needed
  + Failure to advance the needle far enough into the joint space is a common mistake
  + When using the radiocarpal approach, avoid the anatomic snuff box that contains the radial artery and superficial radial nerve
  + Avoid the ulnocarpal approach whenever possible to avoid injury to tendons traveling into the hand

☐ **Cognitive**
  + Send aspirated fluid for cell count with differential, Gram stain and culture, and microscopic evaluation of crystals. See Chapter 61 (Arthrocentesis Appendix: Joint Fluid Analysis) for a guideline of fluid analysis.
  + Septic arthritis may mimic overlying cellulitis. It is imperative that this distinction be made so that this clinical imitator is not seen as a contraindication to arthrocentesis, which is essential to the timely diagnosis of a septic joint.
  + Plain radiographs should be obtained if trauma is part of the history to rule out underlying fracture

☐ **Acknowledgment**
Thank you to prior author Sadie Johnson.

Suggested Readings

Burton JH. Acute disorders of the joints and bursae. In: Tintinalli JE, Stapczynski J, Ma O, et al. eds. *Tintinalli's Emergency Medicine: A Comprehensive Study Guide.* New York, NY: McGraw-Hill; 2011.

Marx JA, Hockberger RS, Walls RM, et al. *Rosen's Emergency Medicine: Concepts and Clinical Practice.* Vol 2. 5th ed. St. Louis, MO: Mosby; 2002.

Partin W, Dorroh C. Emergency procedures. In: Stone C, Humphries RL. eds. *Current Diagnosis & Treatment Emergency Medicine.* 7th ed. New York, NY: McGraw-Hill; 2011. http://accessmedicine.mhmedical.com/content.aspx?bookid=385&Sectionid=40357220. Accessed March 8, 2014.

Rheumatology. In: Simon RR, Sherman SC. eds. *Emergency Orthopedics. 6th ed.* New York, NY: McGraw-Hill; 2011:42–75.

Schwartz GR, Cayten CG, Mangelsen MA, et al. *Principles and Practice of Emergency Medicine.* Vol 1. 3rd ed. Philadelphia, PA: Lea & Febiger; 1992.

61

Arthrocentesis Appendix: Joint Fluid Analysis

Naomi Jean Baptiste

- **Normal Fluid**
  - An ultradiasylate of plasma with protein and hyaluronic acid
  - Clear to straw colored
  - Viscosity of oil
- **Crystals**
  - Gout
    - Monosodium urate (MSU) crystals
    - Negative birefringence
    - Needle shaped
  - Pseudogout
    - Calcium pyrophosphate dihydrate (CPPD) crystals
    - Weak positive birefringence
    - Rhomboid and/or polymorphic
- **Septic Arthritis**
  - Leukocyte counts as low as 5,000 have been associated with early septic joints
  - Most septic joints have a white cell count >50,000, with more than 75% polymorphonuclear leukocytes (TABLE 61.1)

SAFETY/QUALITY TIPS

- If only a small sample is obtained, it is most important to send for Gram stain and culture to rule out infectious arthritis
- About 1 to 2 mL is enough for Gram stain, culture, and wet prep for crystals
- Mucin clot and string test are physical tests of viscosity and inflammation, which are less reliable than laboratory analyses and are therefore not widely used
  For septic arthritis, a review by Carpenter et al[1] calls into question the long-standing practice of measuring fluid glucose and lactate dehydrogenase (LDH). Joint fluid lactate may be useful; however, the data is not conclusive.
- Although leukocyte count and differential will generally distinguish noninflammatory, inflammatory, and septic arthritides, leukocyte counts as low as 5,000 have been associated with early septic joints
- Rarely, crystal arthritis and septic arthritis can occur concomitantly
- Patients with **sickle cell disease** who are being evaluated for the possibility of joint infection are at increased risk for Salmonella species being the causative organism
- Patients who are active **intravenous drug abusers** are at risk for Pseudomonas species being the causative organism
- Patients with negative cultures and synovial fluid suspicious for inflammatory arthritis should be evaluated for **Lyme disease,** especially if they have a potential exposure within 1 year and a history of asymmetric, recurrent, and remitting joint pains (TABLE 61.2)

TABLE 61.1. SYNOVIAL FLUID COLLECTION

Synovial fluid test	Laboratory tube
Gram stain and culture	Sterile tube or specific culture medium
Cell count and differential	EDTA: Lavender top tube
Crystals	Heparin: Green top tube
Chemistries (e.g., glucose, ANA, anti-Lyme Ab, RF)	SST: Gold top tube or Plain: Red top tube

ANA, antinuclear antibody; EDTA, ethylenediaminetetraacetic acid; RF, rheumatoid factor; SST, serum separator tube.

TABLE 61.2 SYNOVIAL FLUID ANALYSIS

	Normal	Noninflammatory	Inflammatory	Septic	Traumatic
Color	Colorless	Yellow	Yellow	Yellow	Red
Appearance	Clear	Clear	Turbid	Purulent	Turbid
WBC/mL	<200	<4,000	<50,000	>50,000	<10,000
%PMNs	<25	<25	>75	>75	<25
Glucose	Same as serum	Same as serum	Less than serum	Much less than serum	Same as serum
Crystals	None	None	May be present	None	None
Culture	Negative	Negative	Negative	Positive	Negative
Common conditions		OA, trauma, viral infection, drug-induced	Crystal-induced arthritides, Lyme disease, acute rheumatic fever, RA, JRA, SLE, spondyloarthopathies, sarcoidosis	Bacterial including GC arthritis	Fracture, ligament injury, hemophilia

GC, gonococcus; JRA, juvenile rheumatoid arthritis; OA, osteoarthritis; PMN, polymorphonuclear cells; RA, rheumatoid arthritis; SLE, systemic lupus erythematosus; WBC, white blood cell.
Drug-induced arthritis: Procainamide, hydralazine, or isoniazid treatment.
Crystal-induced arthritis: Gout vs pseudogout.
Mahadevan SV Garmel GM. *An Introduction to Clinical Emergency Medicine: Guide for Practitioners in the Emergency Department.* New York, NY: Cambridge University Press; 2005.

✚ Acknowledgment
Thank you to prior author Wallace A. Carter.

Reference

1. Carpenter CR, Schurr JD, Everett WW, et al. Evidence-based diagnostics: adult septic arthritis. *Acad Emerg Med.* 2011;18(8):782–796.

62

Shoulder Dislocation and Reduction

Olabiyi Akala and Maureen Gang

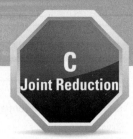

C
Joint Reduction

INDICATIONS

- History and clinical examination consistent with shoulder dislocation
  - **Anterior Dislocation (~95%)**
    - Mechanism
      - Force applied to an externally rotated, abducted, and extended arm
      - Rarely secondary to a blow to the posterior shoulder
    - Examination
      - Prominent humeral head anteriorly and a shallow depression inferior to the acromion may be observed
      - Affected extremity usually held in abduction and external rotation
  - **Posterior Dislocation (2%–4%)**
    - Mechanism
      - Axial loading of adducted and internally rotated arm
      - Less commonly due to direct blow to anterior shoulder or fall on an outstretched arm
      - May result from violent muscle contractions: e.g., seizures, electric shock, psychiatry patients
    - Examination
      - Prominence of posterior shoulder with flattening anteriorly; may be subtle
      - Affected extremity typically held in adduction and internal rotation
      - Patient usually unable to externally rotate affected extremity
  - **Inferior dislocation (luxatio erecta)—rare**
    - Mechanism
      - Forceful hyperabduction of the affected extremity
    - Examination
      - Affected arm is held above the head
      - Patient is unable to adduct the affected extremity
- Radiographs demonstrate glenohumeral dislocation

CONTRAINDICATIONS

- Any associated fracture—particularly fracture of the humeral neck
  - Obtain orthopedic consultation
- Any associated neurologic deficit
  - Closed reduction may still be attempted but multiple attempts should be avoided

RISKS/CONSENT ISSUES

- Recurrent dislocation
  - Risk dependent on age at initial dislocation, with recurrence risk up to 90% for those <20, up to 70% for those between 20 and 40 and between 2% and 4% for those older than 40
- Increased risk of associated rotator cuff injuries in patients >40 years of age
- Complications of reduction
  - Risks associated with procedural sedation
  - Neurovascular injury
  - Fracture of humerus and glenoid

⬚ **General Basic Steps**
  ✚ **Thorough examination of affected extremity, including neurovascular status**
  ✚ **Analgesia/sedation/muscle relaxation**
  ✚ **Reduction via preferred technique**
  ✚ **Postreduction care and follow-up**

LANDMARKS—FIGURE 62.1

⬚ **Technique**
  ✚ **Physical Examination**
    ✚ Compare both the affected and unaffected extremities
    ✚ Perform a thorough neurovascular examination of the injured extremity
      ▪ A sensory deficit over the deltoid (the so-called sergeant's-stripe pattern) or an impaired deltoid contraction implies an axillary nerve injury
      ▪ All major nerves to the arm should be assessed as injuries to the brachial plexus, ulnar, and radial nerves have been reported
  ✚ **Radiographs**
    ✚ Obtain before reduction if the clinician is unsure of the position/type of dislocation or if there is concern for an associated fracture
    ✚ May defer prereduction films if the clinician is confident of an anterior dislocation based on physical examination, the patient is <40, with a history of recurrent dislocations, and the mechanism of the dislocation is not associated with direct trauma
    ✚ Anteroposterior (AP), scapular Y, and axillary lateral view should be obtained
      ▪ A single x-ray view should never be used to diagnose a shoulder dislocation

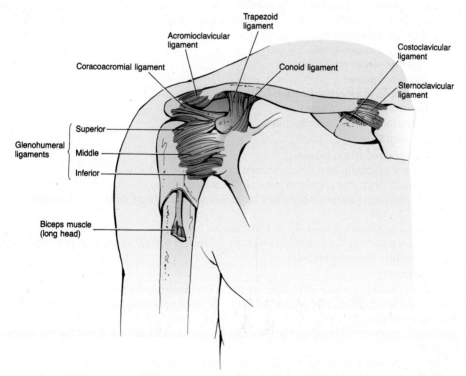

FIGURE 62.1 The essential anatomy of the shoulder. (From Sherman S. Shoulder injuries. In: Wolfson AB, ed. *Harwood-Nuss' Clinical Practice of Emergency Medicine.* 6th ed. Philadelphia, PA: Lippincott Williams & Wilkins; 2015:248, with permission.)

+ In anterior dislocations, the humeral head is anterior in the axillary view (using the coracoid process as a point of orientation, and anterior to the center of Y in the trans-scapular view
+ In posterior dislocations, the AP view may be diagnostic if it shows a partial vacancy of the glenoid fossa (vacant glenoid sign) and >6 mm space between the glenoid rim and humeral head (positive rim sign). The humeral head is posterior on axillary view and posterior to center Y on trans-scapular view.

+ **Sedation, Analgesia, and Muscle Relaxation**
    + Adequate analgesia, muscle relaxation, and/or sedation help facilitate successful reduction
        ▬ A recent systematic review of intra-articular lidocaine vs procedural sedation showed no significant difference in reduction success rates, pain during reduction, and pain after reduction
        ▬ It is reasonable to attempt initial reduction with intra-articular local anesthetic; if unsuccessful, the clinician may consider procedural sedation for subsequent attempts
        ▬ Ensure that the patient relates the use of intra-articular lidocaine to the orthopedic surgeon during follow-up
    + Intra-articular Injection of Lidocaine
        ▬ Cleanse the shoulder with povidone–iodine solution
        ▬ Insert the needle 2 cm inferiorly and directly lateral to the acromion, in the lateral sulcus left by the absent humeral head
        ▬ Fill a 20-mL syringe with 1% lidocaine. Attach a 1.5-inch 20-gauge needle to the syringe (**FIGURE 62.2**).
        ▬ Withdraw to ensure you are not in a blood vessel prior to the injection of 15 to 20 mL of lidocaine into the joint space

+ **Shoulder Reduction**
    + The guiding principle for all methods of reduction should be a gradual and gentle application of technique (**FIGURE 62.3**)
    + The treating physician should be comfortable with several methods of reduction because no technique is 100% effective. The following techniques are described in this chapter:
        ▬ Stimson maneuver
        ▬ Scapular manipulation
        ▬ Traction–countertraction
        ▬ Milch technique
        ▬ Hennepin or external rotation method
        ▬ Cunningham technique
        ▬ Posterior dislocation reduction

+ **Postreduction Care**
    + Obtain postreduction x-rays
    + Perform a postreduction neurovascular assessment and document the findings
    + Position at discharge is controversial. Evidence regarding external rotation splinting is still evolving. Patients should be placed in a shoulder immobilizer or sling and swath for 2 to 3 weeks.
    + Arrange orthopedic follow-up in 1 to 2 weeks
        ▬ Older patients (<40) should have early follow-up within ~1 week to prevent adhesive capsulitis (frozen shoulder)

▣ **Stimson Maneuver**
    + Patient is positioned prone with dislocated arm overhanging the bed
    + Weight of 5 to 15 lb (initially supported by the physician) is strapped to the wrist of the affected extremity
    + Traction is gradually exerted on the shoulder by slow and steady release of the physician's support
    + Up to 30 minutes of sustained, steady traction may be necessary for reduction
    + Reduction may be facilitated by delicate external rotation of the affected extremity
    + Advantages: Can be performed by the lone practitioner without assistance
    + Disadvantages: Often requires more time and materials (weights and straps) than may be readily available (**FIGURE 62.4**). Not appropriate for all patients, particularly those with respiratory compromise.

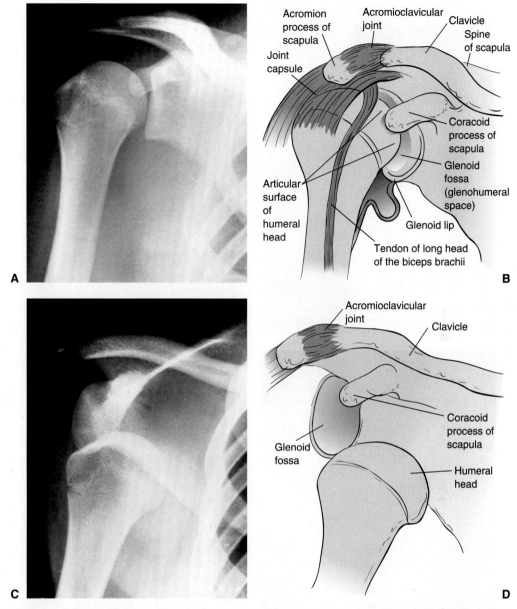

FIGURE 62.2 A, B: Normal shoulder joint. **C, D:** Anterior dislocation of the shoulder. (From Young GM. Reduction of common joint dislocations and subluxations. In: Henretig FM, King C, eds. *Textbook of Pediatric Emergency Procedures.* Philadelphia, PA: Williams & Wilkins; 1997:1083, with permission.)

- ◘ **Scapular Manipulation**
  - ✚ Place the patient in either a prone or seated position
  - ✚ Palpate the inferior tip of the scapula. Manipulate the scapula by pushing the scapular tip medially with one hand and push the superior scapula laterally with the other hand.
  - ✚ An assistant should exert gentle traction on the injured extremity (alternatively weights can be used). Simultaneous external rotation of the humerus may also aid in the reduction effort.
  - ✚ Advantages: Easy to perform with a high degree of safety, efficacy, and patient tolerance
  - ✚ Disadvantages: Requires two people (**FIGURE 62.5**)
- ◘ **Traction–Countertraction Method**
  - ✚ Position the patient supine with a sheet wrapped around the upper torso and under the axilla of the injured extremity. Have an assistant hold the sheet to apply countertraction.

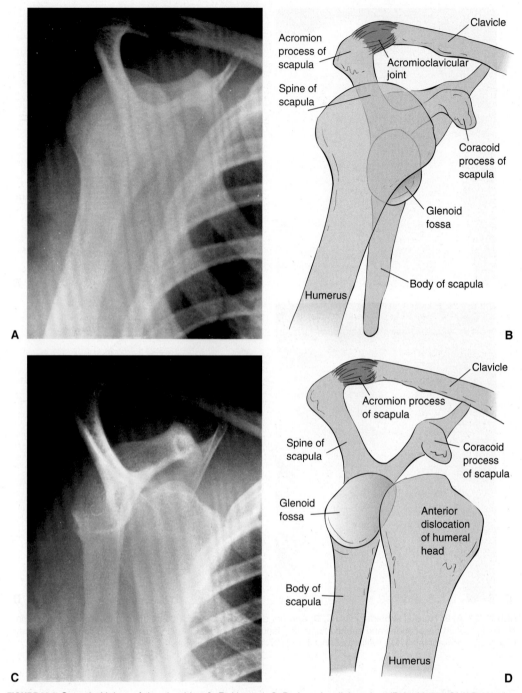

FIGURE 62.3 Scapular Y-view of the shoulder. **A, B:** Normal. **C, D:** Anterior dislocation. (From Young GM. Reduction of common joint dislocations and subluxations. In: Henretig FM, King C, eds. *Textbook of Pediatric Emergency Procedures.* Philadelphia, PA: Williams & Wilkins; 1997:1085, with permission.)

- ✛ Apply gentle traction to the injured, extended extremity
  - ✛ Consider placing a second sheet around the flexed elbow of the patient and tying it around your back. Then lean back while holding the patient's forearm and elbow (above and below the sheet) to apply traction gently (**FIGURE 62.6**).
- ✛ The practice of placing a foot in the axilla of the patient to gain leverage for traction (the so-called Hippocratic technique) should be avoided

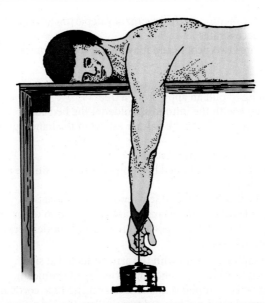

FIGURE 62.4 The Stimson technique for reducing an anterior shoulder dislocation. (From Simon RR, Brenner BE. *Emergency Procedures and Techniques.* 4th ed. Philadelphia, PA: Lippincott Williams & Wilkins; 2002:279, with permission.)

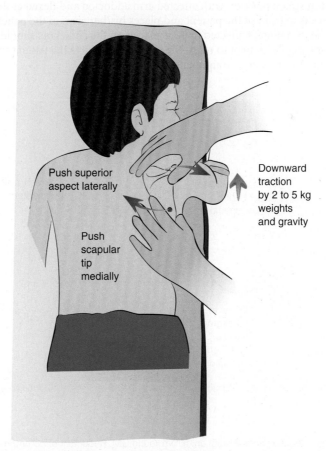

Push superior aspect laterally

Downward traction by 2 to 5 kg weights and gravity

Push scapular tip medially

FIGURE 62.5 Reduction by scapular manipulation. (From Young GM. Reduction of common joint dislocations and subluxations. In: Henretig FM, King C, eds. *Textbook of Pediatric Emergency Procedures.* Philadelphia, PA: Williams & Wilkins; 1997:1086, with permission.)

- Advantages: A popular method in the emergency department where familiarity has resulted in reportedly high success rates
- Disadvantages: Requires two people and may take several minutes of slow gentle traction to be efficacious

◘ **Milch Technique**
- Described as "reaching to pull an apple from a tree"
- Place the patient supine with the injured shoulder at the bed edge
- Abduct the injured arm and bring the palmar aspect of the hand up toward the head slowly and gently
- Apply gentle traction and external rotation
- Stubborn reductions may be facilitated by applying pressure on the humeral head upward, in the direction of the glenoid fossa
- Advantage: High patient tolerance and few reported side effects
- Disadvantages: Patient cooperation is important compared to other techniques. May take several minutes to complete, taking special care to avoid sudden jerky movements.

◘ **Hennepin/External Rotation Method**
- Place patient in the supine position with the arm adducted at side
- With the elbow flexed to 90 degrees and supported by the clinician, externally rotate the arm
- Typically, reduction will occur before the arm has reached the coronal plane, but gentle elevation of the humeral head can be used to complete the reduction
- Advantages: Especially useful for those with prior dislocations. Shoulder muscles permit relocation with minimal manipulation and analgesia **(FIGURE 62.7)**.

◘ **Cunningham Technique**
- Place patient in seated position with affected arm adducted and flexed at the elbow
- The clinician sits in front of the patient and places his/her arm on the patient's proximal forearm, while the patient's affected hand is placed on the clinician's shoulder
- While encouraging the patient to relax, the clinician instructs the patient to pull his/her shoulder blades together and straighten their back

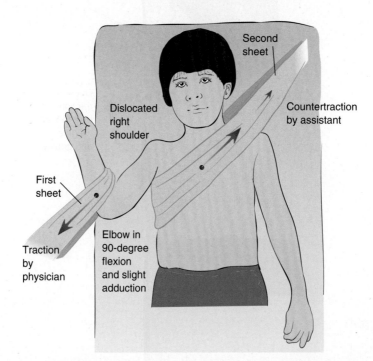

FIGURE 62.6 Reduction by traction/countertraction. (From Young GM. Reduction of common joint dislocations and subluxations. In: Henretig FM, King C, eds. *Textbook of Pediatric Emergency Procedures*. Philadelphia, PA: Williams & Wilkins; 1997:1086, with permission.)

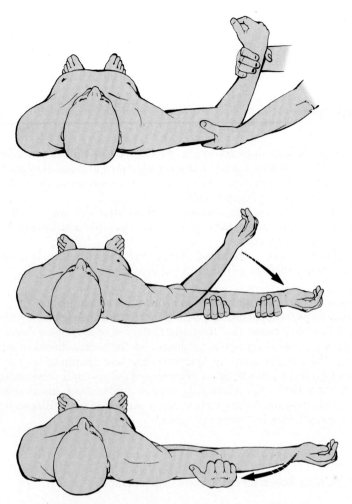

FIGURE 62.7 Hennepin technique for anterior shoulder dislocation reduction. (From Schaider J, Simon RR. Shoulder injuries. In: Wolfson AB, ed. *Harwood-Nuss' Clinical Practice of Emergency Medicine.* 4th ed. Philadelphia, PA: Lippincott Williams & Wilkins; 2005:1037, with permission.)

+ The biceps (level of midhumerus), deltoid, and trapezius muscles are massaged by the clinician to relax the muscles and facilitate reduction
+ Advantages: May be attempted by single provider. Usually requires minimal analgesia and manipulation.
+ Disadvantages: Requires relatively high patient cooperation

◘ **Posterior Dislocation Reduction**

+ With the patient lying supine, place axial traction on the humerus
+ The assistant should apply gentle anterior pressure at the posterior humeral head
+ Slow internal and external rotations in addition to gentle traction will facilitate reduction
+ Advantages: Well-known technique for posterior reduction
+ Dislocation: Success rate not uniformly high, particularly in cases of delayed presentation

COMPLICATIONS

◘ Orthopedic

+ Fracture of the greater tuberosity, glenoid rim (bony Bankart lesion), humeral head (Hill–Sachs deformity) or humeral neck
+ Rotator cuff tear

- ✦ Residual shoulder stiffness
- ✦ Recurrent dislocation
- ☐ Neurovascular
  - ✦ Brachial plexus injury (especially axillary nerve palsies)
  - ✦ Laceration or thrombosis of vascular structures (especially axillary artery)

SAFETY/QUALITY TIPS

☐ **Procedural**

- ✦ Uncomplicated shoulder dislocations can often be reduced without procedural sedation, and most cases should have a quick maneuver attempted in the awake patient. If unsuccessful, the vast majority of shoulder dislocations will easily reduce with complete muscle relaxation achieved by brief deep sedation.
- ✦ Apply persistent, gentle traction and avoid excessive force with any reduction maneuver
- ✦ The ability to place the palm of the injured extremity on the contralateral shoulder is often indicative of reduction success
- ✦ Rotator cuff tears are easier to evaluate after several days when there is resolution of the pain and swelling associated with the original dislocation

☐ **Cognitive**

- ✦ Clearly document pre- and postreduction neurovascular examinations
- ✦ Older patients (>40) should be immobilized for *less* time than younger patients, and should be followed up *sooner* (5–7 days) due to the risk of developing frozen shoulder
- ✦ Nerve injuries generally have a good prognosis, but the patient should be informed of the findings and the need for follow-up. Symptoms may take months to resolve.
- ✦ Patients with posterior dislocation are often missed due to subtle presentations, often in combination with other problems (e.g., seizure, electric shock, intoxication). Careful physical examination and complete radiographs will assure timely diagnosis (should get axillary view and Y-view in addition to AP view).

☐ **Acknowledgment**

Thank you to prior author Robert J. Preston and David J. Berkoff.

Suggested Readings

Cunningham NJ. Techniques for reduction of anteroinferior shoulder dislocation. *Emerg Med Australas* 2005;17:463–471.

Horn AE, Ufberg JW. Management of common dislocations. In: Roberts JR, Hedges JR, eds. *Roberts & Hedges' Clinical Procedures in Emergency Medicine.* 6th ed. Philadelphia, PA: Elsevier Saunders; 2014:954–988.

Ufberg JW, McNamara RM. Management of common dislocations. In: Roberts JR, Hedges JR, eds. *Clinical Procedures in Emergency Medicine.* Philadelphia, PA: Saunders; 2004:949–960..

Ufberg JW, Vilke GM, Chan TC, et al. Anterior shoulder dislocations: beyond traction-countertraction. *J Emerg Med.* 2004;27(3):301–306.

Wakai A, O'Sullivan R, McCabe A. Intra-articular lignocaine versus intravenous analgesia with or without sedation for manual reduction of acute anterior shoulder dislocation in adults. *Cochrane Database of Syst Rev.* 2011; (4): CD004919. doi:10.1002/14651858.CD004919.pub2.

63

Knee Dislocation and Reduction

Amie M. Kim and Maureen Gang

INDICATIONS

- Clinical suspicion of knee dislocation with neurovascular compromise (FIGURE 63.1)
- Radiographic evidence of knee dislocation; anterior (associated with popliteal artery traction and intimal tears) more common than posterior (associated with popliteal artery compression and transection), lateral, medial, and rotary knee dislocations

CONTRAINDICATIONS

- Multiple failed reduction attempts with adequate sedation prompts urgent orthopedic consult

RELATIVE CONTRAINDICATIONS

- Dimple or pucker sign of the skin of the anteromedial knee.

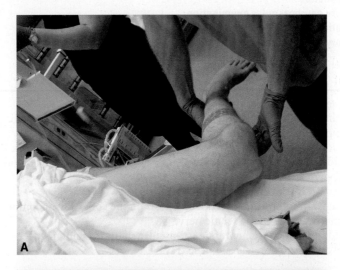

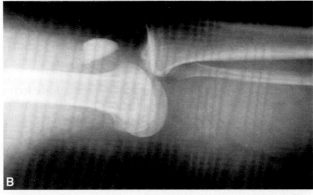

FIGURE 63.1 Clinical suspicion of knee dislocation with neurovascular compromise. (From Silverberg M. Knee dislocations. In: Greenberg MI, ed. *Greenberg's Text-Atlas of Emergency Medicine.* Philadelphia, PA: Lippincott Williams & Wilkins; 2005:522, with permission).

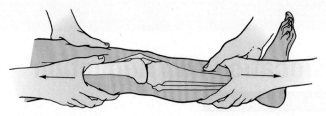

FIGURE 63.2 Gentle and persistent axial traction is applied by the second practitioner, while the first practitioner maintains countertraction. (From Irish CB, Bowe CT. Knee injuries. In: Wolfson AB, ed. *Harwood-Nuss' Clinical Practice of Emergency Medicine.* 6th ed. Philadelphia, PA: Lippincott Williams & Wilkins; 2015:289, with permission.)

RISKS/CONSENT ISSUES

- Knee reduction is a limb-saving procedure and as such it may be performed if informed consent cannot be obtained
- Reduction attempts may result in connective tissue injury, neurovascular compromise, and iatrogenic fractures

- **General Basic Steps**
  - **Neurovascular examination**
  - **Analgesia**
  - **Traction reduction**
  - **Confirmatory neurovascular examination**
  - **Immobilization**
  - **Confirmatory imaging test**

TECHNIQUE

- Neurovascular examination is critical!
  - Document the presence and character of tibialis posterior and dorsalis pedis pulses bilaterally
  - Document presence and character of popliteal pulse, bruit, thrill, and/or hematoma
  - Consider using Doppler acoustics to check pulses and ankle-brachial index (ABI). ABI is the systolic blood pressure of the injured extremity, divided by the systolic blood pressure of an uninjured upper extremity.
  - ABI ratio of <0.9 is concerning for arterial injury
  - Document sensorimotor function with emphasis on the condition of common peroneal and posterior tibial branches of the sciatic nerve
  - Consider additional management if neurovascular status is maintained
  - Obtain anteroposterior and lateral knee x-rays

KNEE REDUCTION

- An assistant stabilizes the distal femur and applies countertraction
- Practitioner applies gentle and persistent axial traction to the ankle/distal tibia **(FIGURE 63.2)**
- If reduction is not achieved within 1 minute, apply an additional attempt while axial traction/countertraction is maintained **(FIGURE 63.3)**
- Anterior dislocation: A second assistant applies gentle anterior force to the distal femur
- Posterior dislocation: Operator applies gentle anterior force to the proximal tibia
- Medial, lateral, or rotatory dislocation: Operator applies gentle force to the proximal tibia in the opposite direction of the dislocation deformity

POSTREDUCTION

- Document a repeat neurovascular examination. Complete the examination for open injuries, associated fractures, or ligamentous laxity.
- Immobilize the reduced knee
- Apply a long leg posterior splint with the knee in 15 to 20 degrees of flexion to prevent posterior subluxation of the tibia

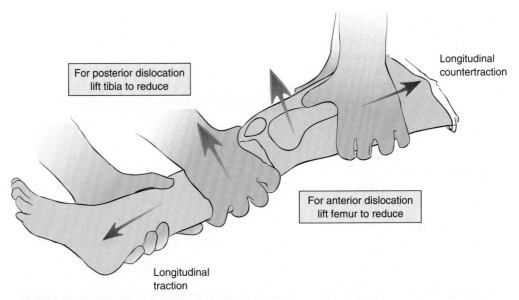

For posterior dislocation
lift tibia to reduce

Longitudinal
countertraction

For anterior dislocation
lift femur to reduce

Longitudinal
traction

FIGURE 63.3 Technique for reduction of knee joint dislocation. (From Young GM. Reduction of common joint dislocations and subluxations. In: Henretig FM, King C, eds. *Textbook of Pediatric Emergency Procedures.* Philadelphia, PA: Williams & Wilkins; 1997:1098, with permission.)

- ✦ Avoid circumferential casting or occlusive dressings
- ✦ Obtain postreduction radiographs
- ✦ Emergent arteriography, duplex ultrasonography, and/or surgical exploration is indicated if:
  - ✦ There is evidence of vascular compromise pre- or postreduction
  - ✦ The reduction cannot be obtained, maintained, or is incomplete
- ✦ All patients are admitted for neurovascular reassessments every 1 to 2 hours

COMPLICATIONS

- ✚ Popliteal vessel disruption
- ✚ Compartment syndrome, occurs 24 to 48 hours after the injury
- ✚ Pseudoaneurysms, occur hours to months after the injury
- ✚ Skin necrosis
- ✚ Articular surface damage
- ✚ Deep vein or arterial thrombosis
- ✚ Common peroneal or tibial nerve dysfunction
- ✚ Multiple concomitant ligament sprains/ruptures
- ✚ Chronic osteoarthritis and knee dysfunction

SAFETY/QUALITY TIPS

✚ **Procedural**
  - ✦ Adequate analgesia and sedation is essential in these high-force injuries
  - ✦ The pucker or dimple sign is a characteristic dimpling of the skin along the anteromedial knee seen in posterolateral knee dislocations. It indicates entrapment of tissues within the joint space and extrusion of the medial femoral condyle from the joint capsule; dislocations with a pucker sign are associated with skin necrosis and peroneal nerve injury, and emergent open reduction with ligamentous repair is indicated.
  - ✦ In addition to the notorious vascular complications of knee dislocation, important neurologic complications include common peroneal nerve and posterior tibial nerve injury. Common peroneal nerve function is tested by the strength of ankle dorsiflexion and sensation at the dorsum of the foot, whereas tibial nerve function is tested by the strength of ankle plantar flexion and sensation at the plantar surface of the foot.

◻ Cognitive

✤ Common presentation with multisystem trauma makes detection difficult; spontaneous reduction is the rule—examine the knee ligaments for laxity.

✤ Vascular injury must be fully evaluated when knee dislocation is suspected

✤ Closed reduction should always be attempted with emergent priority if the injured extremity has clinical evidence of ischemia; prompt joint reduction can restore perfusion and improve outcomes

◻ Acknowledgment

Thank you to prior author James E. Rodriguez.

Suggested Readings

Antosia RE, Robert E, Lyn E, et al. *Rosen's Emergency Medicine: Concepts and Clinical Practice.* 5th ed. St Louis, MO: Mosby; 2002:689–692.

Robert DM, Stallard TC. Emergency department evaluation and treatment of knee and leg injuries. *Emerg Med Clin North Am.* 2000;15:67–84.

Ulfberg JW, McNamara RM. Management of common dislocations. In: Roberts JR, Hedges JR, eds. *Clinical Procedures in Emergency Medicine.* 4th ed. Philadelphia, PA: WB Saunders; 2004:977–998.

64

Patellar Dislocation and Reduction

Meagan Lewis and Moira Davenport

INDICATIONS

- Clinical suspicion of patellar dislocation
  - The knee is held in 20 to 30 degrees of flexion
  - An obvious deformity is typically seen
  - Dislocated patella on x-ray (anteroposterior [AP] or sunrise views; lateral view less helpful)

CONTRAINDICATIONS

- Fracture
- Effusion (hemarthrosis)

TECHNIQUE

- Patellar dislocations frequently relocate spontaneously before the patient seeks treatment
- **Intravenous Sedation and Muscle Relaxation**
  - Often the procedure may be accomplished without use of sedation or muscle relaxation
- **Reduction Procedure**
  - Reduction is performed by manually applying pressure to the patella in an anteromedial direction while extending the extremity
    - A palpable relocation should be felt and confirmed by relief of the patient's symptoms
  - Reduction may be difficult due to the medial patellar facet being locked on to the lateral femoral condyle
    - In these cases, apply downward pressure to the lateral patella which creates the external rotational force needed to unlock the facet (**FIGURE 64.1**). Continue with the standard reduction technique.

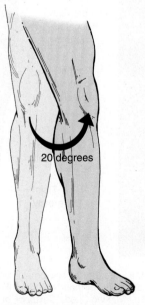

FIGURE 64.1 Apprehension test.

✛ Postprocedure

- ✛ Postreduction films should include an anteroposterior, lateral, and sunrise (Merchant) patellar view to evaluate for any fractures or osteochondral avulsion fragments which may need arthroscopic removal at a later time (FIGURE 64.2)
- ✛ Immobilization in full leg extension for 3 to 6 weeks is warranted, preferably in a commercially available knee immobilizer or a Jones-type compression dressing
- ✛ Patients should be instructed to elevate the extremity and apply ice to the area to reduce swelling

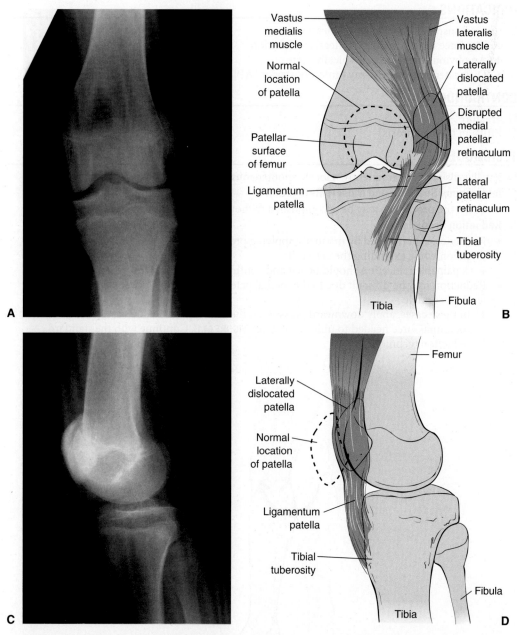

FIGURE 64.2 Patella dislocation. **A:** P x-ray of the knee. **B:** Key anatomic landmarks of the anteroposterior x-ray. **C:** Lateral x-ray of the knee. **D:** Key anatomic landmarks of the lateral x-ray. (From Young GM. Reduction of common joint dislocations and subluxations. In: Henretig FM, King C, eds. *Textbook of Pediatric Emergency Procedures*. Philadelphia, PA: Williams & Wilkins; 1997:1089, with permission.)

✦ Provide and prescribe appropriate analgesia for pain
✦ Crutches maybe used as an aid for weight bearing as tolerated
✦ Orthopedic follow-up should be given within 2 weeks of event
✦ Patients may be instructed to do straight-leg raises to strengthen the quadriceps muscle; however, this should be deferred until the patient is seen by an orthopedic surgeon and proper physical therapy regimens are arranged
✦ Patellar-stabilizing braces may be worn at a later time

COMPLICATIONS

⊞ Pain
⊞ Inability to relocate, requiring surgical treatment
⊞ Moderate rate of recurrence

SAFETY/QUALITY TIPS

⊞ **Procedural**
    ✦ Patellar dislocation reduction can often be accomplished without sedation and analgesia, but if patient is tense with pain, provide as appropriate
⊞ **Cognitive**
    ✦ Patellar dislocations can be confused for knee dislocations. A knee dislocation is an orthopedic emergency, generally the result of a high force mechanism and is strongly associated with popliteal artery injury. Like patellar dislocation, knee dislocation often reduces spontaneously, but the patient is generally left with an unstable knee with multiple ligaments disrupted.
    ✦ Patellar dislocations can easily be missed in a polytrauma patient

⊞ **Acknowledgment**

Thank you to prior author Maria Vasilyadis and Jeffrey Manko.

Suggested Readings

Canale S, Beaty J. *Campbell's Operative Orthopaedics*. 12th ed. (4-vol set). Philadelphia, PA: Elsevier; 2013.
Glaspy JN, Steele MT. *Tintinalli's Emergency Medicine: A Comprehensive Study Guide*. 7th ed. New York, NY: McGraw-Hill; 2011.
Knoop KJ, Stack LB, Storrow AB, et al. *The Atlas of Emergency Medicine*. 3rd ed. New York, NY: McGraw-Hill; 2010.
Marx JA, Hockberger RS, Walls RM. *Rosen's Emergency Medicine Concepts and Clinical Practice*. 8th ed. Philadelphia, PA: Elsevier; 2014.
Roberts JR, Custalow CB, Thomsen TW, et al. *Roberts & Hedges' Clinical Procedures in Emergency Medicine*. 6th ed. Philadelphia, PA: Elsevier; 2014.

65

Elbow Dislocation and Reduction

Tara S. Sexton and Anand K. Swaminathan

INDICATIONS

☐ Clinical suspicion of acute anterior, posterior, lateral, medial, or divergent dislocation with or without neurovascular compromise
  ✛ The clinical presentation depends on the type of dislocation
  ✛ Suspected dislocation is clinically confirmed by disruption of the relationship between the tip of the olecranon and the distal epicondyles of the humerus in comparison with the unaffected elbow
☐ Radiographic evidence of anterior, posterior, lateral, medial, or divergent dislocation (FIGURE 65.1)

CONTRAINDICATIONS

☐ Open dislocations require emergent consultations with an orthopedic surgeon
☐ Multiple failed reduction attempts with adequate sedation should prompt consultation with an orthopedic surgeon
☐ Irreducible elbow dislocations may require operative management
☐ An elbow that has been unreduced for 7 or more days will likely require open reduction with an orthopedic surgeon

RISKS/CONSENT ISSUES

☐ Procedural sedation may be associated with loss of airway reflexes and respiratory arrest (these risks are extremely rare)
☐ Soft-tissue injury may occur with reduction attempts
☐ Fractures and neurovascular injury may occur with reduction attempts

☐ **General Basic Steps**
  ✛ **Obtain necessary x-rays**
  ✛ **Sedation/Analgesia**
  ✛ **Position patient**
  ✛ **Reduction**
  ✛ **Postprocedure exam/x-rays**

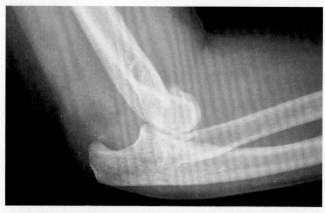

FIGURE 65.1 Posterior dislocation of the olecranon. (From Campbell C. Elbow dislocation. In: Greenberg MI, ed. *Greenberg's Text-Atlas of Emergency Medicine*. Philadelphia, PA: Lippincott Williams & Wilkins; 2005:492, with permission.)

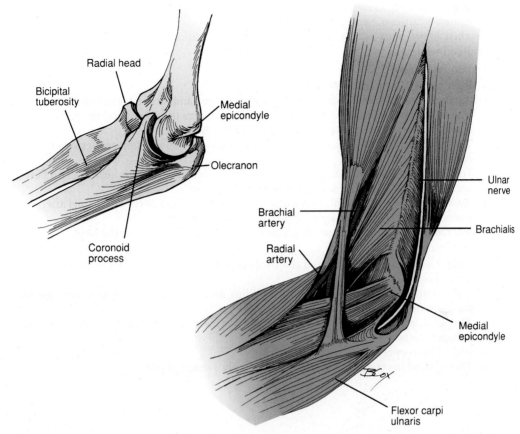

FIGURE 65.2 Elbow anatomy. (From McCue FC III, Sweeney T, Urch S. The elbow, wrist, and hand. In: Perrin DH, ed. *The Injured Athlete*. 3rd ed. Philadelphia, PA: Lippincott Williams & Wilkins; 1999, with permission.)

TECHNIQUE

- Perform a complete neurovascular check before any reduction attempt
- Obtain radiographs of the affected joint and consider radiographs of one joint above and below the injury (shoulder and wrist)
  - Complex dislocations (those with associated fractures) may require consultation with orthopedic surgery
  - Dislocations with neurovascular compromise should be reduced without prior imaging
- Anesthesia/analgesia: Consider parenteral analgesics. Reduction may also be attempted with injection of local anesthetic alone into the elbow joint or an ultrasound-guided brachial plexus block
- Reduction technique is determined by the type of dislocation

TECHNIQUE: POSTERIOR DISLOCATION

- 80% to 90% of all elbow dislocations
- Mechanism of injury: Most commonly caused by a fall on an outstretched hand with the arm in extension
- Clinical presentation: Shortened forearm that is held in flexion with a prominent olecranon posteriorly. In addition, a defect may be palpable above the olecranon **(FIGURE 65.2)**.
- Associated injuries:
  - Fractures including radial head and coronoid process are common
  - Small fractures of the coronoid process may be treated as simple posterior dislocations
  - Neurologic symptoms accompany 15% to 22% of dislocations
    - Ulnar nerve injury is most common followed by median nerve injury
    - Radial nerve injury commonly occurs when the dislocation is complicated by radial head fracture

- + Traction leading to stretch injury, local swelling, and entrapment during reduction are common causes of nerve injury
- + Brachial artery injury occurs in 5% to 13% of posterior dislocations

◻ **Reduction Techniques**
- + **Supine Technique**
  - + Place patient in supine position
  - + An assistant stabilizes the humerus by wrapping both hands around arm just distal to axilla
  - + The physician grasps the wrist with one hand and places the other hand just above the antecubital fossa with the thumb on the olecranon (**FIGURE 65.3**)
  - + The physician applies slow, steady in-line traction while the assistant applies steady countertraction
  - + To minimize additional trauma to the coronoid process, the elbow is held in slight flexion and the wrist is held in supination as traction is applied
  - + Avoid hyperextension as this may cause injury to the median nerve or brachial artery
  - + Reduction is accompanied by a "clunk" that is heard or felt
  - + Alternatively, the forearm may be gently flexed in an effort to reduce the joint
- + **Seated Technique**
  - + Patient is seated in a high backed chair with arm hanging over the back of the chair in a flexed position
  - + The physician applies traction by gently pulling down on the patient's hand while guiding the olecranon into place using the other hand
  - + The physician may also elect to simply apply downward pressure onto the olecranon to reduce the elbow
  - + Reduction is once again signaled by a "clunk"
  - + This method has the advantage of requiring only a single physician

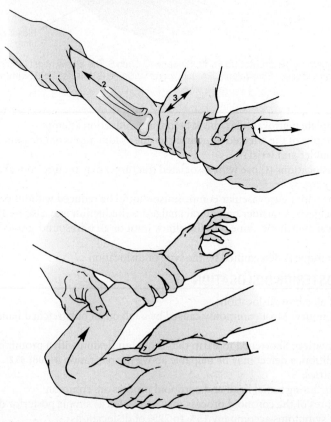

FIGURE 65.3 Technique for reduction of posterior dislocation of the elbow. (From Perron AD, Germann CA. Elbow injuries. In: Wolfson AB. *Harwood-Nuss' Clinical Practice of Emergency Medicine*. 6th ed. Philadelphia, PA: Lippincott Williams & Wilkins; 2015:260, with permission.)

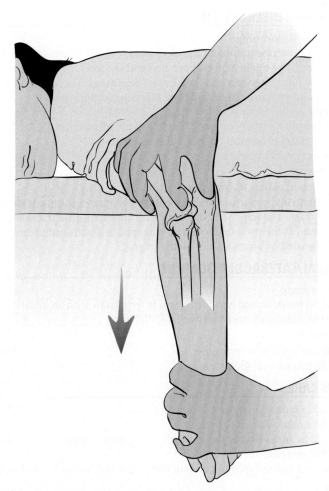

FIGURE 65.4 Technique for reduction of elbow joint dislocation. (From Young GM. Reduction of common joint dislocations and subluxations. In: Henretig FM, King C, eds. *Textbook of Pediatric Emergency Procedures.* Philadelphia, PA: Williams & Wilkins; 1997:1097, with permission.)

+ **Prone Technique**
  + Patient is positioned prone with the arm hanging flexed over the edge of the stretcher **(FIGURE 65.4)**
  + Traction is applied to the forearm, either by the physician or with weights
  + Forward and downward pressure that is applied to the olecranon with the physician's thumbs will facilitate reduction
  + Assistant applying gentle countertraction on the humerus may also help
+ **Leverage Technique**
  + Place the patient in supine position
  + The patient's elbow is flexed and forearm is supinated
  + The physician places his/her elbow on the patient's distal bicep and grasps the patient's wrist or hand
  + The physician's other hand is placed on the dorsal aspect of the patient's forearm
  + The physician's arm acts as a lever guiding the patient's elbow through gradual flexion with the physician's elbow providing steady downward countertraction force
  + Reduction is signaled by an audible or tactile "clunk"
  + This method has the advantage of requiring only a single physician

TECHNIQUE: ANTERIOR DISLOCATION

- 10% to 15% of elbow dislocations
- Mechanism: Direct posterior trauma to the olecranon with the elbow in flexed position
- Clinical presentation: The upper arm is shortened and the forearm appears elongated. Arm is held with the elbow fully extended and the forearm supinated. There is anterior tenting of the proximal forearm and prominence of the distal humerus posteriorly.
- Associated injuries:
  - These injuries require a large amount of force and are often open
  - Brachial artery injury is common in open dislocations
  - Ulnar nerve injury is uncommon
- **Reduction Technique**
  - Patient is positioned supine on stretcher
  - The assistant encircles humerus with both hands and applies countertraction
  - The physician grasps the wrist with one hand and applies in-line traction while the second hand is positioned at the proximal forearm, and applies downward pressure
  - Reduction is signaled by an audible or tactile "clunk"

TECHNIQUE: MEDIAL/LATERAL DISLOCATION

- Epidemiology: Very rare
- Mechanism: Fall on outstretched hand with arm in extension with an additional vector force which displaces the radius/ulna medially or laterally
- **Reduction technique**
  - Same as posterior reduction technique
  - Arm should be placed in slight extension

POSTREDUCTION CARE

- Ensure stability after reduction by gentle range of motion
- Perform a complete neurovascular check
- Immobilize the elbow in 90-degree flexion with a long-arm posterior splint (5–7 days is usually sufficient for stable injuries)
- Obtain postreduction radiographs to confirm reduction and to check for associated injuries

COMPLICATIONS

- Delayed vascular compromise
  - May result from reduction attempts or continued soft-tissue swelling
  - Loosen splint, if already in place
  - Consider arteriogram, surgical consultation
- Median or ulnar nerve injury
- Decreased range of motion
  - Often caused by entrapped medial epicondyle fracture fragment
  - May be secondary to prolonged immobilization
  - Requires surgical intervention
- Anterior dislocations have a high rate of associated vascular injury
  - Emergent orthopedic consultation is required for any open anterior dislocation as well as any anterior dislocation with suspected vascular compromise
- Myositis ossificans may occur when significant hemarthroses accompanies dislocation

SAFETY/QUALITY TIPS

- **Procedural**
  - Adequate analgesia and sedation make success more likely
  - If available, have a colleague help you with countertraction
  - If one technique fails to reduce the joint, try a different technique

⬚ **Cognitive**
+ Examine pre- and postreduction films for fractures
+ Check neurovascular status before and after reduction attempts
+ Treat open dislocations like open fractures—tetanus, antibiotics, early orthopedic consultation

⬚ **Acknowledgment**

Thank you to prior author Elizabeth M. Borock.

Suggested Readings

Geideerman JM. Humerus and elbow. In: Marx JA, Hockberger RS, Walls RM, eds. *Rosen's Emergency Medicine Concepts and Clinical Practice.* 6th ed. Philadelphia, PA: Mosby; 2006:647–670.

Hendrickson RG, Silverberg M. *Greenberg's Text Atlas of Emergency Medicine: A Visual Guide to Diagnosis and Treatment.* Philadelphia, PA: Lippincott Williams & Wilkins; 2005:492–493.

Hildebrand KA, Patterson SD, King GJW. Acute elbow dislocations: simple and complex. *Orthop Clin North Am.* 1999;30(1):63–79.

Horn AE, Ufberg JW. Management of common dislocations. In: Roberts JR, Custalow CB, Thomsen TW, et al. eds. *Roberts and Hedges' Clinical Procedures in Emergency Medicine.* 6th ed. WB Saunders; 2004:954–998.

Kumar A, Ahmed M. Closed reduction of posterior dislocation of the elbow: a simple technique. *J Orthop Trauma.* 1999;13(1):58–59.

Mehta JA, Bain GI. Elbow dislocations in adults and children. *Clin Sports Med.* 2004;23:609–627.

Platz A, Heinzelmann M, Ertel W, et al. Posterior elbow dislocation with associated vascular injury after blunt trauma. *J Trauma.* 1999;46(5):948–950.

Rasool MN. Dislocations of the elbow in children. *J Bone Joint Surg [Br].* 2004;86–B(7):1050–1058.

Simon RR, Brenner BE. *Emergency Procedures and Techniques.* 4th ed. Philadelphia, PA: Lippincott Williams & Wilkins; 2002:281.

Simon RR, Sherman SC. eds. *Emergency Orthopedics.* 6th ed. New York, NY: McGraw-Hill; 2011.

66

Hip Dislocation and Reduction

Brent T. Rau and Mara S. Aloi

INDICATIONS

- ✚ Clinical suspicion of hip dislocation
  - ✚ Hip pain with obvious deformity in the setting of a motor vehicle crash, pedestrian struck by a vehicle, falls, or sports-related injuries
- ✚ Radiographic evidence of hip dislocation

CONTRAINDICATIONS

- ✚ Associated femoral neck fracture
- ✚ Coexistent fracture in dislocated extremity

RISKS/CONSENT ISSUES

- ✚ Inadvertently converting a dislocation to a fracture-dislocation (acetabulum or femoral head fracture)
  - ✚ More common in the elderly with osteoporotic bones
- ✚ Oversedation may lead to inability to protect the airway with subsequent potential risk of aspiration

- ✚ **General Basic Steps**
  - ✚ **Obtain radiographs**
  - ✚ **Sedation/Analgesia**
  - ✚ **Have assistants for help**
  - ✚ **Perform procedure**

LANDMARKS

- ✚ **Posterior Hip Dislocation**
  - ✚ Mechanism of injury—femoral head is forced out of the acetabulum and rests posteriorly
  - ✚ Clinical features—affected extremity shortened, adducted, and internally rotated; patient may hold hip flexed with knee of affected extremity resting on opposite knee (FIGURE 66.1)
  - ✚ Radiographic evidence—femoral head resting posterior to the acetabulum (FIGURE 66.2)
- ✚ **Anterior Hip Dislocation**
  - ✚ Mechanism—forced abduction with the hip in a flexed position or forced hyperextension of the hip
  - ✚ Clinical features—affected extremity abducted, slight flexion, and externally rotated
  - ✚ Radiographic evidence—femoral head dislocated medially toward obturator foramen (obturator dislocation) and femoral head dislocated laterally toward pubis (pubic dislocation) (FIGURE 66.3)

TECHNIQUE

- ✚ Preprocedure
  - ✚ Radiographs
    - ✚ Should be obtained preprocedure only if there is a concern for a fracture or to determine the position of the dislocation

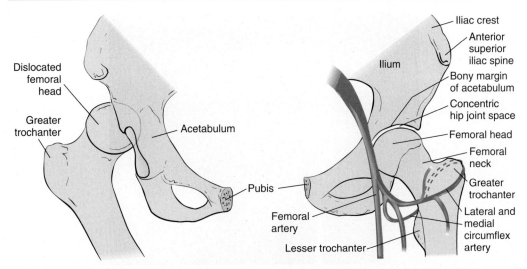

FIGURE 66.1 Normal (left) and dislocated (right) hip. (From Young GM. Reduction of common joint dislocations and subluxations. In: Henretig FM, King C, eds. *Textbook of Pediatric Emergency Procedures*. Philadelphia, PA: Williams & Wilkins; 1997:1093, with permission.)

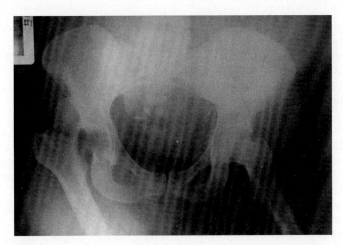

FIGURE 66.2 Anteroposterior pelvis radiograph of a posterior hip dislocation of the right hip. (From Tornetta Paul III. Hip dislocations and fractures of the femoral head. In: Bucholz RW, Heckman JD, Court-Brown C, eds. *Rockwood and Green's Fractures in Adults*. Vol 2. 6th ed. Philadelphia, PA: Lippincott Williams & Wilkins; 2006:1718, with permission.)

☐ Posterior Dislocation Reduction

✛ Allis Maneuver (FIGURE 66.4)

+ Patient is placed supine
+ Downward stabilization of the pelvis is performed by an assistant
+ With the knee flexed, apply traction in-line with the deformity with gentle flexion of the hip to 90 degrees
+ Perform gentle internal-to-external rotation as the hip is flexed
+ Once reduction is achieved, hip is brought to the extended position while traction is maintained
+ Legs are then immobilized in slight abduction through the placement of pillows between the knees

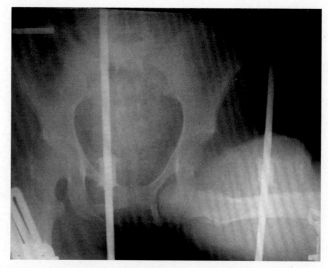

FIGURE 66.3 Anteroposterior pelvis radiograph of an anterior hip dislocation of the left hip. (From Tornetta Paul III. Hip dislocations and fractures of the femoral head. In: Bucholz RW, Heckman JD, Court-Brown C, eds. *Rockwood and Green's Fractures in Adults*. Vol 2. 6th ed. Philadelphia, PA: Lippincott Williams & Wilkins; 2006:1720, with permission.)

+ Repeat physical examination to ensure neurovascular integrity of the affected extremity
+ The reduced hip should be tested for stability by gently placing it through full range of motion to test if the hip will dislocate again
+ Reduction is confirmed by repeat radiographs

+ **Bigelow Maneuver**
    + Patient is placed supine
    + Assistant applies downward pressure on the anterior superior iliac spine
    + Grasp affected extremity at ankle and apply longitudinal traction in-line of deformity
    + Adducted thigh is flexed >90 degrees and internally rotated to relax ligaments
    + While maintaining the traction, the hip is abducted, externally rotated, and then extended as the femoral head relocates to acetabulum
    + The reduced hip should be tested for stability by gently placing it through full range of motion to test if the hip will dislocate again
    + Reduction is confirmed by repeat radiographs

+ **Stimson Technique**
    + Patient is placed prone
    + With affected extremity hanging over bed, the hip and knee are flexed 90 degrees
    + Assistant stabilizes pelvis
    + Perform steady downward traction in-line with femur
    + Assistant pushes greater trochanter anteriorly as femoral head is rotated
    + Once reduced, the hip is brought to extended position while maintaining traction
    + The reduced hip should be tested for stability by gently placing it through full range of motion to test if the hip will dislocate again
    + Reduction is confirmed by repeat radiographs

+ **Captain Morgan Technique**
    + Patient is placed supine
    + Pelvis fixed to bed or backboard with a strap
    + Affected extremity hip and knee are flexed to 90 degrees
    + Physician places his/her own foot on bed or backboard, with a knee behind patient's knee
    + Hold patient's knee in flexion by holding patient's ankle

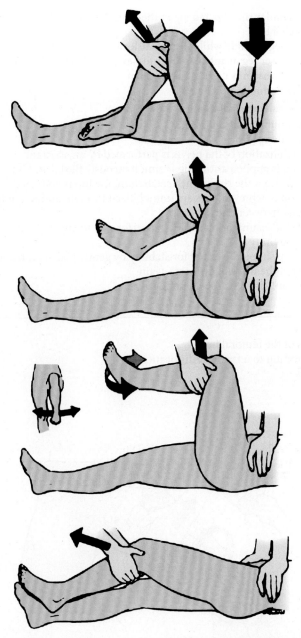

FIGURE 66.4 Allis maneuver for reduction of posterior hip dislocation. (From Tornetta Paul III. Hip dislocations and fractures of the femoral head. In: Bucholz RW, Heckman JD, Court-Brown C, eds. *Rockwood and Green's Fractures in Adults.* Vol 2. 6th ed. Philadelphia, PA: Lippincott Williams & Wilkins; 2006:1730, with permission.)

+ Upward force applied to hip by physician lifting using his/her calf while gently rotating the patient's lower leg
+ The reduced hip should be tested for stability by gently placing it through full range of motion to test if the hip will dislocate again
+ Reduction is confirmed by repeat radiographs
+ **Whistler Technique**
    + Patient is placed supine
    + Assistant stabilizes pelvis and maintains flexion of unaffected leg

+ Place forearm under the affected leg in the popliteal fossa while grasping the knee of the flexed unaffected leg
+ Grasp affected leg at ankle while flexing dislocated hip to 90 degrees
+ Pull down on lower leg, using it as lever to flex knee and pull traction along the femur. The provider's forearm is used as the fulcrum.

◘ **Anterior Dislocation Reduction**
  ✦ **Modified Allis Maneuver (FIGURE 66.5)**
    + Do not use for pubic dislocations
    + Patient is placed supine
    + Downward stabilization of the pelvis is performed by an assistant
    + In-line traction is applied as the hip is simultaneously flexed and internally rotated
    + Once the head clears the rim of the acetabulum, the hip is abducted
    + Once reduction is achieved, legs are immobilized in slight abduction through the placement of pillows between the knees
    + A repeat physical examination should be performed to ensure neurovascular integrity of the affected extremity
    + The reduced hip should be tested for stability by gently placing it through full range of motion to test if the hip will dislocate again
    + Reduction is confirmed by repeat radiographs

COMPLICATIONS

◘ Sciatic nerve injury
◘ Avascular necrosis of the femoral head
◘ Converting a dislocation to a fracture/dislocation
◘ Traumatic arthritis
◘ Joint instability

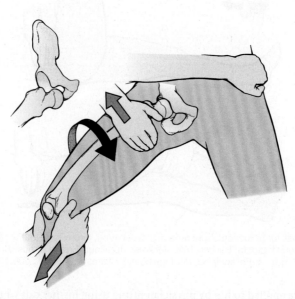

FIGURE 66.5 Modified Allis maneuver for reduction of anterior hip dislocation. (From Tornetta Paul III. Hip dislocations and fractures of the femoral head. In: Bucholz RW, Heckman JD, Court-Brown C, eds. *Rockwood and Green's Fractures in Adults*. Vol 2. 6th ed. Philadelphia, PA: Lippincott Williams & Wilkins; 2006:1730, with permission.)

SAFETY/QUALITY TIPS

⊡ **Procedural**
+ Use adequate analgesia, sedation, and muscle relaxation
+ Hip reduction can require significant force
+ Stabilization of the pelvis by an assistant greatly improves the ease of reduction

⊡ **Cognitive**
+ All native hip dislocations should be considered an orthopedic emergency, especially if clinical evidence of neurovascular injury exists. Avascular necrosis of the femoral head is a major concern in hip dislocations; to minimize the risk, reduction should be performed as soon as possible.
+ Dislocation of a native hip generally requires significant force. Evaluate for associated injuries, especially in the setting of motor vehicle crash.
+ Posterior hip dislocations constitute 80% to 90% of hip dislocations
+ Orthopedic consultation should be obtained for hip dislocation in the presence of a fracture, and for most prosthetic hip dislocations for concern of loosening components of the prosthesis, fracture of the surrounding bone, or movement of the acetabular capsule.

⊡ **Acknowledgment**
Thank you to prior author Tania V. Mariani and Rama B. Rao.

Suggested Readings

Hendey GW, Avila A. The captain morgan technique for the reduction of the dislocated hip. *Ann Emerg Med.* 2011;58:536–540.

Marx JA, Hockberger RS, Walls RM. *Rosen's Emergency Medicine: Concepts and Clinical Practice.* 7th ed. Mosby; 2010:633–638.

Roberts JR, Custalow CB, Thomsen TW, et al. *Roberts & Hedges' Clinical Procedures in Emergency Medicine.* 6th ed. WB Saunders; 2013.

Tintinalli JE, Stapczynski JS, Ma OJ, et al. *Emergency Medicine: A Comprehensive Study Guide.* 7th ed. McGraw-Hill; 2010.

Tornetta P III. Hip dislocations and fractures of the femoral head. In Bucholz RW, Heckman JD, Court-Brown C, eds. *Rockwood and Green's Fractures in Adults.* Vol 2. 6th ed. Philadelphia, PA: Lippincott Williams & Wilkins; 2006:1715–1749.

67

Ankle Dislocation and Reduction

Mara S. Aloi

INDICATIONS

- Dislocated Ankle Joint
  - + Demonstrated on plain radiographs
  - + Clinically dislocated with neurovascular compromise

CONTRAINDICATIONS

- Open dislocations without neurovascular compromise may be better managed in the operating room for cleaning before reduction
- After one or two unsuccessful attempts at reduction, orthopedic consultation should be considered

RISK/CONSENT ISSUES

- Neurovascular damage may result from reduction attempt
- Closed reduction may be unsuccessful and operative repair may be required
- Risks of intravenous (IV) analgesia/sedation
- Risks of regional anesthesia

- **General Basic Steps**
  - + **Patient preparation**
  - + **Obtain radiographs**
  - + **Analgesia/Sedation**
  - + **Reduce joint**
  - + **Check neurovascular status**
  - + **Immobilize joint**
  - + **Postprocedure radiographs**

LANDMARKS

- The ankle joint is a modified saddle joint that comprises the distal fibula, tibia, and the talus bone of the foot
- Is a stable joint with strong ligamentous support
- Dislocations are a result of significant forces applied to the ankle and are often associated with fractures; isolated dislocations are uncommon

TECHNIQUE

- Preprocedure Examination
  - + Search for other injuries, especially if high-energy mechanism
  - + Check neurovascular status of the foot
  - + Get prereduction radiographs of dislocation (anteroposterior [AP], lateral, mortise views)
    - + If there is neurovascular compromise or tenting of the skin, perform immediate reduction before obtaining radiograph
  - + Try to ascertain the mechanism of injury
- Analgesia and Sedation
  - + Procedural sedation
  - + Regional analgesia
    - + Bier block
    - + Hematoma block

☐ **Procedure**
   ✦ Technique depends on type of dislocation but, in general, involves downward traction on heel while a force opposite to the direction of the dislocation is applied
   ✦ Flexion of the hip and knee to 90 degrees may aid reduction by relaxing the gastrocnemius–soleus complex
      ✛ If no assistant is available this can be accomplished by hanging the patient's knee over the end of the bed

LATERAL DISLOCATION (FIGURE 67.1)

☐ Most common ankle dislocation seen in the emergency department (ED)
☐ Usually result of forced inversion of the foot
☐ Associated with malleolar or distal fibula fractures
☐ May be associated with rupture of the deltoid ligament
☐ Presents with foot laterally displaced with the skin very taut over the medial aspect of the ankle joint
☐ **Technique**
   ✦ Place one hand on the heel and the other on the dorsum of the foot
   ✦ Apply longitudinal traction to the foot
   ✦ While assistant applies countertraction to the leg, gently manipulate the foot medially. Successful reduction usually produces a palpable thud.

POSTERIOR DISLOCATION (FIGURE 67.1)

☐ Usually result of forced plantar flexion or a strong forward force applied to the posterior tibia
☐ Most are associated with a fracture of one or more malleoli
☐ Presents with the ankle held in plantar flexion with foot shortened in appearance and resistant to dorsiflexion

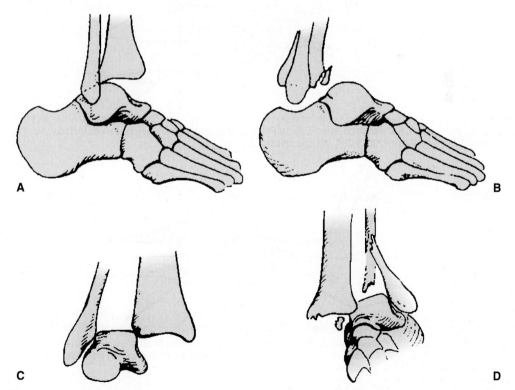

FIGURE 67.1 Four types of ankle dislocations. **A:** Posterior. **B:** Anterior. **C:** Superior. **D:** Lateral. (From Simon RR, Brenner BE. *Emergency Procedures and Techniques.* 4th ed. Philadelphia, PA: Lippincott Williams & Wilkins; 2002:285, with permission.)

○ **Technique**
  ✦ Physician places one hand on the heel and the other on the forefoot
  ✦ Plantar flex the foot while pulling it forward and applying downward traction
  ✦ Dorsiflex the foot and push heel anteriorly
  ✦ Assistant may provide posteriorly directed pressure on the tibia while maintaining flexion of the knee and hip and countertraction of the lower leg (FIGURE 67.2)

ANTERIOR DISLOCATION

○ Usually result of forced dorsiflexion of the foot or a force to the tibia directed posteriorly while the foot is fixed
○ May be associated with loss of dorsalis pedis pulse secondary to pressure from the talus
○ Most common cause is deceleration injuries as seen in motor vehicle accidents
○ Frequently associated with malleolar fractures or a fracture of the anterior lip of the tibia
○ Typically presents with foot held in dorsiflexion with elongated appearance
○ **Technique**
  ✦ Assistant provides countertraction over the calf
  ✦ Physician places one hand on the heel and the other on the forefoot
  ✦ Slightly dorsiflex the foot to free the talus
  ✦ Straight longitudinal traction is applied while the foot is pushed directly backward
  ✦ Assistant provides anteriorly directed pressure on the back of the lower leg (FIGURE 67.3)

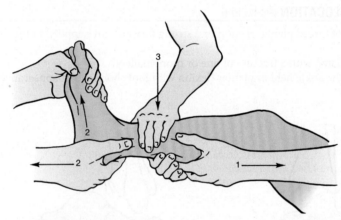

FIGURE 67.2 Technique of reduction of posterior dislocation of the ankle. (From Shah K, Desai N. Ankle and foot injuries. In: Wolfson AB, ed. *Harwood-Nuss' Clinical Practice of Emergency Medicine*. 4th ed. Philadelphia, PA: Lippincott Williams & Wilkins; 2015:294, with permission.)

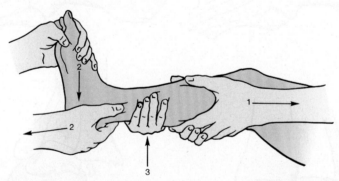

FIGURE 67.3 Technique of reduction of anterior dislocation of the ankle. (From Shah K, Desai N. Ankle and foot injuries. In: Wolfson AB, ed. *Harwood-Nuss' Clinical Practice of Emergency Medicine*. 4th ed. Philadelphia, PA: Lippincott Williams & Wilkins; 2015:294, with permission.)

SUPERIOR DISLOCATION

- Uncommon
- Usually result of significant compresion force which drives the talus upward resulting in diastasis of the tibiofibular joint
- Commonly results from a person landing on feet from a significant height
- Evaluate carefully for concomitant spine injury
- Emergency consultation with an orthopedist is required for open reduction and internal fixation
- **Technique**
  - ✦ Splint, then call for an emergent consultation with an orthopedist

POSTREDUCTION CARE

- Recheck neurovascular status and document the findings
- Order postreduction radiographs
- Adequate immobilization is required for comfort and to prevent redislocation
  - ✦ Ankle is splinted at 90 degrees with a long-leg posterior splint
  - ✦ Splint anterior dislocations in slight plantar flexion
  - ✦ Reconfirm neurovascular status after splint application
- Follow-up for orthopedic consultation is required within 48 to 72 hours for closed fractures without neurovascular compromise
- Open injuries, superior dislocations, and fracture dislocations with neurovascular compromise require emergent orthopedic consultation
- Recommendations for follow-up care are dependent on the injury and its severity. Necessity to admit to the hospital must be determined in consultation with an orthopedic surgeon.
- The patient should not bear weight on that extremity for approximately 6 weeks

COMPLICATIONS

- Nonunion or malunion
- Synostosis—union of two or more bones to form one bone
- Entrapment of the tibialis posterior tendon or of a fracture fragment
- Cartilaginous injury
- Osteochondral fractures of the talar dome
- Joint stiffness and decreased range of motion
- Arterial injury (anterior and posterior tibial, peroneal)
- Avascular necrosis of the talus
- Compartment syndrome (rare)

SAFETY/QUALITY TIPS

- **Procedural**
  - ✦ Use adequate analgesia and sedation to effect muscle relaxation
  - ✦ Assess vascular integrity immediately and repeatedly
  - ✦ If neurovascular function is compromised, do not delay reduction to obtain x-rays
- **Cognitive**
  - ✦ Do not neglect to search for concomitant injuries
  - ✦ Contact an orthopedist if multiple attempts in reduction are needed or if there is an open injury, superior dislocation, or neurovascular compromise

- **Acknowledgment**
Thank you to prior author Cassandra Jo Haddox.

Suggested Readings

Handel DA, Gaines SA. Ankle injuries. In: Tintinalli J, ed. *Emergency Medicine. A Comprehensive Study Guide.* 7th ed. New York, NY: McGraw-Hill; 2011.

Roberts JR, Hedges JR. *Clinical Procedures in Emergency Medicine.* 4th ed. Philadelphia, PA: WB Saunders; 2004.

Shah K. Ankle and foot injuries. In: Wolfson AB, ed. *Harwood-Nuss' Clinical Practice of Emergency Medicine.* 4th ed. Philadelphia, PA: Lippincott Williams & Wilkins; 2005.

Simon RR, Brenner BE. *Emergency Procedures and Techniques.* 4th ed. Philadelphia, PA: Lippincott Williams & Wilkins; 2002:284–285.

Simon RR, Sherman SC. *Emergency Orthopedics: The Extremities.* 6th ed. New York, NY: McGraw-Hill; 2011.

68

Digit Dislocation and Reduction

Amie M. Kim and Moira Davenport

INDICATIONS

- Clinical suspicion of joint dislocation
  - Incidence of dislocations: Dorsal proximal interphalangeal (PIP) >> volar PIP >> dorsal metacarpal (MCP) thumb > dorsal MCP finger >> volar MCP dorsal distal interphalangeal (DIP) >> volar DIP
- Radiographic evidence of dislocation

CONTRAINDICATIONS

- Complex dislocation—rupture of or entrapment in the joint of ligaments or tendons surrounding the joint requires open reduction and repair
- Chronic dislocation (>3 weeks duration)
- Open dislocation
- Unstable joint
- Multiple failed reduction attempts can convert a simple dislocation into a complex dislocation and prompt urgent orthopedic consult

- **General Basic Steps**
  - **Neurovascular examination**
  - **Prereduction radiograph**
  - **Analgesia**
  - **Reduction**
  - **Postreduction neurovascular examination**
  - **Immobilization**
  - **Postreduction radiograph**

LANDMARKS

- Nerves run on the lateral surface of each digit at the 2, 4, 8, and 10 o'clock positions
- Flexor tendons run on the volar surface of the digit
- Extensor tendons run on the dorsal surface of the digit
- PIP joint
  - Dorsal dislocation: The fibrous volar plate resists dorsal dislocations (FIGURE 68.1)
    - Complex dislocation: Head of proximal phalanx or ruptured volar plane can become entrapped in the joint space (FIGURE 68.2)
  - Volar dislocation: Three bands of the extensor tendon (central slip, radial and ulnar lateral bands) resist volar dislocations (FIGURE 68.3)
    - Complex dislocation: Extensor slip tendons can rupture and become entrapped within the joint space (FIGURE 68.4)
  - Lateral dislocation: Radial collateral ligaments resist ulnar dislocation, ulnar collateral ligaments resist radial dislocation
- DIP and thumb IP: Mechanisms of dislocation and reduction are anatomically analogous

RISKS/CONSENT ISSUES

- Risks in joint reduction include swelling with permanent joint enlargement, residual pain, stiffness, or deformity and conversion into complex dislocation including fracture
- Risks in anesthesia

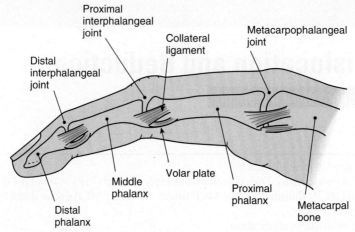

FIGURE 68.1 Fibrous volar plates are found at the MCP and IP joints where they reinforce the joint capsules and limit hyperextension. (From Leggit, JC, Meko CJ. Acute finger injuries: Part I. Tendons and ligaments. *Am Fam Physician.* 2006;73(5):810–816.)

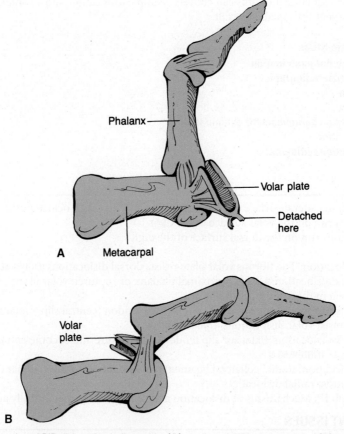

FIGURE 68.2 Complex dorsal PIP dislocation indicated by **(A)** rupture of PIP volar plate and **(B)** entrapment of volar plate fibers and head of proximal phalanx into the joint space. (Jackimczyk K, Shepherd SM, Blackburn P. Hand injuries. In: Wolfson AB, ed. *Harwood-Nuss' Clinical Practice of Emergency Medicine.* 5th ed. Philadelphia, PA: Williams & Wilkins; 2009, with permission.)

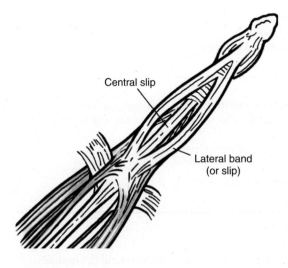

Central slip

Lateral band
(or slip)

FIGURE 68.3 Extensor tendon mechanism trifurcates at the dorsum of the proximal phalanx (Reichman EF. *Emergency Medicine Procedures.* 2013. Permission pending.)

SUPPLIES

- Anesthesia
- Reduction: 3″ Webril or gauze padding, 3″ plaster roll, 3″ Ace bandage, aluminum finger splint, adhesive tape, scissors

NEUROVASCULAR EXAMINATION

Any deficit indicates a complex dislocation and urgent orthopedic consultation
- Inspection
  + Exclude open dislocation
  + Complex dislocation presents with less angulated deformities, with skin dimpling, or rotational deformity of the involved phalanges
- Palpation—frank fracture fragments
- Sensation—normal two-point discrimination on finger pad is between 2 to 4 mm
- Vascular—radial and ulnar pulse-Doppler signal
- Range of motion with stress—assess joint stability with the finger in full extension and in moderate flexion. If displacement occurs, the joint is unstable.

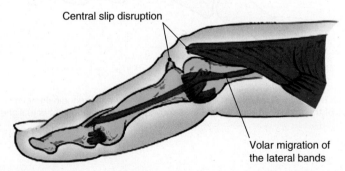

Boutonnière deformity

Central slip disruption

Volar migration of
the lateral bands

FIGURE 68.4 Central slip of the extensor tendon can rupture in sudden IP hyperflexion and can require operative repair. (From Leggit JC, Meko CJ. Acute finger injuries: Part I. Tendons and ligaments. *Am Fam Physician.* 2006;73(5):810–816.)

- ✦ Apply volar stress to assess volar plate integrity
- ✦ Apply dorsal stress to assess extensor slip tendon
- ✦ Apply radial and ulnar stress to assess collateral ligaments

PREREDUCTION RADIOGRAPH

Anteroposterior and lateral views required
- ▢ Dislocation direction—reference the distal segment relative to the proximal segment
- ▢ Concomitant fracture of phalanx or avulsion fractures involving >30% of the articular surface indicates unstable dislocation
- ▢ Significantly widened joint space indicates entrapped structures
- ▢ **Analgesia**
  - ✦ Consider digital block, wrist block, or procedural sedation

TECHNIQUE

- ▢ **PIP Dislocation**
  - ✦ **Dorsal Dislocation**
    - ✦ To disengage the middle phalanx, exaggerate the deformity—hyperextend the middle phalanx and apply longitudinal traction distally **(FIGURE 68.5A)**
    - ✦ Apply ventral force to the dorsal base of the middle phalanx while moving the PIP into flexion **(FIGURE 68.5B)**
    - ✦ Immobilize the reduced PIP in an aluminum finger splint in 30 degrees of flexion for approximately 3 weeks
  - ✦ **Volar Dislocation**
    - ✦ To relax the extensor slip tendons—place the MCP and DIP joints in flexion and the wrist in extension
    - ✦ To disengage the middle phalanx, exaggerate the deformity—hyperextend the middle phalanx and apply longitudinal traction distally **(FIGURE 68.6)**

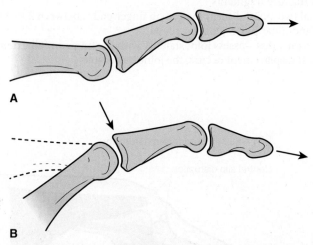

FIGURE 68.5 Dorsal PIP reduction. **A:** Middle phalanx hyperextended with longitudinal traction applied. **B:** Ventral force applied to base of the middle phalanx while PIP is moved into flexion and joint is realigned.

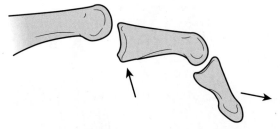

FIGURE 68.6 Volar PIP reduction. Middle phalanx hyperextended with longitudinal traction applied. Dorsal force applied to base of the middle phalanx as joint is realigned.

+ Apply dorsal force to the ventral base of the middle phalanx
+ Immobilize the reduced PIP in extension in an aluminum finger splint for approximately 6 weeks
+ Lateral Dislocation
  + To disengage the middle phalanx, apply longitudinal traction distally. Oppose the deformity and align the distal phalanx with the proximal phalanx.
  + Buddy tape the reduced digit to the adjacent digit for 3 weeks

☐ **MCP Dislocation**
+ Dorsal Dislocation
  + Minimize longitudinal traction—risks entrapping the MCP head in the anterior capsule ("buttonhole effect")
  + Relax flexor tendons—place the wrist and finger joints in flexion
  + Exaggerate the deformity—hyperextend the joint. Apply ventral force to the dorsal base of the proximal phalanx and align it over the MCP head.
  + Splint the reduced MCP in 30 degrees of flexion in a volar splint for approximately 6 weeks
+ Volar Dislocation
  + Minimize longitudinal traction—risks entrapping the torn volar plate dorsally into the joint space
  + Place the MCP joint into flexion while applying dorsal force to the ventral base of the proximal phalanx and align it over the MCP head
  + Splint the reduced MCP into extension for < 3 weeks to prevent stiffness (see Safety and Quality: Procedural)

☐ **DIP Dislocation**
+ Dorsal Dislocation
  + Apply longitudinal traction in DIP hyperextension while applying ventral force to the dorsal base of the distal phalanx (**FIGURE 68.7**)
  + Splint the isolated DIP in extension for 3 weeks
+ Volar Dislocation
  + Apply longitudinal traction in DIP hyperflexion while applying dorsal force to the ventral base of the distal phalanx
  + Splint the isolated DIP in 30 degrees flexion for 3 weeks

POSTREDUCTION NEUROVASCULAR EXAMINATION

☐ Range of motion with stress—if no subluxation or dislocation reoccurs, joint is stable and can be immobilized without orthopedic consultation

POSTREDUCTION RADIOGRAPH

☐ Presentation of occult fractures
☐ Presentation of incomplete reduction

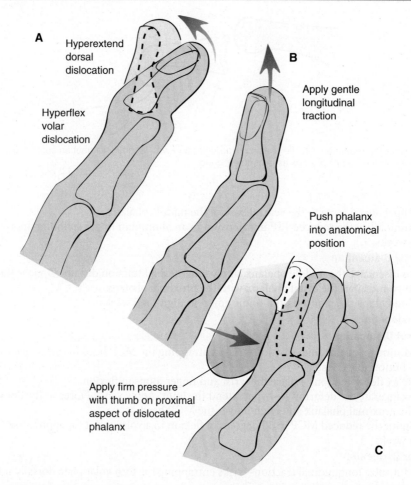

FIGURE 68.7 Dorsal DIP reduction. Longitudinal traction is applied to DIP in hyperextension while ventral force to the base of the distal phalanx is applied. (From Young GM. Reduction of common joint dislocations and subluxations. In: Henretig FM, King C, eds. *Textbook of Pediatric Emergency Procedures*. Philadelphia, PA: Williams & Wilkins; 1997:1080, with permission.)

COMPLICATIONS

☐ Inadequate or delayed reduction—contractures, deformities
☐ Aggressive reduction—fracture, injury to or entrapment of soft tissue, articular trauma
☐ Inadequate immobilization—recurrent instability, ligamentous laxity

SAFETY/QUALITY TIPS

☐ **Procedural**
  ✦ Dorsal dislocations are splinted in moderate flexion to stabilize the injured volar plate. Volar dislocations are splinted in complete extension to stabilize injured extensor slip.
  ✦ Splinted joint should be reassessed at <3 weeks to prevent joint stiffness
  ✦ MCP collateral ligaments provide tighter support in flexion. Immobilize MCP joints in flexion and IP joints in extension.
  ✦ Failure of closed reduction with adequate anesthesia can indicate complex dislocation
☐ **Cognitive**
  ✦ Thumb MCP dislocation—early recognition of gamekeeper's or skier's thumb (laxity of the ulnar collateral ligament of the thumb) is critical. Partial tear requires thumb spica immobilization for 6 weeks. Complete tear requires surgical repair.

+ PIP dislocation—if the joint is reduced prior to evaluation, the mechanism must be identified. Errant splinting of volar deformity in slight flexion or with buddy taping can result in permanent boutonniere deformity.
+ DIP dislocation—do not confuse with Mallet finger (extensor digitorum tendon injury at the DIP). Splint the DIP in extension.
+ Toe dislocations including metatarsophalangeal and IP—dislocation mechanism and reduction technique are anatomically analogous to those of finger PIP and DIP
+ All dislocations are at risk for long-term disability and warrant orthopedic follow-up

Acknowledgment

Thank you to prior authors Taylor J. Kallas and David J. Berkoff.

Suggested Readings

Reichman EF. *Emergency Medicine Procedures*. 2nd ed. New York, NY: McGraw Hill, 2013.

Simon RR, Brenner BE. *Emergency Procedures and Techniques*. 4th ed. Philadelphia, PA: Lippincott Williams & Wilkins; 2002.

69

Wound Closure and Suture Techniques

Anthony Berger

INDICATIONS

- Goals are to optimize wound strength, reduce inflammation, avoid infection, and minimize scar formation
  - Time to wound cleaning is the most important factor
  - To preserve viable tissue and restore continuity and function of tissue

CONTRAINDICATIONS

- Heavily contaminated wounds
- Presentation time for primary closure is after 12 hours for standard lacerations
- Presentation time for primary closure is after 24 hours for lacerations of the face, scalp, or other highly vascular areas
- Wounds under high tension should not be closed by skin adhesives alone
- Animal or human bite and most puncture wounds should not be closed on initial presentation

RISK/CONSENT ISSUES

- Cleaning and repair of wounds cause pain
  - Local anesthetics are indicated for all wound repairs in conscious, alert patients
- Infection is always a risk in wound repair
- Wound repair always results in some scarring and can affect cosmetic appearance permanently
- Tendon, nerve, and vascular injuries can occur at time of initial injury or at time of repair
- Risk of retained foreign body exists despite best methods of foreign body identification and removal, such as local exploration, radiographs, ultrasonography, and irrigation
  - Thorough exploration for foreign bodies must be performed and documented

- **General Basic Steps**
  - **Anesthetize wound**
  - **Clean wound**
  - **Explore wound**
  - **Consider radiography**
  - **Repair wound**

TECHNIQUE

- **Patient and Wound Preparation**
  - Position the patient to prevent falling or fainting during wound repair
  - Practice universal precautions
  - Prepare the surrounding skin with povidone–iodine solution and cover with sterile drapes before manipulation of any kind
- **Local Anesthesia:** Lidocaine (1% or 2%) with or without epinephrine
  - Epinephrine is contraindicated in areas of high risk for ischemia, such as fingers, ears, nose, toes, and penis

+ Use small-gauge needle (25 or 27 gauge) to directly inject into subcutaneous (SQ) tissue within the laceration
+ To decrease pain, inject through the wound and not through the skin
+ Use adequate amount for anesthesia but avoid high volumes that will lead to significant tissue distortion, possible cosmetic embarrassment, or systemic toxicity
    + Maximum dose: 3 to 5 mg/kg 1% lidocaine, 7 mg/kg 1% lidocaine with epinephrine.
+ Consider regional blocks for repairs in cosmetically important areas (face, hands, etc.) to avoid distortion of tissue
- **Wound Cleansing**
    + Copious amounts of sterile water or sterile saline via high-power irrigation with a large syringe and splatter shield or an 18-gauge catheter. Tap water equally effective.
- **Wound Exploration**
    + After cleansing, the true depth of the wound is appreciated
    + Look for deeper tissue involvement and explore the wound
    + If tendon or vascular structures are visualized, inspect through full range of motion, test for state of function, and document findings
- **Radiography and/or Sonography**
    + If the possibility of underlying fracture and/or foreign body exists, image the affected area and document
- **Select Method of Repair**
    + 2-Octyl cyanoacrylate
    + Staples
    + Sutures

DERMABOND (LIQUID ADHESIVE)

- Indicated for simple wounds under low tension
- **Advantages**
    + Ease of use, speed, and safety
    + No return visit necessary (sloughs off in 5 to 10 days and serves as own dressing)
    + Much less painful
- **Disadvantages**
    + Moderate closure strength—cannot be used on joints or areas with high tension
    + Cannot be used in areas with excessive hair
- Caution when using around eyes to prevent accidental runoff into eyes
- Equivalent tensile strength at 7 days when compared to sutures
- **Procedure**
    + Clean the wound
    + Approximate wound edges with forceps or fingers
    + Apply three to four layers along the wound length or perpendicularly to it (as strips)
    + Maintain manual support for 60 seconds

STAPLES

- Indicated for superficial scalp lacerations, linear lacerations on extremities, trunk, and wounds under low tension
- **Advantages**
    + Ease of use, speed, and safety
    + Easily removed and excellent tensile strength
- **Disadvantages**
    + Less refined closure
    + Possible greater scarring
    + Uncomfortable removal **(TABLE 69.1)**
- No significant differences found with infection, healing, or patient acceptance when compared to suturing

TABLE 69.1. SUTURE SIZE AND LOCATION		
Size	**Superficial (nonabsorbable)**	**Deep (absorbable)**
2-0	Suture chest tube	
3-0	Foot	Chest, abdomen, back
4-0	Scalp, chest, abdomen, foot, extremity	Scalp, extremity, foot
5-0	Scalp, brow, mouth, chest, abdomen, hand	Brow, nose, lip, face, hand
6-0	Ear, lid, brow, face, mouth, nose	

◻ **Procedure**
+ Anesthetize, clean, and debride wound as necessary
+ If necessary, close deep fascia with absorbable sutures with a buried knot
+ Evert wound edges before placing staple, if possible utilizing the services of an assistant with forceps. Do not press too hard.
+ Allow the staple crossbar to sit 1 to 2 mm above wound edge
+ Place enough staples to adequately appose tissue edges

SUTURES

◻ **General Rules**
+ Deep stitches require 3-0 or 4-0 absorbable sutures
+ Skin closure requires 4-0 or 5-0 nonabsorbable sutures
+ Face, lips, and eyelid wounds: Consider 6-0 sutures
+ High skin tension areas: Consider 3-0 or 4-0 sutures
+ Always select the smallest size that will hold the skin edges together

◻ **Nonabsorbable Sutures**
+ **Silk**: Has the best knot security, the best tie ability, the least tensile strength, and causes significant tissue reactivity. Used in intraoral mucosa.
+ **Ethilon**: Has good knot security, good tensile strength, minimal tissue reactivity, and good tie ability. Best suited suture material for typical wound closure.
+ **Prolene**: Poorest knot security, best tensile strength, least tissue reactivity, and fair tie ability

◻ **Absorbable Sutures**
+ **Vicryl**: Good knot security, good tensile strength, minimal tissue reactivity, best tie ability, and 30-day suture duration. Used for deep repair to reduce wound tension.
+ **Surgical and chromic gut**: Fair knot security, fair tensile strength, greatest tissue reactivity, poor tie ability, and 5- to 7-day suture duration. Used for intraoral wounds.

◻ **Procedure**
+ Anesthetize, clean, and debride wound as necessary
+ Prepare the skin with povidone–iodine or chlorhexidine solution
+ Minimize trauma by handling skin with toothed forceps and by using small sutures
+ Relieve tension by undermining with a scissor and by using layered sutures (FIGURE 69.1)
+ **Subcutaneous Layer Closure**
  + Reapproximate fascia as needed
  + Close the SQ layer in sections, starting in the middle and then bisecting adjacent sections until adequate tension has been relieved from the skin edges
  + Insert the suture at the bottom of the layer and draw it through to just beneath the dermis on the same side of the wound
  + Reenter beneath the dermis on the adjacent side and draw through to the bottom of the SQ layer
  + Tie the knot such that it remains at the bottom of the wound, thereby preventing a palpable knot near the skin surface
+ **Interrupted Stitch**
  + Most commonly used stitch. If one fails, the rest will maintain closure.
  + Insert the needle at 90 degrees to the skin surface and include sufficient SQ tissue in the bite and carry the suture through to the opposite side

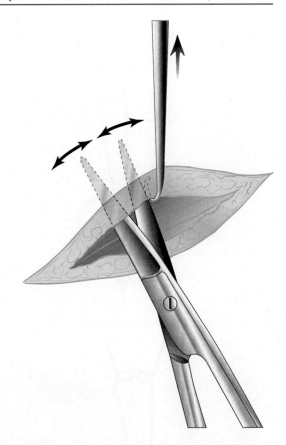

FIGURE 69.1 Undermining a wound reduces the degree of tension present after the repair. (From McNamara R, Loiselle J. Laceration repair. In: Henretig FM, King C, eds. *Textbook of Pediatric Emergency Procedures*. Philadelphia, PA: Williams & Wilkins; 1997:1152, with permission.)

+ Generally, the distance between sutures should equal the distance from the wound to the needle insertion site for each stitch
+ The stitch depth should be greater than its width to produce eversion of wound edges **(FIGURES 69.2 and 69.3)**
+ Tying the knot requires an initial double loop around the needle driver, and then only one loop for the next three to four ties, alternating directions with each one for a strong durable knot **(FIGURE 69.4)**

+ **Mattress Stitch**
  + Variation of the interrupted stitch, which can be vertical or horizontal
  + Used when approximation of wound edges requires more tensile strength
  + Vertical mattress stitch
    - The first stitch is made by passing the needle more widely separated from the wound edges and deeper into the wound than usual
    - The needle is then passed back through the epidermis and lower dermis taking a small bite of the skin from both sides and approximating the edges
    - Tie the suture as an initial double loop around the needle driver, then one loop for the next three to four ties, alternating directions with each throw **(FIGURE 69.5)**
  + Horizontal mattress stitch
    - The first stitch is made 0.5 to 1 cm away from the wound edge
    - Pass the needle through the opposite side
    - Then enter the skin perpendicularly to the last motion and exit on the other side of the wound
    - Tie the suture as an initial double loop around the needle driver, then one loop for the next three to four ties, alternating directions with each throw **(FIGURE 69.6)**

+ **Continuous or "Running" Stitch**
  + Used for linear wounds that require minimal debridement
  + Advantages include speed of repair, strength, and minimal knot tying

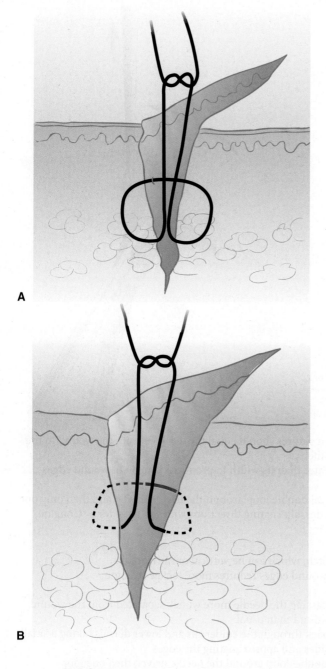

A

B

FIGURE 69.2 A: The buried subcutaneous suture. **B:** The horizontal dermal stitch. (From McNamara R, Loiselle J. Laceration repair. In: Henretig FM, King C, eds. *Textbook of Pediatric Emergency Procedures*. Philadelphia, PA: Williams & Wilkins; 1997:1155, with permission.)

+ Disadvantages
  - One break in the stitch will cause the entire repair to unravel
  - Sutures with differing tensions along the wound
+ Technique
  - Begin with a single suture that is tied to anchor the rest of the suture
  - Do not cut the stitch
  - Pass the needle perpendicular to the skin edge (the same distance and depth as interrupted stitches) continuously, until the edge of the wound is reached
  - After each pass, pull the suture thread to keep the wound closed
  - Close the running stitch by leaving a loop on one end of the wound that can be tied to the remaining suture thread as you would in a simple interrupted stitch **(FIGURE 69.7)**

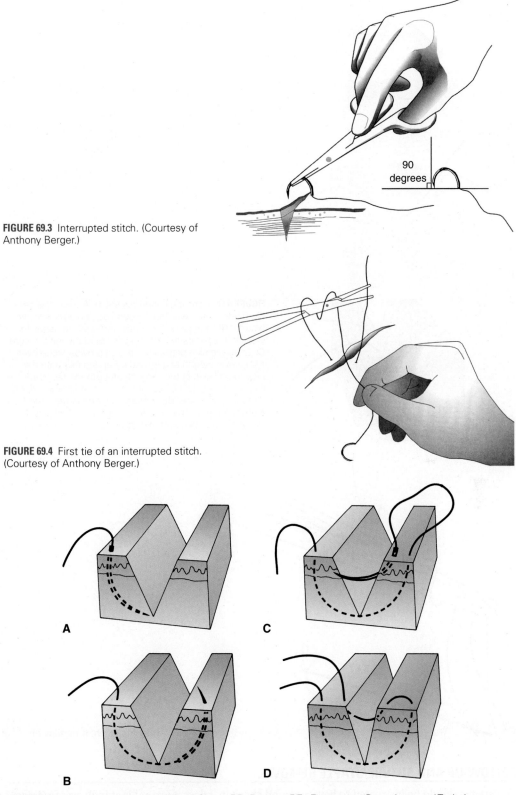

FIGURE 69.3 Interrupted stitch. (Courtesy of Anthony Berger.)

FIGURE 69.4 First tie of an interrupted stitch. (Courtesy of Anthony Berger.)

FIGURE 69.5 Vertical mattress stitch. (From Simon RR, Brenner BE. *Emergency Procedures and Techniques.* 4th ed. Philadelphia, PA: Lippincott Williams & Wilkins; 2002:379, with permission.)

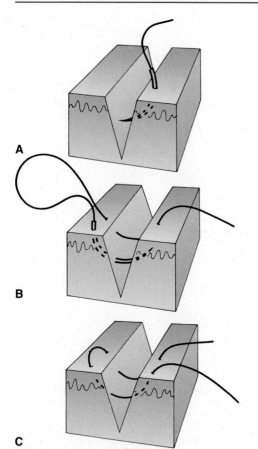

A

B

C

FIGURE 69.6 Horizontal mattress stitch. **A:** Pass the needle 0.5 to 1 cm away from wound edge deeply into the wound. **B:** Then pass the needle through the opposite side so it reenters the wound parallel to the initial suture. **C:** Enter the skin perpendicularly to provide some eversion of the wound edges, and enter and exit both the wound and skin at the same depth; otherwise, "buckling" and irregularities occur in the wound margin. (From Simon RR, Brenner BE. *Emergency Procedures and Techniques.* 4th ed. Philadelphia, PA: Lippincott Williams & Wilkins; 2002:381, with permission.)

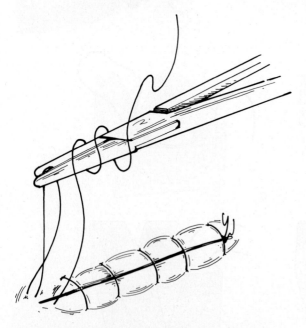

FIGURE 69.7 Running stitch. (Courtesy of Anthony Berger.)

FOLLOW-UP AND SUTURE/STAPLE REMOVAL

✚ Patients should be instructed to have a wound check in 2 days if wound is at high risk for infection or if patient is at high risk, such as a diabetic or immunocompromised patient

TABLE 69.2. REMOVAL TIME OF SUTURES

Area	Length of time (days)
Face	3–5
Scalp	7–9
Chest	8–10
Back	10–14
Forearm	10–14
Fingers and hand	8–10
Lower extremity	8–12
Foot	10–12
Overlying joint	14

- Consider antibiotics for patients with high-risk wounds
  + Antibiotic selection varies by institution and region and should be chosen on the basis of likely pathogen
- The proper removal time of sutures/staples should be conveyed to the patient because it affects wound closure and cosmetics **(TABLE 69.2)**
- Tetanus immunization should be updated if required
  + In general, if >5 years since last tetanus shot, give Td booster
- Patients should be instructed to return if signs of symptoms of infection occur
  + Increasing pain, redness, or warmth
  + Fever
  + Purulent drainage

COMPLICATIONS

- **Infection**
  + Incidence of wound infection (assuming proper irrigation and sterile technique) is still 2% to 3%
  + Lowest incidence of infection—scalp, face, neck, trunk
  + Higher incidence of infection—extremities, especially hands and feet and in large, complex lacerations
- **Cosmesis**
  + Keloid formation
  + Larger suture material causes more scarring
  + Poor alignment (i.e., vermilion border) leads to poor cosmetic result

SAFETY/QUALITY TIPS

- **Procedural**
  + When suturing, adhere to the principles of minimizing trauma to tissues, relieving tension by undermining, using deep sutures, and realigning skin edges accurately
  + The key to effective wound exploration is adequate anesthesia
  + Be mindful of anesthetic toxicity when managing large wounds. Consider regional anesthesia techniques in these circumstances.
  + Use absorbable sutures for pediatrics and when return for suture removal not assured
- **Cognitive**
  + Wounds should be evaluated systematically, specifically considering the likelihood of damage to underlying structures, retained foreign body, as well as the need for prophylactic antibiotics, rabies and tetanus prophylaxis
  + There is no specific delay to presentation beyond which a wound cannot be closed—the likelihood of wound infection must be weighed against the likelihood of improved cosmetic outcome for each case individually
  + Even if studies are negative, advise patients who have foreign body-prone wounds that a foreign body could still be present, and develop a follow-up plan

✚ Acknowledgment

Thank you to prior author Brenda L. Liu.

Suggested Readings

Roberts JR, Hedges JR. *Clinical Procedures in Emergency Medicine*. 4th ed. Philadelphia, PA: WB Saunders; 2004.

Simon RR, Brenner BE. *Emergency Procedures and Techniques*. 4th ed. Philadelphia, PA: Lippincott Williams & Wilkins; 2002:335–395.

Singer AJ, Hollander JE. *Lacerations and Acute Wounds: an Evidence-Based Guide*. Philadelphia, PA: FA Davis; 2003.

70

Perianal Abscess: Incision and Drainage

Brian Chung and Todd A. Mastrovitch

INDICATIONS

⊕ To drain infection of the soft tissue surrounding the rectum, which is caused by obstruction of the anal crypts and ducts

CONTRAINDICATIONS

⊕ Perianal abscesses with fistula-in-ano should be drained in the operating room (OR)

LANDMARKS

⊕ Most perianal abscesses form in the soft tissue adjacent to the anal sphincter
⊕ Ischiorectal, intersphincteric, external sphincter, and supralevator abscesses form internally underneath the subcutaneous tissue adjacent to the rectum (FIGURE 70.1)

⊕ **General Basic Steps**
  ✦ **Analgesia**
  ✦ **Incision**
  ✦ **Blunt dissection**
  ✦ **Packing and dressing**

TECHNIQUE

⊕ **Supplies**
  ✦ Adhesive tape
  ✦ 1% Lidocaine with epinephrine (1:100,000)
  ✦ 25- and 22-guage needles, 10-mL syringes

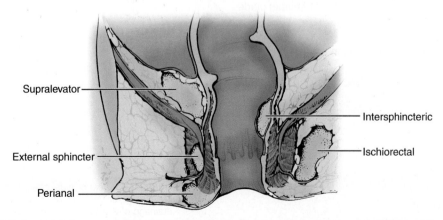

FIGURE 70.1 Anorectal abscesses. (From Coates WC. Perianal, rectal, and anal diseases. In: Wolfson AB, ed. *Harwood-Nuss' Clinical Practice of Emergency Medicine.* 6th ed. Philadelphia, PA: Lippincott Williams & Wilkins; 2014:609, with permission.)

- ✚ No. 11 scalpel blade
- ✚ Hemostat
- ✚ Saline
- ✚ Sterile packing
- ✚ 4 × 4 gauze pads

Preparation

- ✚ Consider mild oral sedative or anxiolytic for the patient before procedure
- ✚ Place patient in the prone position
- ✚ Separate buttocks with adhesive tape to the lateral aspect of the hip **(FIGURE 70.2)**

Analgesia

- ✚ Infiltrate area around the abscess with 1% lidocaine with epinephrine (1:100,000)

Incision

- ✚ Using a no.11 blade, a linear or elliptical incision is made over the most fluctuant part of the abscess
- ✚ Express as much as possible from the abscess with gentle squeezing pressure **(FIGURE 70.3)**

Blunt Dissection

- ✚ Explore abscess with a hemostat to break loculations
- ✚ Irrigate the abscess with normal saline **(FIGURE 70.4)**

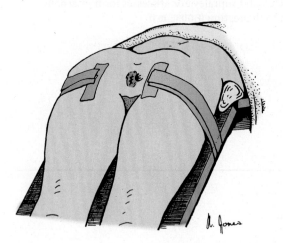

FIGURE 70.2 When excising a thrombosed external hemorrhoid or performing incision and drainage of an anal abscess, separate the buttocks by using 3-inch adhesive tape, as shown, to provide optimal exposure. (From Simon RR, Brenner BE. *Emergency Procedures and Techniques.* 4th ed. Philadelphia, PA: Lippincott Williams & Wilkins; 2002:33, with permission.)

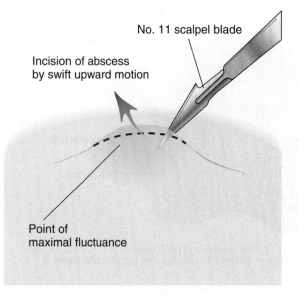

No. 11 scalpel blade

Incision of abscess by swift upward motion

Point of maximal fluctuance

FIGURE 70.3 Linear incision of a cutaneous abscess. (From Young GM. Incision and drainage of a cutaneous abscess. In: Henretig FM, King C, eds. *Textbook of Pediatric Emergency Procedures.* Philadelphia, PA: Williams & Wilkins; 1997:1202, with permission.)

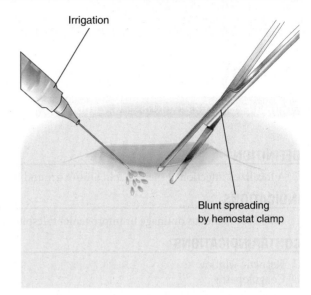

Irrigation

Blunt spreading
by hemostat clamp

FIGURE 70.4 Removal of loculations and irrigation of an abscess. (From Young GM. Incision and drainage of a cutaneous abscess. In: Henretig FM, King C, eds. *Textbook of Pediatric Emergency Procedures*. Philadelphia, PA: Williams & Wilkins; 1997:1203, with permission.)

☐ **Packing and Dressing**
+ Pack cavity lightly with sterile packing material to allow incision to stay open, thereby allowing continuous drainage
+ Dress wound for patient comfort

COMPLICATIONS

☐ Fistula formation
☐ Systemic infection

SAFETY/QUALITY TIPS

☐ **Procedural**
+ The most important predictor of a successful abscess drainage is adequate anesthesia; generously infiltrate the region
+ The most common procedural mistake is making the initial skin incision too small. Err on the side of larger to facilitate further steps in the incision and drainage (I&D), especially in cosmetically unimportant areas.
+ The wound should be loosely packed—overpacking will not allow for proper drainage and healing

☐ **Cognitive**
+ Abscesses drainable in the emergency department should be able to be fully visualized. If the extent of the abscess cannot be appreciated (usually because it extends into and around the rectum), utilize advanced imaging and surgical consultation.
+ Antibiotics are generally not required unless overlying cellulitis is present
+ If adequate analgesia cannot be achieved, consider I&D in the OR with general anesthesia
+ Packing is to be replaced at 48-hour intervals until infection has cleared
+ Advise the patient to take sitz baths daily for comfort until healing is complete

Suggested Readings

Coates WC. Perianal, rectal, and anal diseases. In: Wolfson AB, ed. *Harwood-Nuss' Clinical Practice of Emergency Medicine*. 6th ed. Philadelphia, PA: Lippincott Williams & Wilkins; 2014:609.

Simon RR, Brenner BE. *Emergency Procedures and Techniques*. 4th ed. Philadelphia, PA: Lippincott Williams & Wilkins; 2002:33.

Young GM. Incision and drainage of a cutaneous abscess. In: King C, Henretig FM, eds. *Textbook of Pediatric Emergency Procedures*. 2nd ed. Philadelphia, PA: Williams & Wilkins; 2008.

71

Paronychia: Incision and Drainage

Alison E. Suarez and Kris E. C. Zaporteza

DEFINITION
- A localized infection at the nail fold and/or around the nail plate

INDICATIONS
- Failed spontaneous drainage or improvement despite warm soaks

CONTRAINDICATIONS
- Herpetic whitlow
- Coagulopathy

- **General Basic Steps**
  - **Analgesia**
  - **Incision and drainage**
  - **Irrigation**
  - **Packing and dressing**
  - **Ensure follow-up**

TECHNIQUE
- Perform digital block under sterile setting
- Using a no. 11 blade make an incision parallel to the nail at the area of maximal fluctuance **(FIGURE 71.1)**
- For large paronychia, elevate the nail fold from skin and express pus
- Irrigate cavity with isotonic saline under pressure, using a splash guard
- Insert a small piece of packing gauze, creating a wick to allow drainage
- Apply gentle nonadhesive dressing and ensure follow-up in 24 to 48 hours

COMPLICATIONS
- Osteomyelitis
- Abscess
- Extension of infection
- Destruction of nail matrix, compromising nail growth

SAFETY/QUALITY TIPS
- **Procedural**
  - Drainage can sometimes occur by lifting the nail fold skin with a sterile 18-gauge needle
  - The proximal part of the nail may need to be removed to ensure maximal drainage of pus
  - Extensive infections may require surgical debridement
- **Cognitive**
  - Provide antistaphylococcal/antistreptococcal antibiotic coverage with overlying cellulitis, especially in patients with underlying diabetes or other immunocompromising condition
  - Hand surgical consultation is appropriate in the setting of extensive cellulitis, osteomyelitis, or tumor

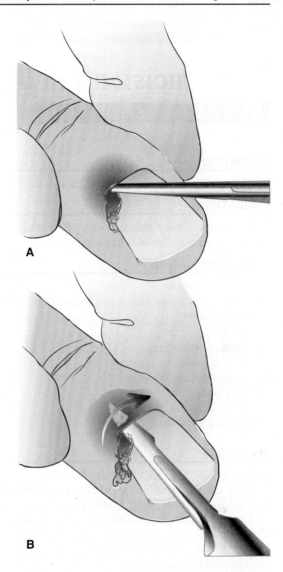

FIGURE 71.1 Drainage of the paronychia. (From Henretig FM. Incision and drainage of a parony-chia. In: Henretig FM, King C, eds. *Textbook of Pediatric Emergency Procedures*. Philadelphia, PA: Williams & Wilkins; 1997:1207, with permission.)

✦ Paronychia can be difficult to distinguish from herpetic whitlow, and draining whitlow is contraindicated. See Chapter 72 (Felon: Incision and Drainage) for tips on identifying whitlow.
✦ Chronic infection is most likely due to candida
✦ Chronic infections that do not respond to conservative therapy need to be evaluated for possible underlying malignancy

◘ **Acknowledgment**

Thank you to prior author Audrey Paul.

Suggested Readings

Fleisher G, Ludwig S, eds. *Textbook of Pediatric Emergency Medicine*. 6th ed. Philadelphia, PA: Lippincott Williams & Wilkins; 2010:1478.

Wolfson AB, ed. *Harwood-Nuss' Clinical Practice of Emergency Medicine*. 6th ed. Philadelphia, PA: Lippincott Williams & Wilkins; 2014:720–722.

72

Felon: Incision and Drainage

Alison E. Suarez and Kris Zaporteza

DEFINITION

- An infection or abscess of the fingertip pulp

INDICATIONS

- Fluctuance of the distal pulp with pain worsened by pressure
- Failure of resolution of infection after conservative therapy

CONTRAINDICATIONS

- Herpetic whitlow
- Infection extending proximally to distal interphalangeal (DIP) joint
- Coagulopathy

- **General Basic Steps**
  - **Analgesia**
  - **Incision and drainage**
  - **Irrigate**
  - **Packing and dressing**
  - **Ensure follow-up**

TECHNIQUE

- Perform digital block under sterile setting
- Make small longitudinal incision at area of maximal fluctuance
- Disrupt loculations using blunt curved hemostat without disrupting the vertical septa
- Irrigate wound with sterile saline under pressure
- Insert a small piece of packing gauze, creating a wick to allow drainage
- Apply gentle nonadhesive dressing and ensure follow-up in 24 to 48 hours to remove packing
- Splint the involved finger
- Ensure tetanus is updated
- Encourage elevation to minimize pain and follow up with the hand surgeon

COMPLICATIONS

- Digital nerve injury
- Osteomyelitis
- Painful neuroma **(FIGURE 72.1)**
- Flexor tenosynovitis
- Skin necrosis
- Septic arthritis
- Fingertip deformity

SAFETY/QUALITY TIPS

- **Procedural**
  - Incisions should not be within 3 mm of the DIP joint to prevent flexion contracture and deformity
  - Transverse incisions can injure the neuromuscular bundle causing ischemia and anesthesia

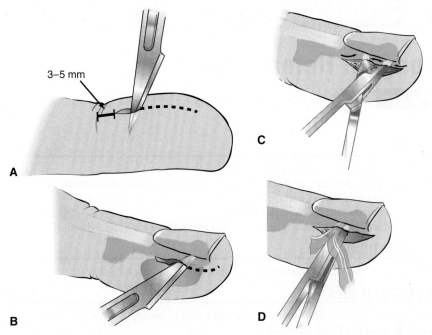

3–5 mm

A

B

C

D

FIGURE 72.1 A: Longitudinal incision on the palmar surface of the distal finger. **B:** J-shaped lateral incision of a felon. **C:** Disruption of loculations within a felon. **D:** Wick placement. (From Bethel CA. Incision and drainage of a felon. In: Henretig FM, King C, eds. *Textbook of Pediatric Emergency Procedures*. Philadelphia, PA: Williams & Wilkins; 1997:1214, with permission.)

✦ Use of a fish-mouth incision is associated with a higher rate of complications
✦ The longitudinal incision at the area of maximal fluctuance is associated with the lowest rate of complications

⊕ **Cognitive**

✦ Provide antistaphylococcal/antistreptococcal antibiotic coverage if felon is associated with overlying cellulitis; especially in patients with underlying diabetes or other immunocompromised condition
✦ Incision is contraindicated in the setting of herpetic whitlow as it may result in delayed resolution, viremia, or bacterial superinfection. Herpetic whitlow features vesicles that coalesce with pus, mimicking a felon or paronychia; look for and ask about vesicles. Whitlow is more common in health care workers (exposed to the saliva of herpes-infected patients). The pulp of the distal phalanx should be soft with whitlow, tense with a felon.

⊕ **Acknowledgment**

Thank you to prior author Audrey Paul.

Suggested Readings

Clark D. Common acute hand infections. *Am Fam Physician*. 2003;68:2167–2176.
Jebson PJ. Infections of the fingertip. Paronychias and felons. *Hand Clin*. 1998;14:547–555.
King C, Henretig FM, eds. *Textbook of Pediatric Procedures*. 2nd ed. Philadelphia, PA: Lippincott Williams & Wilkins; 2008:1090–1094.
Rockwell P. Acute and chronic paronychia. *Am Fam Physician*. 2001;63:1113–1116.
Simon RR, Brenner BE. *Emergency Procedures and Techniques*. 4th ed. Philadelphia, PA: Lippincott Williams & Wilkins; 2002.
Wolfson AB, ed. *Harwood-Nuss' Clinical Practice of Emergency Medicine*. 6th ed. Philadelphia, PA: Lippincott Williams & Wilkins; 2014:722–723.

73

Subungual Hematoma

David Barlas

INDICATIONS

- ☐ Trephination: To create a fistula through the nail to the hematoma
  - ✦ Decompression, drainage, and pain relief of small subungual hematomas
- ☐ Nail removal and nail bed laceration repair
  - ✦ Large hematomas and nail bed lacerations
  - ✦ Partial nail avulsion or subluxation with nail instability or nail fold disruption

CONTRAINDICATIONS

- ☐ Significant crush injuries or missing/destroyed nail matrix warrant specialty consultation

RISKS/CONSENT ISSUES

- ☐ Germinal matrix injuries and open tuft fractures should be documented and referred to a specialist to ensure optimal outcome

LANDMARKS

- ☐ Hematomas typically collect on the sterile matrix under the nail
- ☐ Germinal matrix
  - ✦ Region where new nail is formed
  - ✦ Avoid injury during the procedure

- ☐ **General Basic Steps**
  - ✦ **X-ray digit if fracture possible**
  - ✦ **Prepare patient**
  - ✦ **Consider anesthesia**
  - ✦ **Perform procedure** (FIGURE 73.1)

- ☐ **Trephination**
  - ✦ Goal is to form a hole through the nail of sufficient size to drain the hematoma
  - ✦ Personal protection (including an eye shield) as blood may spurt out when released
  - ✦ Needle or scalpel method: Apply gentle pressure with the tip of the instrument perpendicular to the surface of the nail, twisting until blood is released
  - ✦ Heated paper clip method: Creates a wider hole but may tattoo the nail bed
  - ✦ Disposable electrocautery device method: Quick and effective (FIGURE 73.2)
  - ✦ Discharge instructions are to soak the finger in warm water twice a day for 7 days to allow the blood to continue to drain
- ☐ **Nail Bed Laceration Repair**
  - ✦ Supplies: Iris scissors, hemostats, and suture set with fine absorbable sutures (5-0 to 7-0 chromic or Vicryl)
  - ✦ Perform digital block under sterile conditions
  - ✦ Apply tourniquet for hemostasis
  - ✦ Remove the nail from the nail bed matrix
    - ✛ Insert closed Iris scissors horizontally under the nail
    - ✛ Gently spread scissors and advance in repeated movements, gradually progressing to the nail root and separating the entire nail from the nail bed
    - ✛ Once the nail is free from the nail bed and eponychium, grasp with hemostat and gently pull longitudinally to free the nail

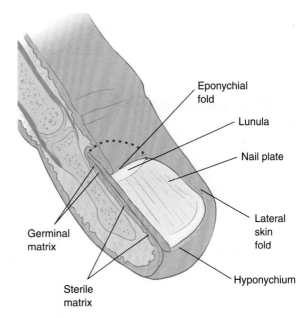

FIGURE 73.1 Anatomy of the finger and nail bed. (From Eberlein R. Hand and finger injuries. In: Henretig FM, King C, eds. *Textbook of Pediatric Emergency Procedures*. Philadelphia, PA: Williams & Wilkins; 1997:1048, with permission.)

Labels: Eponychial fold, Lunula, Nail plate, Lateral skin fold, Hyponychium, Sterile matrix, Germinal matrix

- ✦ Repair nail bed laceration
  - ✦ Use interrupted fine, absorbable sutures
  - ✦ Significantly damaged nail beds or germinal matrix involvement should prompt hand surgeon consultation
  - ✦ Gently rinse and reinsert the nail into anatomic position
  - ✦ If necessary, secure the nail with a 5-0 suture
  - ✦ If nail is damaged or missing, gently insert petroleum gauze between the nail matrix and eponychium
- ✦ Dress loosely but securely and splint the finger
- ✦ Discharge instructions are to elevate the digit and return for wound check in 2 days
- ✦ The replaced nail should be left in place for 2 to 3 weeks

COMPLICATIONS

- ▣ Local bleeding
- ▣ Infection
- ▣ Poor cosmetic outcome
  - ✦ Split or deformed nail growth
  - ✦ Adhesions between cuticle and germinal matrix

SAFETY/QUALITY TIPS

- ▣ **Procedural**
  - ✦ The key predictor of a successful procedure is adequate anesthesia
  - ✦ Aggressive or hasty technique can damage the germinal matrix
  - ✦ Be mindful of forceful ejection of blood from trephination—wear eye protection
- ▣ **Cognitive**
  - ✦ Consider the likelihood of a nail bed laceration in all significant subungual hematomas; when uncertain, remove the nail
  - ✦ Have a low threshold to obtain an x-ray to diagnose fracture
  - ✦ Suspect tuft fractures with significant nail bed lacerations
  - ✦ Oral antibiotics are indicated when patients have a concurrent fracture since it is technically an open fracture; however, osteomyelitis of the distal phalanx after tuft fracture and subungual hematoma is uncommon
  - ✦ Set patient's expectations low regarding final cosmetic outcome

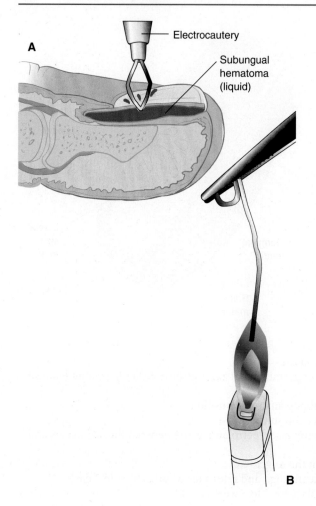

A

Electrocautery

Subungual hematoma (liquid)

B

FIGURE 73.2 Nail trephination. (From Eberlein R. Hand and finger injuries. In: Henretig FM, King C, eds. *Textbook of Pediatric Emergency Procedures.* Philadelphia, PA: Williams & Wilkins; 1997:1051, with permission.)

⊞ Acknowledgment

Thank you to prior author Peter A. Binkley.

Suggested Readings

Lammers RL, Smith ZE. Methods of wound closure. In: Roberts JR, Custalow CB, Thomsen TW, et al. eds. *Roberts & Hedges' Clinical Procedures in Emergency Medicine.* 6th ed. Philadelphia, PA: WB Saunders; 2013:682–685.

74

Escharotomy and Burn Care

Jeffrey P. Green

INDICATIONS

- Used to decompress accumulated edema under tight, unyielding eschar following full-thickness burn (classic and modern classifications of burns are given in **TABLE 74.1**)
- Circumferential extremity burn with evidence of neurovascular compromise:
  - Cyanosis
  - Deep tissue pain
  - Progressive paresthesia
  - Decreased or absent pulses
  - Elevated compartment pressure
  - Decreased arterial flow on Doppler ultrasonography
  - Pulse oximetry <95% of affected extremity (without systemic hypoxia)
- Thoracic burn with evidence of respiratory compromise due to eschar
- Circumferential neck burn
- Abdominal burn with evidence of increased intra-abdominal pressure (usually estimated by bladder pressure)
- Circumferential penile burn

CONTRAINDICATIONS

- No evidence of tissue hypoperfusion on physical examination
- Normal findings on arterial Doppler ultrasonography
- Adequate respiration despite eschar
- No evidence of increased intra-abdominal pressure

RISK/CONSENT ISSUES

- Often difficult to obtain consent from major burn victims; escharotomy is a life-saving procedure and should be performed even if informed consent from the patient cannot be obtained
- Procedure can cause pain (local and systemic analgesia will be provided)
- Risk of bleeding (minimized with proper technique)
- Whenever the skin is broken, there is potential for introducing infection (sterile technique will be utilized)

TABLE 74.1. BURN DEPTH CLASSIFICATION

Classic classification	Modern classification	Burn depth	Appearance	Healing
First degree	Superficial	Epidermis only	Painful, dry, red Blanch with pressure	3–6 days No scarring
Second degree	Superficial partial thickness	Epidermis and superficial dermis	Red, weeping, usually blister Blanch with pressure	7–21 days Scarring unusual
	Deep partial thickness	Epidermis and deep dermis	Usually blister, waxy, and dry, white to red color Nonblanching	>21 days Scarring severe
Third degree	Full thickness	Extends through and destroys dermis	Waxy-white to charred black, dry, inelastic skin Nonblanching	No spontaneous healing Severe scarring with contractures

LANDMARKS

Escharotomy sites are depicted in **FIGURE 74.1**.

TECHNIQUE

⊞ **General Basic Steps**
  ✚ **Airway, breathing, and circulation (ABC)**
  ✚ **Consider early intubation**
  ✚ **Fluid resuscitation**
  ✚ **Analgesia**
  ✚ **Tetanus prophylaxis**
  ✚ **Wound care**
  ✚ **Escharotomy**

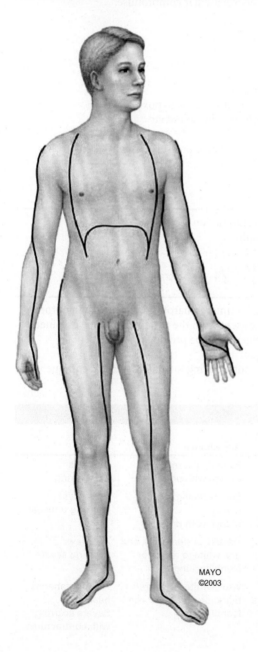

MAYO
©2003

FIGURE 74.1 Escharotomy sites. (From Haro LH, Miller S, Decker WW. Burns. In: Wolfson AB, ed. *Harwood-Nuss' Clinical Practice of Emergency Medicine*. 6th ed. Philadelphia, PA: Lippincott Williams & Wilkins; 2014:315, with permission.)

BURN MANAGEMENT

- ☐ First ensure ABC and administer supplemental oxygen
- ☐ Strongly consider endotracheal intubation if:
  - ✚ Burns to the face and neck are present
  - ✚ Soot in and around the mouth and nose
  - ✚ Hoarseness, stridor, wheezing, or development of acute coughing
  - ✚ Carbonaceous sputum
- ☐ Give intravenous fluids for resuscitation (for moderate to major burns)
  - ✚ Use Parkland formula: Ringer lactate 4 mL × weight (kg) × % of total body surface area (TBSA) burned (excluding superficial burns)
    - ✦ Give ½ of total volume over the first 8 hours from time of burn injury
    - ✦ Give second ½ of total volume over the following 16 hours
    - ✦ Titrate to maintain blood pressure and urine output of at least 1 mL/kg/hour
    - ✦ Continue maintenance fluids in addition
  - ✚ Place urinary catheter to monitor adequate resuscitation **(FIGURE 74.2)**
- ☐ Provide pain management with frequent pain assessment
  - ✚ Acetaminophen and nonsteroidal anti-inflammatory drugs (NSAIDS) with or without opioids for superficial burns
  - ✚ Opioids are necessary for partial-to-full thickness burns
- ☐ Administer tetanus prophylaxis
- ☐ Wound care, if not delaying transfer to burn unit:
  - ✚ Use sterile technique
  - ✚ Clean with mild soap and tap water
  - ✚ Debride sloughed or necrotic skin; avoid extensive debridement
  - ✚ Remove ruptured blisters
    - ✦ Intact blister management is controversial; it is recommended to unroof cloudy blisters or those where rupture is imminent (e.g., over joints)

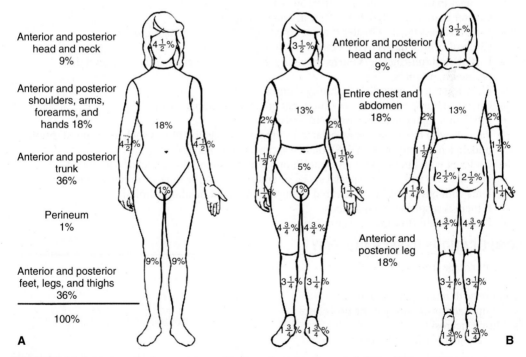

FIGURE 74.2 Methods to evaluate percentage of body surface area burned. **A:** Rule of Nines. **B:** Lund and Browder chart. (From Haro LH, Miller S, Decker WW. Burns. In: Wolfson AB, ed. *Harwood-Nuss' Clinical Practice of Emergency Medicine.* 6th ed. Philadelphia, PA: Lippincott Williams & Wilkins; 2014:1103, with permission.)

+ Superficial burns do not need dressings; application of aloe vera cream is sufficient
+ Deeper burns require chemoprophylaxis to prevent infection:
    + Apply silver sulfadiazine (Silvadene) to a thickness of 1/16 of an inch on burns other than the face where bacitracin is preferred
    + Over the silver sulfadiazine, place three layers of gauze: First, a nonadherent gauze, ideally with a nonpetroleum-based lubricant. Then, a fluffed gauze layer capable of absorbing exudates. Finally, place an outer wrap with elastic gauze with enough pressure to keep the dressing in place.
        - Wrap all fingers and toes individually to prevent maceration and adherence
        - *Caveat*: If transferring to a nearby burn unit, covering wounds with sterile moist dressings is appropriate

ESCHAROTOMY

- Do not delay procedure for transfer to Burn Center
- Make incision to subcutaneous level so that eschar is released, preferably with Bovie cautery device to minimize bleeding
- Thoracic escharotomy
    + Make longitudinal incisions along each midclavicular line from 2 cm below the clavicle to the 10th rib; connect with two transverse incisions across the chest, forming a square
- Extremity eschar
    + Make incision to subcutaneous layer only
    + Cut through the entire length of the burn eschar

DISPOSITION

- Patients with superficial burns may be safely discharged home
- For burns beyond superficial, apply American Burn Association Minimal Criteria for Transfer to Burn Center:
    + Partial-thickness and full-thickness burns: Greater than or equal to 10% TBSA in patients younger than 10 years or older than 50 years
    + Greater than or equal to 20% TBSA in other age-groups
    + Full-thickness burns: Greater than or equal to 5% TBSA in all age-groups
    + Circumferential burns of the extremities or chest
    + Partial- and full-thickness burns involving the face, eyes, ears, hands, feet, genitalia, perineum, or joints
    + Electrical burns, including lightning injuries
    + Chemical burns with threat of functional or cosmetic impairment
    + Inhalation injury in association with burns
    + Patients with burns having associated trauma or preexisting illness such as acquired immunodeficiency syndrome (AIDS), diabetes, cancer, and alcoholism
    + Children with burns seen in hospitals not having qualified personnel or equipment
    + Patients who will require special social or emotional care or long-term rehabilitation
- Patients with burns not being referred to Burn Center, but needing admission:
    + If there is suspicion of child abuse
    + Patients unable to care for wounds at home

COMPLICATIONS OF ESCHAROTOMY

- Hemorrhage from superficial veins
- Infection
- Damage to underlying structures
- Complications of poorly done procedure
- Muscle necrosis
- Nerve injury, such as foot drop

SAFETY/QUALITY TIPS

🔲 **Procedural**
+ Never apply silver sulfadiazine to the face because it can cause skin discoloration
+ Always give tetanus prophylaxis
+ Individually wrap toes and fingers
+ For sulfa allergic patients, bacitracin is appropriate for initial burn infection prophylaxis
+ Use a Bovie cautery for escharotomy to minimize bleeding
+ Escharotomy incision must go through entire burn and to subcutaneous level to ensure releasing the eschar
+ Escharotomy should not be delayed for transfer to Burn Center

🔲 **Cognitive**
+ Do not underestimate the extent of the burn; often burns will not fully declare their penetration for 24 to 72 hours
+ Remember to frequently reevaluate airway patency
+ Consider concomitant carbon monoxide poisoning and obtain a carboxyhemoglobin level for all closed space burns
+ Suspect cyanide poisoning for burns involving wool, silk, nylon, and polyurethane found in furniture or paper

🔲 **Acknowledgment**

Thank you to prior author Steven Shuchat.

Suggested Readings

American Burn Association. Practice guidelines for burn care. *J Burn Care Rehabil.* 2001;i-67S.

Simon RR, Brenner BE. *Emergency Procedures and Techniques.* 4th ed. Philadelphia, PA: Lippincott Williams & Wilkins; 2002:395–397.

Wolfson AB. *Harwood-Nuss' Clinical Practice of Emergency Medicine.* 6th ed. Philadelphia, PA: Lippincott Williams & Wilkins; 2014:310–315.

75

Epistaxis

Carey C. Li

INDICATION

Nasal bleeding that does not stop with a topical vasoconstrictor and direct pressure applied by the patient (described below in the "Technique" section).

PROCEDURES

- ☐ **Cauterization**
  - ✦ Anterior source bleeding that can be visualized
- ☐ **Anterior Nasal Packing**
  - ✦ Anterior source bleeding that cannot be visualized
  - ✦ Cauterization fails
- ☐ **Posterior Nasal Packing or Balloon Tamponade**
  - ✦ Anterior source cannot be identified *and*
    - ✚ Bleeding from both nares *or*
    - ✚ Blood draining into the posterior pharynx
  - ✦ Anterior packing of both nares fails to control bleeding

CONTRAINDICATIONS

- ☐ None

RISKS

- ☐ Nasal packing can cause pain or discomfort
- ☐ Risk of infection, septal damage, and ulceration
- ☐ Risk of balloon migration, airway obstruction, or aspiration with posterior packing

LANDMARKS

- ☐ The choice of procedure depends on the source of bleeding. The source can be identified by direct visualization, or with use of a nasal speculum (described in more detail in the "Technique" section).
- ☐ Nosebleeds are most commonly anterior (80% to 90%), originating from the Kiesselbach plexus in the septum
- ☐ Most posterior nosebleeds originate from branches of the sphenopalatine artery in the posterior nasal cavity or nasopharynx. A posterior source is likely when an anterior source cannot be identified, when bleeding is from both nares, or when blood is draining into the posterior pharynx.

- ☐ **General Basic Steps**
  - ✚ **Patient preparation**
  - ✚ **Analgesia**
  - ✚ **Visualization**
  - ✚ **Cauterization**
  - ✚ **Anterior packing**
  - ✚ **Posterior packing**

TECHNIQUE

◘ **Patient Preparation**

+ Ask the patient to blow his or her nose, which decreases the effects of local fibrinolysis and removes clots (FIGURE 75.1)

+ Ask the patient to lean forward and apply continuous pressure to the alae of both nares for 10 to 20 minutes. If this stops bleeding, consider sending patient home with follow-up to ear, nose, and throat (ENT) specialist or Primary Medical Doctor (PMD).

◘ **Analgesia**

+ Apply a topical anesthetic and vasoconstrictor

  + Soak cotton or gauze in 2% lidocaine with or without topical epinephrine or 4% topical cocaine. Place in the nasal cavity for 15 to 20 minutes.

  + Alternatively, a topical anesthetic with a decongestant (2% lidocaine and 4% phenylephrine mixed 1:1) or oxymetazoline hydrochloride (Afrin) nasal spray may be used

+ Because patients may be apprehensive and packing is uncomfortable, opiates or benzodiazepines may be given before the examination (strongly recommended in cases of posterior packing)

◘ **Visualization**

+ Position the patient sitting upright, facing forward in the sniffing position

+ Insert a nasal speculum so that one blade moves superiorly and the other inferiorly and spread the nares vertically. Suction all remaining clots and blood. This permits visualization of most anterior sources.

◘ **Cauterization**

+ If an anterior source is visualized, cauterization should be attempted. To be effective, cautery should be performed after bleeding is controlled. Only cauterize one side of the septum at a time to prevent perforation or necrosis of the septum.

+ Chemical cauterization can be performed using silver nitrate sticks. Apply the tip of a silver nitrate stick to the bleeding site until a white precipitate forms (usually a few seconds, rarely more than 10).

+ If bleeding is vigorous, electrocauterization can be used. Apply the device to the bleeding site for up to 10 seconds or until a white precipitate forms.

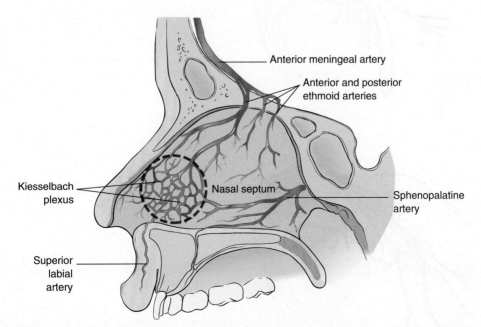

FIGURE 75.1 Anatomy of nasal septum. (From Kost SI, Post JC. Management of epistaxis. In: Henretig FM, King C, eds. *Textbook of Pediatric Emergency Procedures.* Philadelphia, PA: Williams & Wilkins; 1997:663, with permission.)

✦ If cautery is successful, patients should apply a daily topical antibiotic ointment to the area for 1 week

Anterior Packing

✦ If the source of an anterior bleed cannot be identified, or if bleeding persists despite cauterization, an anterior pack can be placed

✦ A Merocel nasal tampon can be used. Lubricate the tip with lidocaine or a topical antibiotic and insert the device along the floor of the nasal cavity. Expand the tampon with 10 to 20 mL of saline via syringe.

✦ A Rapid Rhino balloon tampon can also be used. Soak the catheter in sterile water, then insert it along the floor of the nasal cavity. When the plastic fabric lies within the nares, inflate it with up to 20 mL of air via syringe until the cuff is firm.

✦ Ribbon (Xeroform) gauze ½-inch wide (dispensed in 72-inch strip) can also be used. Using forceps, grab 4 to 5 inch of gauze and advance into the nasal cavity as far as possible, then grasp another 4 to 5 inch and layer on top. Continue to layer in an accordion manner until the nose is tightly packed **(FIGURE 75.2)**.

✦ If bleeding persists despite initial packing, the contralateral naris can be packed. If bleeding still persists, it is likely coming from a posterior source.

✦ Instructions if nasal packing is successful are:
  + Packing should be left in for 2 to 3 days
  + Consider prescribing antibiotics with staphylococcus coverage (such as trimethoprim/sulfamethoxazole (TMP/SMX), cephalexin, or amoxicillin/clavulanic acid) for the duration of packing

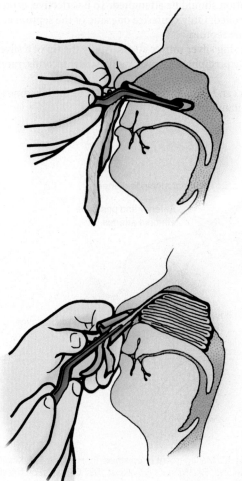

FIGURE 75.2 Anterior nasal packing. (From Simon RR, Brenner BE. *Emergency Procedures and Techniques.* 4th ed. Philadelphia, PA: Lippincott Williams & Wilkins; 2002:313, with permission.)

+ Avoid nasal manipulation and nose blowing, as well as vasodilating actions such as physical exertion, spicy foods, and alcohol
+ Follow up with ENT specialist

Posterior Packing
  + Rolled gauze method
    + Prepare 3 × 3-inch or 2 × 2-inch gauze rolled and bound tightly around the middle with umbilical tape/silk (no. 0) tie. Ten inches of umbilical tape/silk tie should be left on each end.
    + Lubricate a rubber catheter with lidocaine or a topical antibiotic and feed it through the nose, pulling it through the mouth
    + Tie the rolled gauze to the catheter at the oral end, and pull the gauze back into the mouth by pulling on the catheter from the nasal end
    + Once the pack lodges in the posterior portion of the nose, secure the tie anteriorly by tying it around a piece of gauze
    + Apply an anterior pack to the same side, because bleeding may resume anterior to the posterior pack **(FIGURE 75.3)**
  + Epistat device (balloon tamponade)
    + Composed of anterior and posterior balloons
    + Lubricate the catheter and advance it along the floor of the nasal cavity

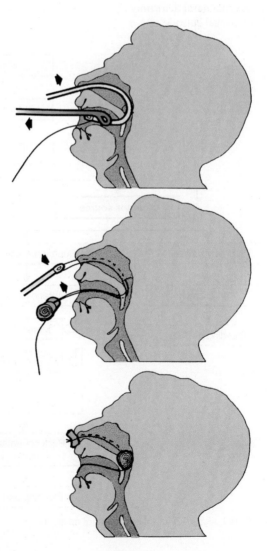

FIGURE 75.3 Posterior nasal packing. (From Simon RR, Brenner BE. *Emergency Procedures and Techniques.* 4th ed. Philadelphia, PA: Lippincott Williams & Wilkins; 2002:314, with permission.)

+ Inflate the posterior balloon with 7 to 10 mL of saline, then pull forward gently until it lodges in the posterior portion of the nose
+ Inflate the anterior balloon with 15 to 30 mL of saline
+ Apply an anterior pack to the same side
+ Foley catheter
    + Catheter size (10- to 16-French) should be approximately the diameter of the external nares
    + Check the balloon for an air leak
    + Cut catheter tip distal to the balloon to prevent irritation of the posterior pharynx
    + Lubricate the catheter and advance it along the floor of the nasal cavity until it is visible in the mouth
    + Inflate the balloon with 15 mL of saline and then pull forward until it lodges in the posterior portion of the nose
    + Apply an anterior pack to the same side

Note: Because of possible multiple complications with posterior packing (see following text), these patients should be admitted with involvement of ENT specialist.

COMPLICATIONS

See **FIGURE 75.4** for algorithm for management of epistaxis.
⊞ Infection (sinusitis, otitis media, abscess formation)
⊞ Septal hematoma, ulceration, or perforation
⊞ External nasal deformity
⊞ Vasovagal episode

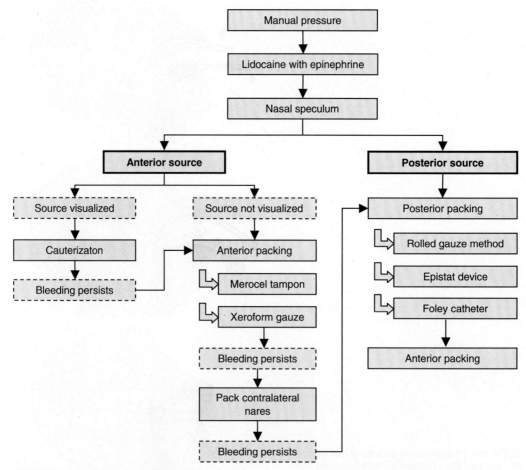

FIGURE 75.4 Algorithm for management of epistaxis.

- Aspiration
- Balloon migration and airway obstruction with posterior packing
- Hypoxia and hypoventilation with posterior packing

SAFETY/QUALITY TIPS

- **Procedural**
  - Many anterior nosebleeds can be managed by first having the patient aggressively blow out clots from each naris, then hold firm pressure for 10 minutes. Patients commonly erroneously apply pressure cephalad the nasal bone.
  - Septal perforation is an important complication of cauterization. Do not blindly cauterize, and never cauterize both sides of the septum.
  - When applying a posterior pack, place an anterior pack on the same side
- **Cognitive**
  - When bleeding is from both nares, or when bleeding persists despite bilateral anterior packing, the source is likely posterior
  - Large posterior bleeds may require airway control with endotracheal intubation. Most patients who require posterior packing should be admitted to a monitored setting.
  - Patients often have vasovagal episodes while being packed—be prepared to bring patient to a supine or semisupine position if needed
  - Although evidence is poor, most otolaryngologists recommend prophylactic antibiotics for patients discharged with nasal packs

- **Acknowledgment**

Thank you to prior author James Hsiao.

Suggested Readings

Alter H. Approach to the adult with epistaxis. *UpToDate*. http://www.uptodate.com. Accessed Feb 17, 2014.

Bamimore O. Acute epistaxis. *Medscape*. http://emedicine.medscape.com. Accessed March 3, 2014.

Patel PB, Kost SI. Management of epistaxis. In: King C, Henretig F, eds. *Textbook of Pediatric Emergency Procedures*. 2nd ed. Philadelphia, PA: Williams & Wilkins; 2007:604.

Rosen P. *Atlas of Emergency Procedures*. St. Louis, MO: Mosby; 2001:194–197.

Simon RR, Brenner BE. *Emergency Procedures and Techniques*. 4th ed. Philadelphia, PA: Lippincott Williams & Wilkins; 2002:309–316.

76

Peritonsillar Abscess

Jennifer Sedor

INDICATIONS

- ⊡ Clinical suspicion
  - ✤ Swollen/red peritonsillar region causing uvular shift
  - ✤ Fluctuance of area
- ⊡ Interim treatment for peritonsillar closed space infection until tonsillectomy

CONTRAINDICATIONS

- ⊡ Extension into the deep neck tissue
- ⊡ Septicemia/toxic appearance
- ⊡ Airway obstruction
- ⊡ Severe trismus
- ⊡ Coagulopathy

- ⊡ **General Basic Steps**
  - ✤ **Patient preparation**
  - ✤ **Analgesia**
  - ✤ **Visualization**
  - ✤ **Needle aspiration/incision and drainage (I&D)**

LANDMARKS

- ⊡ Superior lateral border of affected tonsil, or area of most fluctuance
- ⊡ Aspirate peritonsillar abscess' (PTA's) superior pole first, then middle pole, and finally the inferior pole (FIGURE 76.1)

TECHNIQUE

- ⊡ **Patient Preparation**
  - ✤ **Cooperative** patient sitting upright in a chair with occipital support
  - ✤ Consider intravenous analgesia or sedation
  - ✤ Digital exam key: Must feel abscess!
  - ✤ Use ultrasound (endocavitary probe) to assess volume, location, and relationship to the carotid artery (FIGURE 76.2)
- ⊡ **Needle Aspiration**
  - ✤ Anesthetize with benzocaine spray or have patient gargle viscous lidocaine
  - ✤ Have patient depress own tongue by holding laryngoscope, insert as you would for intubation. Patient will be less likely to trigger own gag reflex while pulling down on blade (FIGURE 76.3)
  - ✤ Anesthetize locally with 1 to 2 mL of 1% lidocaine via 27-gauge needle
  - ✤ Use a long spinal needle so visualization is not obscured by syringe
  - ✤ Cut the distal 1 cm off of the needle cover and recap the needle, thereby preventing the needle from penetrating >1 cm (FIGURE 76.4)
  - ✤ Insert spinal needle at area of greatest fluctuance (usually the superior pole) and aspirate the pus

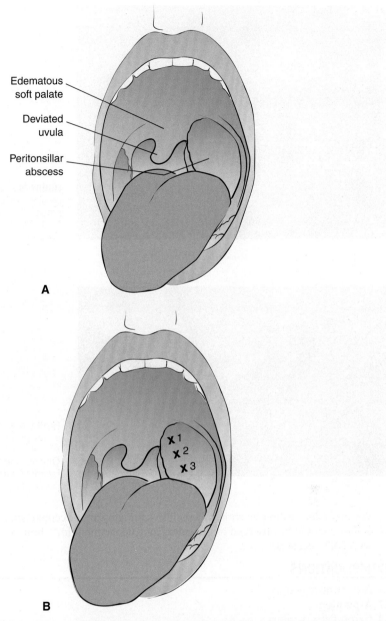

FIGURE 76.1 A: Peritonsillar abscess. The tonsil is displaced forward and inferomedial, the uvula is deviated toward the unaffected tonsil, and the soft palate is edematous and ruborous. **B:** Recommended sites for three-point needle aspiration of a peritonsillar abscess. (From Saladino RA. Pharyngeal procedures. In: Henretig FM, King C, eds. *Textbook of Pediatric Emergency Procedures*. Philadelphia, PA: Williams & Wilkins; 1997:692, 696, with permission.)

➕ **Incision and Drainage**
   ✛ If a large amount of pus is aspirated or continues to drain from aspiration site, an incision can be made
   ✛ Obtain a no. 11 blade and tape the blade leaving only the distal 0.5 cm free, thereby preventing the scalpel from penetrating too deep (Figure 76.3)
   ✛ Incise the mucosa at the area of aspiration horizontally
   ✛ Suction the area with a Frazier suction tip
   ✛ Insert a Kelly clamp to break up loculations
   ✛ Have patient rinse and gargle with saline

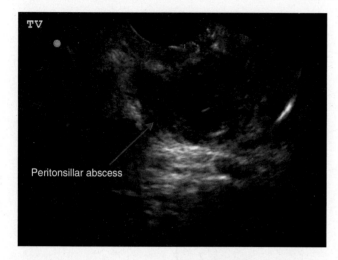

FIGURE 76.2 Ultrasound image of peritonsillar abscess using endocavitary probe. (Courtesy of Turandot Saul, M.D., RDMS, RDCS, FACEP; St. Luke's Roosevelt; New York, NY, with permission.)

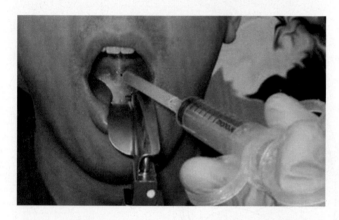

FIGURE 76.3 Peritonsillar abscess drainage technique. (Courtesy of Hagop Afarian, MD; Chief Medical Informatics Officer; Community Medical Centers; Fresno, California, with permission.)

- ☐ Postprocedure antibiotic choice: Penicillin, clindamycin, or cephalosporin
- ☐ Patients should be observed in the emergency department for 1 hour and next day follow up with ENT specialist

COMPLICATIONS

- ☐ Airway obstruction
- ☐ Aspiration
- ☐ Carotid artery injury

SAFETY/QUALITY TIPS

- ☐ **Procedural**
  - ✚ Patient must be relatively cooperative to safely perform this procedure without procedural sedation
  - ✚ Lighting and space are key—use laryngoscope with bright light and have assistant (or patient) pull corner of the mouth
  - ✚ Safeguard needles and scalpel blades as described above to avoid penetrating too deep; the carotid artery is nearby
  - ✚ Always have suction available and on. The patient can hold and control suction if cooperative.

☐ **Cognitive**
+ Do not attempt drainage on patients with severe trismus
+ Unlike most other abscesses, needle aspiration and I&D are thought to be equally effective
+ About 80% of PTAs can be palpated. There are a variety of other deep space neck infections that may require consultative management. If diagnostic uncertainty exists, use advanced imaging (computed tomography or ultrasound), especially in sicker patients.

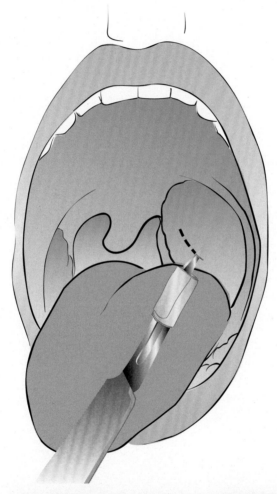

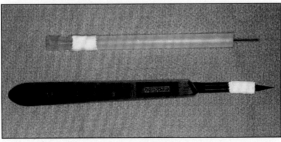

FIGURE 76.4 The depth of the needle and blade are controlled using a needle guard or an adhesive tape blade guard. (From Saladino RA. Pharyngeal procedures. In: Henretig FM, King C, eds. *Textbook of Pediatric Emergency Procedures*. Philadelphia, PA: Williams & Wilkins; 1997:695, with permission.)

⬚ **Acknowledgment**

Thank you to prior author Jenice Forde-Baker.

Suggested Readings

Johnson RF, Stewart MG. The contemporary approach to diagnosis and management of peritonsillar abscess. *Curr Opin Otolaryngol Head Neck Surg.* 2005;13(3):157–160.

Knoop KJ, Dennis WR. Otolaryngologic procedures. In: Roberts JR, Hedges JR, Chanmugam AS, et al., eds. *Clinical Procedures in Emergency Medicine.* 4th ed. Philadelphia, PA: WB Saunders; 2013:1298.

Lin M. Trick of the trade: peritonsillar abscess needle aspiration. http://www.aliem.com/trick-of-the-trade-peritonsillar-abscess-needle-aspiration/ Published September 9, 2009. Accessed February 20, 2014.

77

Auricular Hematoma Drainage

Eric Ingulsrud

INDICATIONS

- A subperichondrial hematoma that separates the perichondrium from the underlying auricular cartilage
  - Result of a shearing force to the ear, but can also develop after blunt trauma
  - The hematoma disrupts normal blood supply provided by the overlying perichondrium causing necrosis, fibrosis, and disfigurement of the auricle
  - Commonly seen in wrestlers
  - Early diagnosis and treatment is the key—necrosis begins within 24 hours
  - In general, needle aspiration is sufficient. However, if a hematoma reaccumulates, incision and drainage (I&D) may be indicated.

CONTRAINDICATIONS

- There are no absolute contraindications
- Anticoagulation is a relative contraindication. Consult with ear, nose, and throat (ENT) specialist if there are any concerns.

RISKS/CONSENT ISSUES

- Risk of infection is low. If clinical suspicion is high, an antistaphylococcal antibiotic may be prescribed.
- Recurrent and untreated injuries allow new cartilage to develop, which leads to deformity of the auricle (cauliflower ear) (FIGURES 77.1 and 77.2)

LANDMARKS

- The pinna is most commonly involved
- The needle/scalpel is used in the area of greatest fluctuance

- **General Basic Steps—Aspiration**
  - **Cleanse**
  - **Aspirate**
  - **"Milk" hematoma**
  - **Pressure dressing**

TECHNIQUE

- For needle aspiration, a 10-mL syringe and a 20-gauge needle are required
  - Cleanse the outer ear with a topical antiseptic (Betadine or chlorhexidine)
  - Local anesthesia is seldom required. If used, avoid epinephrine (causes tissue necrosis).
  - Stabilize pinna with thumb and fingers
  - Puncture area of greatest fluctuance with needle
  - "Milk" hematoma with thumb and index finger until completely evacuated
  - Maintain pressure on ear for 3 minutes after needle has been withdrawn
  - Apply antibiotic ointment and a pressure dressing
  - Patient should be advised to avoid strenuous activity
  - Check ear again in 24 hours for reaccumulation of hematoma
  - Reaspiration may be required, whereas persistent reaccumulation warrants I&D

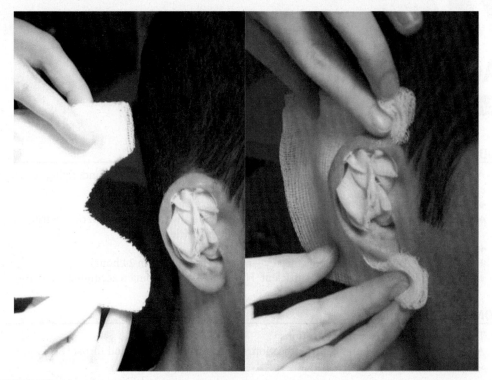

FIGURE 77.1 Compression dressing.

➕ **General Basic Steps—Incision and Drainage**
  ✚ **Cleanse**
  ✚ **Analgesia**
  ✚ **Incise**
  ✚ **Evacuate**
  ✚ **Irrigate**
  ✚ **Pressure dressing**

TECHNIQUE

➕ Cleanse the outer ear with a topical antiseptic (Betadine or chlorhexidine)
➕ Local anesthesia with 1 to 3 cc of 1% lidocaine (*without* epinephrine)
➕ Using a no. 15 blade, incise the skin at the edge of the hematoma following the natural curvature of the pinna
➕ With the use of forceps, gently peel the skin and perichondrium off and evacuate the hematoma completely
➕ Irrigate the pocket with sterile normal saline **(FIGURE 77.3)**

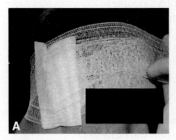
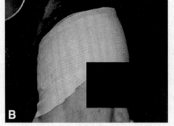
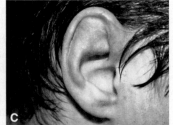

FIGURE 77.2 Pressure dressing.

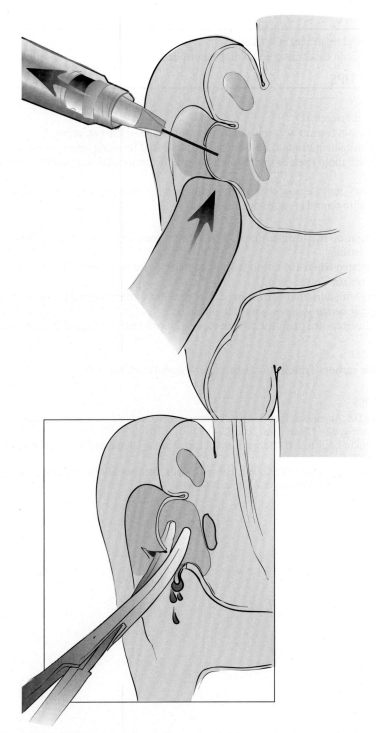

FIGURE 77.3 Evacuation of auricular hematoma. (From Pierce MC. External ear procedures. In: Henretig FM, King C, eds. *Textbook of Pediatric Emergency Procedures*. Philadelphia, PA: Williams & Wilkins; 1997:655, with permission.)

- Apply antibiotic ointment and a securely placed pressure dressing
- Patient should be advised to avoid strenuous activity
- Reevaluate ear in 24 hours for recurrence of hematoma

PRECAUTIONS

⊡ Early diagnosis and treatment is the key
⊡ For severe or difficult cases, involve ENT specialist early

SAFETY/QUALITY TIPS

⊡ **Procedural**
  ✛ Drains are not necessary
  ✛ Pressure dressings must securely conform to the shape of the ear, minimizing the risk of reaccumulating hematoma. This may be accomplished by using conventional casting plaster, which will mold itself to the ear architecture. A thermoplastic splint may also be used, if available.
  ✛ A "beanie hat" may be used to keep the splint and surrounding gauze in place; this is fashioned by pulling tubular gauze over the head
⊡ **Cognitive**
  ✛ Needle aspiration may be attempted two to three times (in one procedural session) and is largely successful
  ✛ I&D is indicated when aspiration fails, or sometimes for hematomas lasting >6 hours (as they may contain clotted blood)
  ✛ All patients with auricular hematoma drainage require mandatory 24 to 48 hour follow-up to ensure that hematoma has not reaccumulated
  ✛ If I&D is unsuccessful, then the patient should be promptly evaluated by a facial surgeon

⊡ **Acknowledgment**

Thank you to prior authors Timothy C. Loftus and Joseph P. Underwood.

Suggested Readings

Brickman K, Adams DZ, Akpunonu P, et al. Acute management of auricular hematoma: a novel approach and retrospective review. *Clin J Sport Med.* 2013;23(4):321.

Greywoode JD, Pribitkin EA, Krein H. Management of auricular hematoma and the cauliflower ear. *Fac Plast Surg.* 2010;26(6):451.

Pierce MC. External ear procedures. In: King C, Henretig F, eds. *Textbook of Pediatric Emergency Procedures.* 2nd ed. Philadelphia, PA: Williams & Wilkins; 2007:593.

78

Intercostal Nerve Block

Jennifer V. Pope and Jason A. Tracy

INDICATIONS

- Used to provide analgesia for acute and chronic pain conditions affecting the thorax including the following:
  - Significant rib fractures causing hypoventilation, splinting respirations, or atelectasis
  - Chest wall/upper abdominal surgery: Thoracotomy, thoracostomy, gastrostomy tube placement
  - Neuralgia: Posttraumatic, postherpetic (acute herpes simplex virus [HSV] infection), metastatic neoplasm of vertebral body

CONTRAINDICATIONS

- Contralateral pneumothorax
  - Inadvertant creation of bilateral pneumothorax puts the patient at unnecessarily high health risk
- Relative contraindications
  - Routine rib fracture that is tolerating oral analgesia
  - Local infection
  - Lack of surgical expertise
  - Serious hemostasis disorders, such as platelets <50,000 or international normalized ratio (INR) >1.0

RISK/CONSENT ISSUES

- Procedure can cause local pain. Local anesthesia will be given.
- Needle puncture can cause local bleeding, which is usually minimal. More significant bleeding can occur if the intercostal artery is punctured but care will be taken to avoid the artery.
- The needle could puncture the lung and cause a collapsed lung (pneumothorax). The risk is <1.5% and we have definitive treatment to reinflate the lung if the situation arises.
- Potential for introducing infection exists; however, this is extremely rare. Sterile technique will be utilized.

LANDMARKS

- The following landmarks are useful to determine the position of the desired rib:
  - 7th rib is the lowest rib covered by the angle of the scapula
  - 12th rib is the last rib palpable (FIGURE 78.1)
- The intercostal nerves (ICNs) course in the subcostal groove parallel to the ribs. Within the subcostal groove, the ICNs lie inferior to the intercostal arteries (**v**ein, **a**rtery, **n**erve).
- Most ICN blocks are performed between the posterior and midaxillary line at a point proximal to the origin of the lateral cutaneous nerve. In adults, this correlates with 6 to 8 cm from the spinous process at the angle of the rib.

TECHNIQUE

- **Collect Equipment**
  - Standard 25-gauge needle and 22-gauge 1.5-inch short-bevel needle
  - Sterile draping and sterile gloves
  - Povidone–iodine solution or chlorhexidine

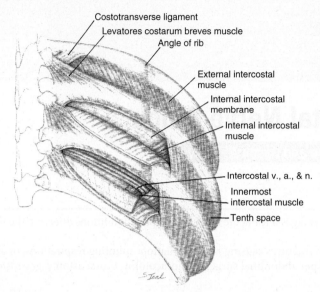

Costotransverse ligament
Levatores costarum breves muscle
Angle of rib

External intercostal
muscle

Internal intercostal
membrane

Internal intercostal
muscle

Intercostal v., a., & n.

Innermost
intercostal muscle

Tenth space

FIGURE 78.1 Exposure of the posterior part of intercostal spaces 8, 9, and 10. Note that the intercostal vein (*v.*), artery (*a.*), and nerve (*n.*) lie between the internal intercostal muscle and the innermost intercostal muscle layers. From the intervertebral foramen to the angle of the rib, the intercostal vessels and nerves are covered by the internal intercostal membrane. (Reprinted with permission from Blevins CE. Anatomy of the thorax. In: Shields TW, LoCicero J III, Ponn RB, et al. eds. *General Thoracic Surgery*. Vol 1. 6th ed. Philadelphia, PA: Lippincott Williams & Wilkins; 2005:11.)

⊡ **Select Anesthetic of Choice**
+ The levels of local anesthetic in the blood are highest after ICN block as compared to any other block; therefore, the risk of systemic toxicity needs to be considered
+ Bupivacaine 0.25% to 0.50% or lidocaine 1% to 2% with or without epinephrine can be used. Duration of analgesia is 12 to 18 hours and 3 to 4 hours respectively. A 1:1 mixture of the two can also be used.
+ While bupivacaine has a longer duration of action, it can cause central nervous system (CNS) toxicity at smaller doses than lidocaine
+ Because of the increased systemic absorption, stay within the recommended dosing range (bupivacaine 3 mg/kg maximum, lidocaine 4.5 mg/kg and 7 mg/kg when used with epinephrine)

⊡ **Patient Preparation**
+ The patient may be in a sitting position, prone, or lying with the unaffected side down. Ensure that the arms are forward in any position to pull the scapulae laterally to expose the posterior ribs.
+ Intravenous sedation with benzodiazepines, opioids, or ketamine may be needed and appreciated
+ Prepare the chest wall in a sterile manner with povidone–iodine solution or chlorhexidine

⊡ **Skin Entry/Injection**
+ Find the angle of the rib (costovertebral junction); in adults, this correlates with 6 to 8 cm from the spinous process (**FIGURE 78.2**). Anesthetize the skin surface by creating a wheal with 25-gauge needle and then switch to the 22-gauge needle.
+ Use the index finger of the nondominant hand to retract the skin at the lower edge of the rib, cephalad, and over the rib
+ With the syringe hand resting on the chest wall, advance the 22-gauge needle pointing cephalad at a 20-degree angle. The needle is advanced until it touches the lower border of the rib (<1 cm in depth).

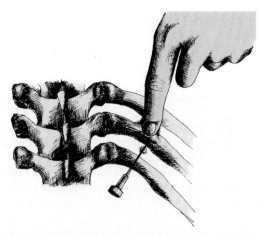

FIGURE 78.2 The intercostal nerve block. With the index finger of the left hand, palpate the rib to be injected and pull the skin overlying the rib cephalad. Insert the needle at a right angle to the skin and touch the rib. (Reused with permission from Simon RR, Brenner BE. *Emergency Procedures and Techniques.* 4th ed. Philadelphia, PA: Lippincott Williams & Wilkins; 2002:143.).

- ✚ Inject local anesthetic to anesthetize the periosteum
- ✚ With the nondominant hand, release the skin and hold the needle firmly while the syringe hand walks the needle caudally to just below the rib. Advance the needle 3 mm to reach the nerve in the intercostal space **(FIGURE 78.3)**
- ✚ After a negative aspirate, inject 3 to 5 mL of anesthetic
- ✚ Repeat the above procedure on one to two ICNs above and below to cover overlapping innervation
- ⊞ Postprocedure chest x-ray is recommended especially if the patient develops symptoms of a pneumothorax including new cough, new pain, and/or shortness of breath
    - ✚ This procedure can also be performed ultrasound-guided using a high-frequency linear transducer

COMPLICATIONS

- ⊞ Pneumothorax
    - ✚ In a large study of 100,000 ICN blocks performed by anesthesia residents, the rate of pneumothorax was 0.073%
    - ✚ Another study of ICN blocks after rib fracture alone found the rate of pneumothorax (PTX) to be 1.4%

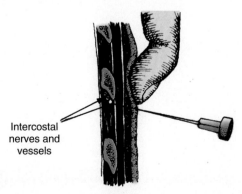

Intercostal
nerves and
vessels

FIGURE 78.3 The intercostal nerves lie beneath the rib margin, accompanied by the intercostal arteries. "Walk" the needle cautiously down the rib until it passes just beneath the inferior margin. Deposit the anesthetic solution here. Exercise caution not to go too deeply when passing the needle beneath the rib margin. (Reused with permission from Simon RR, Brenner BE. *Emergency Procedures and Techniques.* 4th ed. Philadelphia, PA: Lippincott Williams & Wilkins; 2002:143.)

- Systemic toxic reaction to the local anesthetic: Confusion, paresthesias, seizures
- Vasovagal reaction
- Hematoma formation
- Infection at the site

SAFETY/QUALITY TIPS

- **Procedural**
  - Consider using a skin marker to identify the proper landmarks
  - Aspirate prior to injection to avoid systemic toxicity, especially when using bupivacaine, which is both neurotoxic and, more dangerously, cardiotoxic
  - Patient should be on cardiac monitor when performing a nerve block with bupivacaine, and the antidote (20% lipid emulsion) should be available in case of overdose or inadvertent intravascular injection
- **Cognitive**
  - When compared with opiates, ICN blocks have been shown to improve pulmonary function after rib fractures and chest surgery
  - ICN block is an attractive alternative to opiates for pain control in the elderly, as it does not impair respiratory function, mentation, or balance
  - Exercise particular caution in patients with diminished pulmonary function, as pneumothorax will be poorly tolerated
  - Patients with chronic obstructive pulmonary disease (COPD) or other structural lung disease have altered lung and pleural anatomy, which increases the risk of pneumothorax

Suggested Readings

Shanti CM, Carlin AM, Tyburski JG. Incidence of pneumothorax from intercostal nerve block for analgesia in rib fractures. *J Trauma*. 2001;51:536–539.

Spektor M, Kelly JJ. Nerve blocks of the thorax and extremities. In: Roberts RJ, Custalow CB, Thomsen TW, et al. eds. *Roberts & Hedges Clinical Procedures in Emergency Medicine*. 6th ed. Philadelphia, PA: Elsevier Saunders; 2014:519–540.

Stone MB, Carnell J, Fischer JW, et al. Ultrasound-guided intercostal nerve block for traumatic pneumothorax requiring tube thoracostomy. *Am J Emerg Med*. 2011;29(6):697e1–697e2.

Watson DS, Panian S, Kendall V, et al. Pain control after thoracotomy: bupivacaine versus lidocaine in continuous extrapleural intercostal nerve block. *Ann Thorac Surg*. 1999;67:825–829.

79

Dental Nerve Blocks

Julie A. Zeller and Peter B. Smulowitz

INDICATIONS

- To provide temporary analgesia for intraoral or facial pain related to the following:
  - Trauma requiring intraoral or facial laceration repair
  - Dental trauma resulting in fractured teeth
  - Infection (tooth abscess, root impaction, gum disease) **(TABLE 79.1)**

CONTRAINDICATIONS

- **Absolute Contraindications**
  - Hypersensitivity/allergic reaction to local anesthetic agents
- **Relative Contraindications**
  - Coagulopathy
  - Uncooperative or obtunded patients

LANDMARKS AND TECHNIQUE

- **Equipment and Patient Positioning**
  - Adjust examination chair to accommodate patient height
  - Ensure adequate lighting to visualize oral landmarks
  - Assemble the necessary tools
    - Sterile "thumb-control" Monoject aspirating dental syringe
    - 1½-inch 25- to 27-gauge needle
    - Carpule cartridges containing anesthetic (either 2% lidocaine or 0.5% bupivacaine each with epinephrine 1:100,000 and 1:200,000 respectively)
    - Cotton-tipped applicators for administering topical anesthetic and controlling bleeding
  - Apply topical anesthetic (20% benzocaine or 5% to 10% lidocaine ointment) to mucosa before injection
  - Use lidocaine for laceration repairs and bupivacaine for dental blocks; 0.5% bupivacaine provides roughly 1 to 3 hours of dental pulp analgesia and 4 to 9 hours of soft-tissue analgesia
  - Buffering with bicarbonate is not recommended

SUPRAPERIOSTEAL NERVE BLOCK

- Apply topical anesthetic to apex of mucobuccal fold adjacent to the affected tooth
- Lift the patient's upper lip and pull the tissue taut
- Orient needle and syringe parallel to the long axis of the tooth
- Insert needle into the target area with the bevel facing the bone
- Advance and aspirate until the needle is a few millimeters beyond the apex of the tooth
- If aspiration is negative then inject approximately 2 mL of anesthetic **(FIGURE 79.1)**

INFRAORBITAL NERVE BLOCK

See Chapter 80 (Facial Nerve Blocks)

POSTERIOR SUPERIOR ALVEOLAR NERVE BLOCK

- Apply topical anesthetic to apex of mucobuccal fold above the second maxillary molar
- Have the patient partially open the mouth and deviate the mandible toward the side of the pain to create more room
- Use your index finger to retract the patient's cheek on the side being injected and pull the tissue taut

TABLE 79.1. TYPES OF DENTAL BLOCKS

Block	Area anesthetized	Comments
Supraperiosteal (local or apical)	Any individual maxillary tooth	⊞ Straightforward, high success rate ⊞ Not recommended for more than two adjacent teeth ⊞ Works poorly on mandible because of bone density
Infraorbital (includes middle and anterior superior alveolar nerves)	⊞ Maxillary teeth from midline through canine ⊞ Buccal soft tissue of upper lip, lateral aspect of nose, lower eyelid	⊞ Ideal for repairing upper lip lacerations ⊞ Poor landmark identification could result in needle insertion into globe
Posterior superior alveolar	⊞ Entire second and third maxillary molars ⊞ First maxillary molar fully anesthetized in approximately 70% of patients	⊞ Preferred block for pain in several maxillary molars ⊞ Significant risk of hematoma, avoid overpenetration with needle; aspiration is crucial
Inferior alveolar	⊞ All mandibular teeth to midline ⊞ Anterior two-thirds of tongue (lingular branch) ⊞ Floor of oral cavity ⊞ Distribution of mental nerve	⊞ Most widely used block, very effective when successful ⊞ Failure rate high: 20%
Mental	⊞ Mandibular teeth from midline to second premolar ⊞ Buccal soft tissues from second premolar to midline, skin of lower lip and chin	⊞ High success rate ⊞ Ideal for repairing lower-lip and chin lacerations

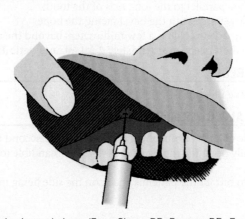

FIGURE 79.1 Supraperiosteal injection technique. (From Simon RR, Brenner BE. *Emergency Procedures and Techniques*. 4th ed. Philadelphia, PA: Lippincott Williams & Wilkins; 2002:326, with permission.)

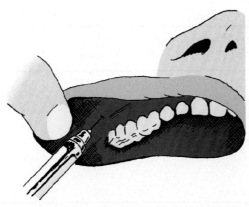

FIGURE 79.2 Posterior superior alveolar nerve injection technique. (From Simon RR, Brenner BE. *Emergency Procedures and Techniques*. 4th ed. Philadelphia, PA: Lippincott Williams & Wilkins; 2002:326, with permission.)

- Insert needle into the apex of the second maxillary molar, bevel facing bone
- Advance needle through the soft tissue superiorly and medially (at a 45-degree angle to the plane of occlusion) and then posteriorly (at a 45-degree angle to the long axis of the second maxillary molar); approximately 15 mm in depth
- If aspiration is negative, inject approximately 2 mL of anesthetic **(FIGURE 79.2)**

INFERIOR ALVEOLAR NERVE BLOCK

- Stand opposite to the side to be injected
- Apply topical anesthetic to mucosa at the site of the pterygomandibular triangle approximately 1 cm above the occlusal surface of the molars
- Locate the anterior and posterior aspects of the mandibular ramus. Place thumb of the nondominant hand intraorally and the index finger extraorally. The mandibular foramen is located between the index finger and the thumb, slightly above the level of the mandibular molars and midway between the anterior and posterior borders of the ramus **(FIGURE 79.3)**.
- Orient syringe so the barrel is in the opposite corner of the mouth, resting on the premolars
- Aim toward your index finger and slowly penetrate the mucosa at the pterygomandibular triangle until you hit bone (approximately 2.5 cm)
- Failure to reach bone generally results from directing the needle too far posteriorly, toward the parotid gland. This risks temporary paralysis of the facial nerve.
- Once bone is contacted, withdraw slightly and aspirate. If no blood is aspirated, inject up to 2 mL of anesthetic.

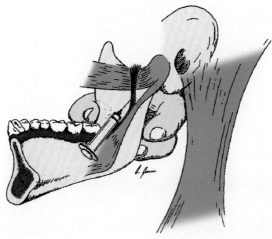

FIGURE 79.3 Inferior alveolar nerve injection. (From Simon RR, Brenner BE. *Emergency Procedures and Techniques*. 4th ed. Philadelphia, PA: Lippincott Williams & Wilkins; 2002:327, with permission.)

MENTAL NERVE BLOCK

See Chapter 80 (Facial Nerve Blocks)

COMPLICATIONS

☐ Nerve damage
☐ Localized hematoma
☐ Incomplete analgesia
☐ Infection
☐ Allergic reaction to anesthetic
☐ Intravascular injection
☐ Vasovagal syncope

SAFETY/QUALITY TIPS

☐ **Procedural**
  + Use adequate topical anesthesia before needle insertion
  + A common error is to insufficiently advance the needle to reach the tooth apex
  + Injection pain is reduced if smaller needle is used and anesthetic injected slowly (over 30 seconds)
☐ **Cognitive**
  + Dental blocks are relatively easy, safe, and more effective than systemic analgesics for tooth pain. Dental blocks should be offered to most patients with tooth pain, especially as an alternative to opiates when opiate misuse is suspected.
  + Convey to patient that dental blocks are intended for temporary pain relief; the procedure is not a substitute for prompt follow-up with a dentist

Suggested Readings

Amsterdam JT, Kilgore KP. Regional anesthesia of the head and neck. In: Roberts JR, Custalow CB, Thomsen TW, et al. eds. *Roberts & Hedges Clinical Procedures in Emergency Medicine*. 6th ed. Philadelphia, PA: Elsevier Saunders; 2014:541–553.

Powell SL, Robertson L, Doty BJ. Dental nerve blocks: toothache remedies for the acute-care setting. *Postgrad Med*. 2000;107(1):229–245.

Trott AT. *Wounds and Lacerations: Emergency Care and Closure*. 2nd ed. St. Louis, MO: Mosby; 1997.

80

Facial Nerve Blocks

Catherine H. Horwitz and Jason A. Tracy

INDICATIONS

- To anesthetize portions of the face and ears
- Areas of distributions:
  - Supraorbital and supratrochlear: Forehead
  - Infraorbital: Upper lip, upper cheek, lateral portion of the nose, and anterior maxillary teeth
  - Inferior alveolar: Lower jaw, lower lip, lower teeth, and anterior two-thirds of the tongue
  - Mental: Lower jaw, lower teeth, anterior tongue, and floor of the mouth
  - Auricular: External ear

CONTRAINDICATIONS

- **Absolute Contraindications**
  - Anaphylaxis to local anesthetic agents
- **Relative Contraindications**
  - Coagulopathy
  - Infection at the injection site
  - Uncooperative or obtunded patients

SUPPLIES

- 25-gauge to 30-gauge needle
- Syringe
- Topical anesthetic (optional)
  - Eutectic mixture of local anesthetics (EMLA), 20% benzocaine, or 5% to 10% lidocaine ointment can be used to decrease the pain of needle insertion
- Bicarbonate (optional)
  - 1:10 dilution with injectable anesthetic to decrease the pain of infiltration
- Anesthetic agent
  - Lidocaine 1% to 2%
    - Onset of action: 4 to 10 minutes
    - Duration of action: 1 to 2 hours
    - Maximum one time dose: 4.5 mg/kg
  - Bupivacaine 0.25%
    - Onset of action: 8 to 12 minutes
    - Duration of action: 4 to 8 hours

- **General Basic Steps**
  - **Preparation**
  - **Identify landmarks**
  - **Injection of anesthetic**

PREPARATION

- Position patient and adjust lighting for optimal visualization
- Apply topical local anesthetic
- Prepare nonmucosal injection sites with povidone–iodine solution or chlorhexidine
- Use sterile gloves

LANDMARKS AND TECHNIQUES

☐ **Forehead Nerve Block (Supraorbital and Supratrochlear Nerve Blocks)**
  ✦ Locate the supraorbital notch which is at the intersection of the superior edge of the orbit and a vertical line through the middle of the pupil when the eyes are looking forward
  ✦ Insert the needle slightly superior and medial to the supraorbital notch and inject 2 to 4 mL of anesthetic
  ✦ Move 0.5 to 1.0 cm medially and inject an additional 2 to 4 mL of anesthetic to block the supratrochlear nerve (FIGURE 80.1)

☐ **Infraorbital Nerve Block**
  ✦ Locate the infraorbital foramen which is at the intersection of the inferior edge of the orbit and a vertical line through the middle of the pupil when the eyes are looking forward
  ✦ Extraoral or intraoral approaches can be used
    + Extraoral
      ▪ Insert the needle 1 cm below the infraorbital foramen and inject 2 to 4 mL of anesthetic
    + Intraoral
      ▪ Place one finger on the infraorbital foramen and retract the upper lip
      ▪ Identify the first maxillary premolar and insert the needle into the mucobuccal fold with the bevel facing the bone
      ▪ Advance the needle toward the apex of the tooth or 1 cm below the infraorbital foramen
      ▪ Take caution to avoid entering the orbit or the infraorbital foramen. If the patient feels paresthesias, retract the needle.
      ▪ Inject 2 to 4 mL of anesthetic

☐ **Mental Nerve Block**
  ✦ Locate the mental foramen which lies in the plane of the supraorbital and infraorbital foramina (see above) at the apex of the lower second premolar
  ✦ Extraoral or intraoral approaches can be used (FIGURE 80.2)
    + Extraoral
      ▪ Insert the needle 1 cm inferolateral to the foramen
      ▪ Inject 2 to 4 mL of anesthetic
    + Intraoral
      ▪ Retract the patient's lower lip
      ▪ Locate the space between the premolar and molar teeth

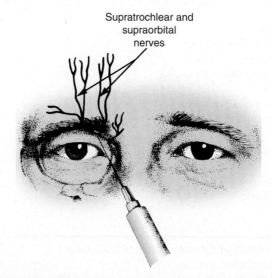

Supratrochlear and supraorbital nerves

FIGURE 80.1 The supraorbital and supratrochlear nerves emerging through the notches at the upper border of the orbital ridge. (From Simon RR, Brenner BE. *Emergency Procedures and Techniques.* 4th ed. Philadelphia, PA: Lippincott Williams & Wilkins; 2002:117, with permission.)

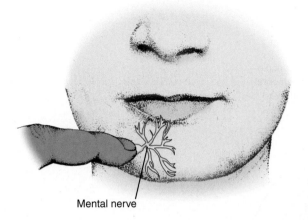

FIGURE 80.2 The mental nerve supplies sensation to the skin and mucous membranes of the lower lip.(From Simon RR, Brenner BE. *Emergency Procedures and Techniques.* 4th ed. Philadelphia, PA: Lippincott Williams & Wilkins; 2002:114, with permission.)

Mental nerve

- Insert the needle into the mucobuccal fold and advance toward the apex of the teeth
- Aspirate. If no blood returns, inject 2 to 4 mL of anesthetic.

◻ **Auricular Block**
- ✚ Begin at the inferior aspect of the pinna and infiltrate along the inferior/posterior aspect and then along the inferior/anterior aspect of the ear **(FIGURE 80.3)**
- ✚ Next, enter the skin superior to the pinna and infiltrate along the superior/posterior aspect and then along the superior/anterior aspect of the ear
- ✚ A total of 10 to 20 mL of anesthetic is injected in a diamond shape around the pinna

◻ **Inferior Alveolar Nerve Block**
See Chapter 79 (Dental Nerve Blocks) **(FIGURE 80.4)**

COMPLICATIONS

◻ Nerve damage
◻ Localized hematoma
◻ Incomplete analgesia
◻ Infection
◻ Allergic reaction to anesthetic
◻ Intravascular injection
◻ Vasovagal syncope

SAFETY/QUALITY TIPS

◻ **Procedural**
- ✚ Aspirate prior to injecting anesthetic to avoid an intravascular injection, especially if using bupivacaine
- ✚ Minimize the pain of needle insertion by using a narrow-gauge needle, applying topical anesthesia prior to the procedure, buffering the injectable anesthetic with bicarbonate, and injecting the anesthetic slowly over 30 seconds
- ✚ Avoid injecting directly into the foramen which can cause nerve damage
- ✚ Do not change the direction of the needle without first withdrawing to avoid damaging tissue or breaking the needle
- ✚ Always insert the needle with the bevel toward bone

◻ **Cognitive**
- ✚ Take time to review the method, gather all necessary equipment, ensure adequate lighting, and identify landmarks before procedure
- ✚ EMLA should not be used on mucosal surfaces and requires 30 to 60 minutes to have its desired effect

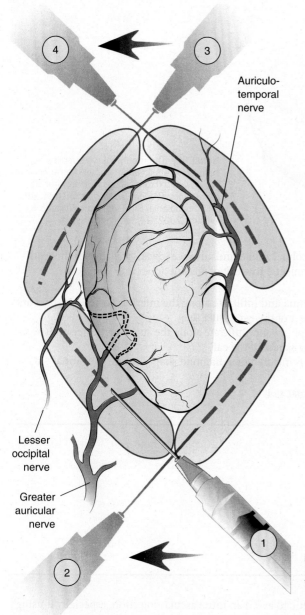

Auriculo-
temporal
nerve

Lesser
occipital
nerve

Greater
auricular
nerve

FIGURE 80.3 Regional auricular block. (From Kassutto Z, Helpin ML. Orofacial anesthesia techniques. In: Henretig FM, King C, eds. *Textbook of Pediatric Emergency Procedures.* Philadelphia, PA: Williams & Wilkins; 1997:719, with permission.)

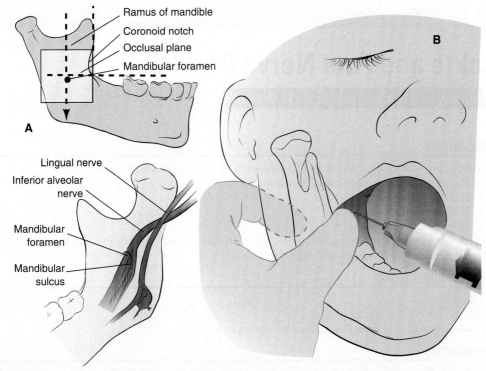

FIGURE 80.4 A: Localization of inferior alveolar nerve. **B:** Hand and needle positions for inferior alveolar nerve block. (From Kassutto Z, Helpin ML. Orofacial anesthesia techniques. In: Henretig FM, King C, eds. *Textbook of Pediatric Emergency Procedures*. Philadelphia, PA: Williams & Wilkins; 1997:719, with permission.)

Suggested Readings

Amsterdam JT, Kilgore KP. Regional anesthesia of the head and neck. In: Roberts JR, Custalow CB, Thomsen TW, et al. eds. *Roberts & Hedges' Clinical Procedures in Emergency Medicine*. 6th ed. Philadelphia, PA: Elsevier Saunders; 2014:541–553.

Simon RR, Brenner BE. *Emergency Procedures and Techniques*. 4th ed. Philadelphia, PA: Lippincott Williams & Wilkins; 2002.

Tintinalli JE, Ruiz E, Krome RL. *Emergency Medicine: A Comprehensive Study Guide*. 4th ed. New York, NY: McGraw-Hill; 1996.

Wolfson AB. *Harwood-Nuss' Clinical Practice of Emergency Medicine*. 6th ed. Philadelphia, PA: Lippincott Williams & Wilkins; 2014.

81

Ankle and Foot Nerve Blocks

Matthew R. Babineau and Scott G. Weiner

INDICATIONS

- Used to provide regional anesthesia to the foot in order to facilitate the following:
    - Primary closure/exploration of foot wounds
    - Incision and drainage
    - Removal of foreign bodies
    - Operative intervention
- Preferred technique because glabrous skin of the epidermis and fibrous septae in the dermis of the foot limit local diffusion of anesthetic

CONTRAINDICATIONS

- Patient refusal
- Infection overlying injection sites
- *Relative contraindications*: Coagulopathy, systemic infection

LANDMARKS

- There are five nerves which supply the entire surface of the foot (FIGURE 81.1); anatomic landmarks to locate individual nerves are found in the text

TECHNIQUE

- Preparation
    - Obtain informed consent
    - Position patient supine with knee in flexion and foot placed flat on the gurney
    - Sterilize the area of injection with povidone–iodine or chlorhexidine solution
    - Drape the area with sterile towels
    - Prepare one to three 10-mL syringes filled with anesthetic of choice
    - Use 25-gauge to 30-gauge needle

- **General Basic Steps**
    - **Identify landmarks**
    - **Prepare for sterile procedure**
    - **Inject anesthetic**

POSTERIOR TIBIAL NERVE BLOCK

- *Innervation*: Divides into medial and lateral plantar nerves to supply most of the plantar aspect of the foot
- *Location*: Medial aspect of the ankle between medial malleolus and Achilles tendon
- *Technique* (FIGURE 81.2)
    - Palpate posterior tibial artery posterior to medial malleolus
    - Direct needle at 45-degree angle to mediolateral plane, posterior to artery
    - At depth of artery (0.5–1 cm deep), move needle slightly to induce paresthesia
    - If elicited, 3 to 5 mL of anesthetic is injected after aspiration
    - Withdraw 1 mm, then infiltrate 5 to 7 mL of anesthetic while withdrawing 1 cm

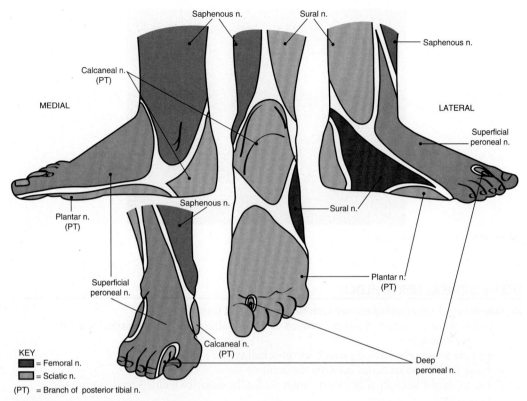

FIGURE 81.1 The sensory nerve supply to the foot. (From Brown DL, ed. *Atlas of Regional Anesthesia*. 4th ed. Philadelphia, PA: Elsevier Saunders; 2010:135–138.)

SURAL NERVE BLOCK

- ⊡ *Innervation*: Lateral edge of foot, variable to fifth toe
- ⊡ *Location*: Lateral aspect of ankle between Achilles tendon and lateral malleolus
- ⊡ *Technique* (FIGURE 81.3)
  - ✦ Infiltrate 3 to 5 mL of local anesthetic in a band between Achilles tendon and lateral malleolus

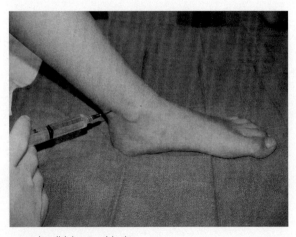

FIGURE 81.2 Approach for posterior tibial nerve block.

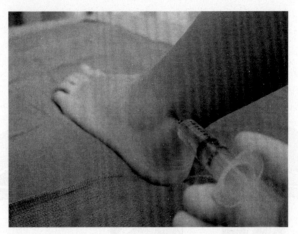

FIGURE 81.3 Approach for sural nerve block.

DEEP PERONEAL NERVE BLOCK

◻ *Innervation*: Dorsal webspace between first and second toes
◻ *Location*: Anterior aspect of ankle, between extensor hallucis and anterior tibial tendons
◻ *Technique* **(FIGURE 81.4)**
   ✚ Palpate tendons by having patient dorsiflex hallux and foot
   ✚ Raise subcutaneous wheal between the tendons
   ✚ Direct needle laterally at 30-degree angle under the extensor hallucis tendon until the tibia is met
   ✚ Withdraw needle 1 to 2 mm and infiltrate 1 mL of local anesthetic

SUPERFICIAL PERONEAL NERVE BLOCK

◻ *Innervation*: Dorsal aspect of foot, except webspace between first and second toes
◻ *Location*: Anterior aspect of ankle between extensor hallucis tendon and lateral malleolus
◻ *Technique*
   ✚ Infiltrate 5 to 10 mL of local anesthetic subcutaneously in a band between extensor hallucis tendon and lateral malleolus

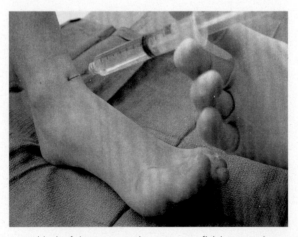

FIGURE 81.4 Approach for nerve block of deep peroneal nerve, superficial peroneal nerve, and saphenous nerve.

SAPHENOUS NERVE BLOCK

- ☐ *Innervation*: Medial aspect of foot, variable to first toe
- ☐ *Location*: Anterior aspect of ankle between anterior tibial tendon and medial malleolus
- ☐ *Technique*
  - ✦ Infiltrate 3 to 5 mL of local anesthetic in a band between anterior tibial tendon and medial malleolus. This can be done while withdrawing the needle from the deep peroneal nerve block (FIGURE 81.4).

COMPLICATIONS

- ☐ Infection
- ☐ Hematoma
- ☐ Vessel puncture with subsequent cardiotoxicity
- ☐ Nerve injury, neuritis

SAFETY/QUALITY TIPS

- ☐ **Procedural**
  - ✦ Proper positioning of patient will allow all nerves to be accessed without repositioning patient or drapes
  - ✦ The superficial nerves (sural nerve, saphenous nerve, and superficial peroneal nerve) have extensive branches and anastomoses, so a generous subcutaneous infiltration will provide better anesthesia
  - ✦ For the deep nerve blocks (deep peroneal nerve and posterior tibial nerve), repeating the described procedures twice while "fanning" the needle 30 degrees medial and lateral will improve anesthesia
  - ✦ Alternatively, all five nerves can be blocked using three injections (FIGURE 81.5)
    - + Block posterior tibial nerve as described
    - + Block sural nerve as described
    - + Block deep peroneal nerve as described; as the needle is withdrawn, fan medially and infiltrate to block the saphenous nerve, then fan laterally and infiltrate to block the superficial peroneal nerve
- ☐ **Cognitive**
  - ✦ Inform patient that technique does not always work on first attempt and may require reinjection (and subsequent pain)
  - ✦ Due to overlap of sensory supply to foot, strongly consider blocking all five nerves for any procedure
  - ✦ The block requires relatively high volume of local anesthetic, so patients may benefit from oral or parenteral analgesia prior to the procedure
  - ✦ Respect maximum doses of anesthetic. Aspirate prior to injection to avoid systemic toxicity, especially when using bupivacaine, which is both neurotoxic and, more dangerously, cardiotoxic.
  - ✦ Patient should be on cardiac monitor when performing a nerve block with bupivacaine, and the antidote (20% lipid emulsion) should be available in case of overdose or inadvertent intravascular injection
  - ✦ Perform and document a thorough sensory examination prior to procedure
  - ✦ Ultrasound guidance may lead to greater analgesic success rates

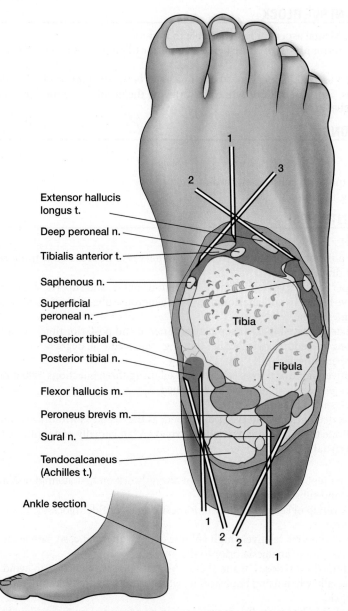

Extensor hallucis
longus t.

Deep peroneal n.

Tibialis anterior t.

Saphenous n.

Superficial
peroneal n.

Posterior tibial a.

Posterior tibial n.

Flexor hallucis m.

Peroneus brevis m.

Sural n.

Tendocalcaneus
(Achilles t.)

Ankle section

Tibia

Fibula

FIGURE 81.5 Three-injection method (transverse view) to block all five nerves (From Brown DL, ed. *Atlas of Regional Anesthesia.* 4th ed. Philadelphia, PA: Elsevier Saunders; 2010:135–138.)

Suggested Readings

Boezaart AP, ed. *Atlas of Peripheral Nerve Blocks and Anatomy for Orthopaedic Anesthesia.* Philadelphia, PA: Elsevier Saunders; 2008:195–203.

Brown DL, ed. *Atlas of Regional Anesthesia.* 4th ed. Philadelphia, PA: Elsevier Saunders; 2010:135–138.

Chin KJ, Wong NW, Macfarlane AJ, et al. Ultrasound-guided versus anatomic landmark-guided ankle blocks: a 6-year retrospective review. *Reg Anesth Pain Med.* 2011;36(6):611–618.

Spektor M, Kelly JJ. Nerve blocks of the thorax and extremities. In: Roberts JR, Custalow CB, Thomsen TW, et al. eds. *Roberts & Hedges' Clinical Procedures in Emergency Medicine.* 6th ed. Philadelphia, PA: Elsevier Saunders; 2014:554–589.

82

Wrist Nerve Blocks

Jayson R. Pereira and Ryan P. Friedberg

INDICATIONS

- Used to provide anesthesia in distribution of median, ulnar, and/or radial nerves for the treatment of complex soft-tissue or bony injuries of the hand
  - Irrigation of deep abrasions with embedded debris
  - Extensive or complex laceration repair
  - Burn injury pain control
  - Incision and drainage of abscess
  - Fracture/dislocation reduction
  - Traumatic amputation

CONTRAINDICATIONS

- Overlying cellulitis at site of anticipated injection
- **Relative Contraindications**
  - Simple laceration or injury that can be easily and adequately anesthetized with local infiltration or digital block

COMPLICATIONS

- Hematoma formation and/or vascular injury
- Nerve injury
- Infection
- Allergic reaction

- **General Basic Steps**
  - **Palpate landmarks**
  - **Sterile prep of skin**
  - **Inject anesthetic**
  - **Consider sensory branches**

ULNAR NERVE BLOCK

- **Landmarks**
  - Flexor carpi ulnaris tendon, pisiform bone, ulnar artery, proximal wrist crease (FIGURE 82.1)
  - Ulnar nerve splits into dorsal and palmar branches approximately 5 cm proximal to the wrist crease
  - Palmar branch runs between the flexor carpi ulnaris tendon and the ulnar artery at the level of the proximal wrist crease
- **Technique**
  - **Patient Preparation**
    - Place the hand comfortably on bedside procedure table with palmar surface up
    - Prepare wrist site in standard sterile manner (povidone–iodine solution or chlorhexidine)
    - Have patient flex wrist against resistance to accentuate landmarks
    - Identify and mark the flexor carpi ulnaris tendon from its insertion site at the pisiform bone to the ulnar nerve branch point (approximately 5 cm proximal to wrist crease)

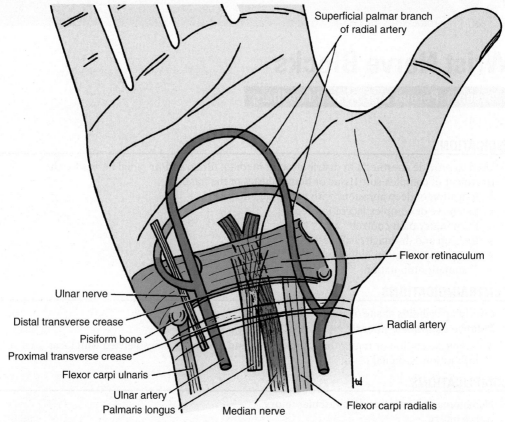

Superficial palmar branch
of radial artery

Flexor retinaculum

Ulnar nerve

Distal transverse crease

Pisiform bone

Proximal transverse crease

Flexor carpi ulnaris

Ulnar artery

Palmaris longus

Radial artery

Median nerve

Flexor carpi radialis

FIGURE 82.1 Surface anatomy of the wrist region. (From Snell RS. *Clinical Anatomy*. 7th ed. Philadelphia, PA: Lippincott Williams & Wilkins; 2004:534, with permission.)

+ **Injection**
  + Approach the wrist medially and insert a small-bore (25-gauge) needle beneath the flexor carpi ulnaris tendon at the level of the proximal wrist crease **(FIGURE 82.2)**
    - Inject approximately 2 mL of anesthetic solution (lidocaine/bupivacaine) beneath the tendon at its radial border
    - Aspirate before injecting anesthetic to ensure that ulnar artery has not been inadvertently entered
  + To anesthetize the dorsal branch of the ulnar nerve use the same initial insertion site and technique. However, redirect needle 3 to 5 cm proximally toward the branch point.
    - Inject approximately 5 mL of anesthetic solution beneath the tendon at this branch point

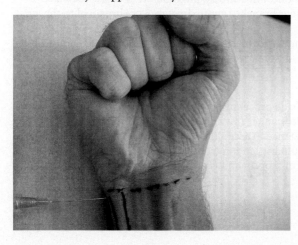

FIGURE 82.2 Injection site of an ulnar nerve block.

SAFETY/QUALITY TIPS

▢ **Procedural**
  ✦ Inadequate anesthesia will result if there is failure to redirect and inject at the dorsal cutaneous branch point
  ✦ A common error is depositing anesthetic solution too medially owing to fear of entering/injuring the ulnar artery
  ✦ If the proximal wrist crease cannot be easily identified, the ulnar styloid can be used as an alternative landmark
  ✦ If tendon is not identified initially, have patient oppose thumb and fifth finger while flexing against resistance
  ✦ If paresthesias are elicited during advancement of the needle, stop and withdraw approximately 5 mm and inject the anesthetic

MEDIAN NERVE BLOCK

▢ **Landmarks**
  ✦ Palmaris longus tendon, flexor carpi radialis tendon, proximal wrist crease (Figure 82.1)
  ✦ Median nerve runs beneath palmaris longus tendon along its radial edge
  ✦ If the palmaris longus tendon is absent (approximately 15% of population) the median nerve can be found approximately 1 cm ulnar to flexor carpi radialis tendon
  ✦ In contrast to the superficial position of the palmaris longus, the median nerve courses deep to the flexor retinaculum

▢ **Technique**
  ✦ **Patient Preparation**
    + Place the hand comfortably on bedside procedure table with palmar surface up
    + Prepare wrist site in standard sterile manner (povidone–iodine solution or chlorhexidine)
    + Have patient flex wrist against resistance to accentuate landmarks
    + Identify and mark palmaris longus tendon and/or flexor carpi radialis tendon at the level of the proximal wrist crease
  ✦ **Injection**
    + Approach the wrist from palmar side and insert a small-bore (25-gauge) needle through the proximal wrist crease at a right angle to the lateral border of the palmaris longus tendon **(FIGURE 82.3)**
      ▪ Inject approximately 5 mL of anesthetic solution (lidocaine/bupivacaine) deep to the flexor retinaculum
    + In patients without a palmaris longus, insert and inject 1 cm medial to flexor carpi radialis using the same approach and technique

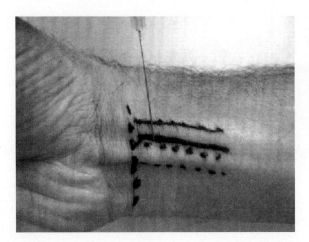

FIGURE 82.3 Injection site of a median nerve block.

SAFETY/QUALITY TIPS

⊕ **Procedural**

+ A common mistake is injecting anesthetic superficial to flexor retinaculum, which then blocks anesthetic solution from contacting the nerve
+ Do not mistake the flexor carpi radialis tendon for the palmaris longus tendon in those patients in whom the palmaris longus is absent
+ If tendons are not identified easily, have patient oppose thumb and fifth finger while flexing against resistance
+ Feel for resistance as needle pierces the flexor retinaculum
+ To ensure that the injection is deep to the flexor retinaculum, insert needle until bone is contacted, then withdraw 0.5 cm and deposit anesthetic solution
+ If paresthesias are elicited during advancement of the needle, stop and withdraw approximately 5 mm and inject the anesthetic

RADIAL NERVE BLOCK

⊕ **Landmarks**

+ Radial styloid, radial artery, proximal wrist crease, anatomic snuff box (**FIGURE 82.4**)
+ Radial nerve follows the course of the radial artery breaking off into multiple deep and superficial branches before entering the hand
+ At the level of the proximal wrist crease all sensory branches of the radial nerve run superficially, providing an access point for complete anesthesia

⊕ **Technique**

+ **Patient Preparation**
    + Place the hand comfortably on bedside procedure table with the ulnar surface down
    + Prepare wrist site in standard sterile manner (povidone–iodine solution or chlorhexidine)
    + Identify and mark the radial artery at the level of the proximal wrist crease
+ **Injection**
    + Palpate for the radial styloid. Approach the wrist from palmar side and insert a small-bore (25-gauge) needle through the proximal wrist crease, immediately lateral to the radial artery.
        ▪ Inject approximately 3 mL of anesthetic solution (lidocaine/bupivacaine) subcutaneously over the palmar aspect of the radial styloid
    + Next ensure anesthesia of all the sensory branches. Using the same initial needle insertion point redirect the needle over the snuff box, and inject approximately 5 mL of the anesthetic solution in a bandlike manner to the dorsal midline.

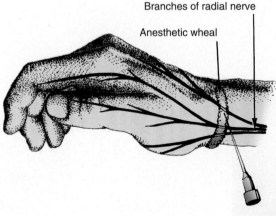

Branches of radial nerve

Anesthetic wheal

FIGURE 82.4 Deposit a subcutaneous wheal of anesthetic in a semicircle manner to block all branches of the radial nerve. (From Simon RR, Brenner BE. *Emergency Procedures and Techniques.* 4th ed. Philadelphia, PA: Lippincott Williams & Wilkins; 2002:132, with permission.)

SAFETY/QUALITY TIPS

▢ **Procedural**

+ Inadequate anesthesia of the dorsal sensory branches will result if bandlike injection is stopped short of the dorsal midline

+ Avoid unnecessary patient discomfort when anesthetizing dorsal sensory branches; new needle insertions should be through areas of already anesthetized skin

▢ **Cognitive**

+ Especially when performing multiple nerve blocks, be mindful of maximum doses to avoid local anesthetic toxicity

+ If a significant amount of local anesthetic (especially bupivacaine) is to be used, have lipid emulsion therapy available in case toxicity develops

Suggested Readings

Mulroy MF, Bernards CM, McDonald SB, Salinas FV. *A Practical Approach to Regional Anesthesia.* 4th ed. Baltimore, MD: Lippincott Williams & Wilkins; 2008.

Roberts RJ, Custalow CB, Thomsen TW, et al. *Roberts & Hedges' Clinical Procedures in Emergency Medicine.* 6th ed. Philadelphia, PA: WB Saunders; 2013.

Rosen P, Chan T, Vilke G, et al. *Atlas of Emergency Procedures.* San Diego, CA: Mosby; 2001.

Simon RR, Brenner BE. *Emergency Procedures and Techniques.* 4th ed. Philadelphia, PA: Lippincott Williams & Wilkins; 2002.

Snell R. *Clinical Anatomy.* 7th ed. Philadelphia, PA: Lippincott Williams & Wilkins; 2004.

83

Anorectal Foreign Body Removal

Heather Huffman-Dracht and Wendy Coates

INDICATIONS

⊞ Anorectal foreign body (FB) in a stable, cooperative patient, which is:
  ✦ Palpable by rectal approach
  ✦ Absence of a sharp edge

CONTRAINDICATIONS

⊞ Obtain surgical consult immediately in following instances:
  ✦ Signs of perforation, obstruction, or severe abdominal pain
  ✦ Nonpalpable FB
  ✦ Broken glass in rectum
  ✦ Uncooperative or intolerant patient
  ✦ Lack of equipment necessary for retrieval

General Basic Steps
  ✦ **Determine type of FB**
  ✦ **Radiography**
  ✦ **Obtain necessary equipment**
  ✦ **Patient preparation**
  ✦ **Analgesia**
  ✦ **FB removal**
  ✦ **Assess for structural damage**

KEY ELEMENTS OF HISTORY

⊞ Ingestion (e.g., bones, toothpicks) versus rectal insertion
⊞ Size and composition of FB
⊞ Time of ingestion/insertion
⊞ Attempts made to remove FB
⊞ Assess for red flags—fever, abdominal pain, hematochezia
⊞ Assess for sexual/physical assault, sexually transmitted disease (STD) risk

LANDMARKS

⊞ Determine the orientation, location, and composition of the anorectal FB and, thereby the appropriate approach to removal by the following:
  ✦ Detailed history
  ✦ Consider radiography
    + Kidney, ureter, and bladder (KUB) x-ray
    + Chest x-ray for free air detection (if concerned about perforation)
  ✦ Physical examination, including digital rectal examination (DRE)
⊞ Visualization of the anorectum is enhanced with the patient in the lateral decubitus position, lithotomy position, or prone with knees tucked into chest

TECHNIQUE

◻ **Equipment**
- ✦ Depends on the composition and locale of the FB but may include:
  - ✦ Anesthesia/analgesia
  - ✦ Light source
  - ✦ Speculum (i.e., vaginal speculum or anoscope) or Parks retractor to improve visualization
  - ✦ Ring and/or tenaculum forceps
  - ✦ Foley catheter and/or endotracheal tube (ETT)
  - ✦ Vacuum extractor

◻ **Patient Preparation**
- ✦ Get informed consent detailing risks, benefits, and alternatives
- ✦ Order KUB x-ray to localize and define FB, and to assess for obstruction or perforation if clinically necessary **(FIGURE 83.1)**
- ✦ Parenteral sedation and analgesia to enable relaxation and tolerance of the procedure. Avoid oversedation because the patient must be alert to assist in the delivery of the FB.
- ✦ Place the patient in the desired position
- ✦ A perianal block may facilitate further sphincter relaxation. This is achieved by superficial injection of local anesthetic (≤1.5 mg/kg of 0.5% bupivacaine or ≤7 mg/kg of 1% lidocaine with 1:100,000 epinephrine) in a ring around the anus.

◻ **Examination**
- ✦ External examination: Assess for signs of trauma
- ✦ DRE
  - ✦ Gauge location and orientation of FB
  - ✦ Assess for discharge or bleeding
  - ✦ Small, blunt FBs may be removed during DRE
- ✦ Anoscopy
  - ✦ Assess for mucosal injury
  - ✦ Visualize FB

◻ **Removal of FB**
- ✦ Attempt delivery of the FB by applying suprapubic pressure in synchrony with the patient bearing down

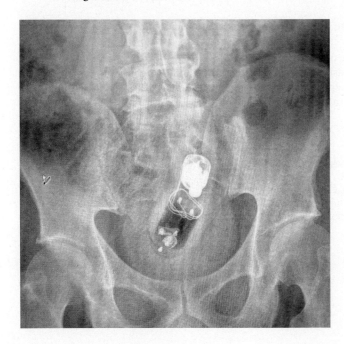

FIGURE 83.1 X-ray of a retained rectal vibrator. (Courtesy of Heather Huffman–Dracht.)

+ If unsuccessful, digitally guide the presenting part of the FB anteriorly (away from the sacrum) and attempt delivery again
+ If still unsuccessful, directly visualize the anorectum via speculum or anoscopy. Use forceps to grasp the presenting portion and apply gentle traction in conjunction with the Valsalva maneuver. The goal is removal of speculum/anoscope, forceps, and FB as a single unit.
+ Glass FBs may prove difficult to remove by traction alone due to the vacuum created by the glass in conjunction with the proximal bowel. The following two additional techniques may prove helpful in the removal of glass FBs:
    + Pass two Foley catheters or ETTs just beyond the FB on opposite sides and inflate the balloons. Attempt removal of FB by gentle traction on the catheters/ETTs.
    + Utilize rigid sigmoidoscopy or Foley catheter to insufflate air in the rectum proximal to the FB, thereby releasing the vacuum and allowing removal by traction with plastic, rubber, or gauze-tipped forceps

☐ **Follow-up**
+ Postprocedure sigmoidoscopy is mandated in following instances:
    + Rectal bleeding/mucosal damage
    + Worsening of rectal pain
+ Surgical consult and admission warranted in following instances:
    + Failed retrieval/uncooperative patient
    + Postretrieval abdominal pain, fever, hematochezia
    + Shattering of glass FB

COMPLICATIONS

☐ Mucosal damage
☐ Bowel perforation
☐ Shattering of glass within the anorectum
☐ Infection

SAFETY/QUALITY TIPS

☐ **Procedural**
+ Only attempt removal of FBs palpable on DRE
+ If using forceps, prevent rectal injury by covering tips and only applying under direct visualization
+ Perform sigmoidoscopy before disposition if concern for mucosal damage
☐ **Cognitive**
+ Consider sexual assault as the mechanism for a rectal FB
+ Take time to plan approach based on the orientation and composition of the FB
+ Impress upon discharged patients the importance of immediate return if signs of infection, rectal bleeding, or perforation

Suggested Readings

Coates WC. Anorectum. In: Marx JA, Hockberger RS, Walls RM, eds. *Rosen's Emergency Medicine*. 6th ed. St. Louis, MO: Mosby; 2006:1521–1522.

Coskun A, Erkan N, Yakan S, et al. Management of rectal foreign bodies. *World J Emerg Surg*. 2013;8:11.

Strear CM, Coates WC. Anorectal procedures. In: Roberts JR, Hedges JR, eds. *Clinical Procedures in Emergency Medicine*. 4th ed. Philadelphia, PA: WB Saunders; 2004:874–876.

84

Foreign Body Removal: Ticks, Rings, and Fish Hooks

Elan S. Levy and Heidi E. Ladner

INDICATIONS

- Indicated only if location of foreign body (FB) is certain
- Removal may be done in 30 minutes or less

RELATIVE CONTRAINDICATIONS

- Involvement of joint—orthopedic consultation may be required
- Coagulopathies or bleeding diathesis
- Allergy to anesthetic
- Chronic medical problems that delay healing, such as diabetes, uremia, or immunocompromised state
- Involvement of abdomen/pelvis/thorax
- Near major vascular structures that are difficult to visualize
- Uncooperative, difficult, or intoxicated patient
- FB not localized

RISKS/CONSENT ISSUES

- Procedure can cause pain (local anesthesia will be given)
- Local bleeding
- There is potential for introducing infection (sterile technique will be utilized)
- Risk of injuring local neurovascular structures
- Scar at site of FB removal
- Patient must be informed that all FBs may not be removed
- Retained wood FBs always develop an inflammatory response, but retained bullets rarely produce inflammation

- **General Basic Steps**
  - **Localize the FB**
  - **Patient preparation**
  - **Decide on method of removal**

TECHNIQUE

- **Localize the FB**
  - Get multiple projections of plain x-ray using a soft-tissue technique (e.g., underpenetrated film); to locate radiopaque FBs, place a marker (i.e., needle) on the skin surface at the wound entrance before the x-ray procedure
  - Although glass and metal are easily located with plain films, ultrasonographic localization may be required for wood and thorns
  - All intraorbital and intracranial FBs must be imaged by computed tomography (CT)
  - If a patient has a previously explored wound demonstrating signs of infection, poor wound healing, or persistent pain, consider doing a CT
- **Patient Preparation**
  - Sterilize and drape the area from where FB will be removed
  - Anesthetize area either via local infiltration or appropriate nerve block

General Removal Techniques

+ Enlarge the entrance to wound with an adequate skin incision
+ Spread the soft tissue with hemostats, avoiding use of fingers
  + Hemostats can help find glass in a wound by creating a clicking sound when tapped against glass
+ If visualization is inadequate, consider excision of small block of tissue, only if no significant neurovascular structures are involved
+ When searching for a thorn or needle, consider an elliptical incision, undermine the skin in all directions, and then compress the sides, expelling the FB
+ Closure of the wound after thorough irrigation is indicated unless exploring a contaminated wound

TICK REMOVAL

- Nonmechanical means of tick removal is not recommended (i.e., drowning the tick in petroleum jelly), because it may cause the tick to regurgitate, increasing infection risk (**FIGURE 84.1**)
- Mechanical removal
  + Using the tip of forceps, grab the tick as close as possible to the patient's skin, and apply steady traction
  + Ensure that all mouth parts are removed. Use an 18-gauge needle to remove retained pieces.
  + Thoroughly cleanse the area with soap and water
- In patients at high risk of Lyme disease, consider administration of 200 mg of doxycycline in a single dose (or amoxicillin in pediatrics) (Figure 84.1)

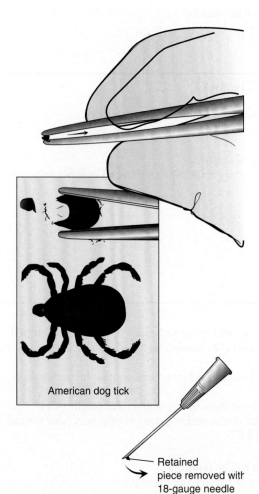

American dog tick

Retained piece removed with 18-gauge needle

FIGURE 84.1 Tick removal. (From Bond GR. Envenomation management and tick removal. In: Henretig FM, King C, eds. *Textbook of Pediatric Emergency Procedures*. Philadelphia, PA: Williams & Wilkins; 1997:1328, with permission.)

RING REMOVAL

- Initial attempt at ring removal should be with soap and water
- **String-wrap Method**
  - Consider a digital block to reduce pain and minimize swelling
  - With 25+ inch of string, umbilical tape, or suture, pass the tip between the ring and finger
  - Using the distal end of the string, wrap clockwise (proximal to distal), including the proximal interphalangeal (PIP) and distal finger, ensuring compression
  - Do not leave gaps between the wraps of string (**FIGURES 84.2** and **84.3**)
  - Unwrap the string from the proximal end, slowly forcing the ring over the PIP and distal finger, unraveling the ring with the string
  - If this technique fails, consider using a ring cutter
- **Ring Cutters**
  - Reassure the patient that the ring cutter will not cut the finger
  - Turn the ring such that the thinnest portion is on the palmar side of the finger
  - Gently slide the ring cutter guard under the ring (this will likely cause some pain due to swelling of the distal finger)
  - Grasp the ring cutter handle firmly such that the cutting wheel is against the ring
  - Turn the wheel until the ring is cut
  - Pull off the ring with hemostats or clamps; alternatively, make another cut in the ring

FISH HOOK REMOVAL

- Determine if fish hook is single, multiple, or trebled, and also note the number and location of the barbs
- Administer 1% lidocaine locally
- Advance the hook through the anesthetized skin
- Clip off the barb, and remove the rest of the hook in a retrograde manner (**FIGURE 84.4**)

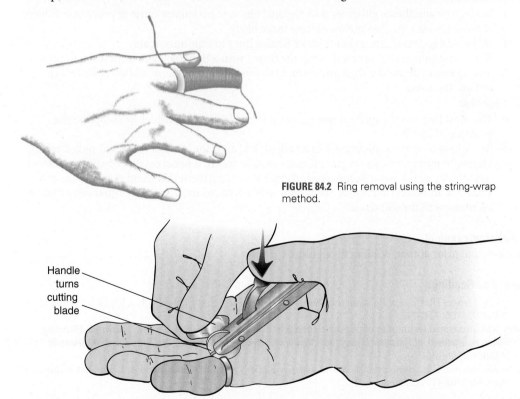

FIGURE 84.2 Ring removal using the string-wrap method.

Handle turns cutting blade

FIGURE 84.3 Ring cutter method of ring removal. (From Fuchs SM. Ring removal. In: Henretig FM, King C, eds. *Textbook of Pediatric Emergency Procedures.* Philadelphia, PA: Williams & Wilkins; 1997:1231, with permission.)

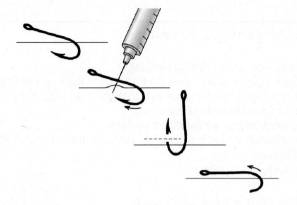

FIGURE 84.4 Hook removal.

COMPLICATIONS

- ✛ Bleeding
- ✛ Infection
- ✛ Scarring
- ✛ Pain
- ✛ Nerve damage
- ✛ Incomplete removal
- ✛ Retained FBs, such as wood, always lead to inflammation
- ✛ Rarely, retained FBs containing lead may lead to systemic lead poisoning

SAFETY/QUALITY TIPS

▣ **Procedural**
- ✛ Inadequate anesthesia, either local or regional block, is a common cause of procedure failure
- ✛ A generous skin incision makes success more likely
- ✛ Make skin incisions along skin folds or Kraissl lines to minimize scars
- ✛ Before attempting ring removal, wrap the finger with a tight bandage from distal to proximal to exsanguinate the digit and reduce swelling. This maneuver is often sufficient to remove the ring.

▣ **Cognitive**
- ✛ The most important cognitive error around FBs is failure to consider or recognize the presence of an FB
- ✛ Be vigilant to remove all parts of an attached tick, after the body of the tick is pulled off
- ✛ Start with multiple views on plain film to localize an FB. If unsuccessful, consider ultrasonography or CT scan. Recognize and explain to the patient that there is always the possibility of an FB that cannot be seen, even with advanced imaging. Never guarantee that no FB remains in the soft tissue.

▣ **Acknowledgment**

Thank-you to prior author William C. Manson.

Suggested Readings

Roberts JR, Hedges JR. *Clinical Procedures in Emergency Medicine*. 4th ed. Philadelphia, PA: WB Saunders; 2004:703–705, 711–713.

Ruddy RM. Illustrated techniques of pediatric emergency procedures. In: Fleisher GR, Ludwig S, Henretig FM, eds. *Textbook of Pediatric Emergency Medicine*. 5th ed. Philadelphia, PA: Lippincott Williams & Wilkins; 2006:1861.

Simon RR, Brenner BE. *Emergency Procedures and Techniques*. 4th ed. Philadelphia, PA: Lippincott Williams & Wilkins; 2002:419–422.

85

Eye Foreign Body Removal

Diana Kim

INDICATIONS

- To remove external foreign bodies (FBs) in the eye
- Symptoms include pain, redness, increased tearing, or FB sensation

CONTRAINDICATIONS

- Caution and care must be taken if globe rupture is suspected especially when the history includes flying particles or high-velocity projectiles

LANDMARKS—FIGURE 85.1

- **General Basic Steps**
  - **Preparation**
  - **Inspection**
  - **Stain**
  - **Slit lamp examination**
  - **Removal of FB**

TECHNIQUE

- **Patient Preparation**
  - Place 0.5% tetracaine or 0.5% proparacaine drops in the eye (may use in both eyes to reduce the blink reflex)
  - In case of intense blepharospasm, administer an ipsilateral facial block
- **Inspection—FIGURE 85.2**
  - Examine the conjunctiva and cornea carefully. Do not assume there will only be one FB.
  - Carefully examine behind both eyelids
    - Lower eyelid: Pull down the lower eyelid and ask the patient to look up
    - Upper eyelid: Using a cotton-tipped applicator as a fulcrum, carefully pull the eyelashes down and out to evert the lid

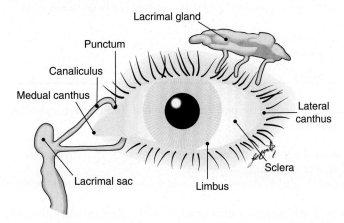

FIGURE 85.1 Periorbital structures. (From Knoop KJ, Dennis W. Eye trauma. In: Wolfson AB, ed. *Harwood-Nuss' Clinical Practice of Emergency Medicine*. 6th ed. Philadelphia, PA: Lippincott Williams & Wilkins; 2015:174, with permission.)

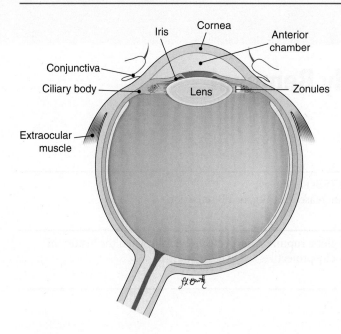

Iris
Cornea
Anterior chamber
Conjunctiva
Ciliary body
Lens
Zonules
Extraocular muscle

FIGURE 85.2 Cross section of the eye. (From Knoop KJ, Dennis W. Eye trauma. In: Wolfson AB, ed. *Harwood-Nuss' Clinical Practice of Emergency Medicine.* 6th ed. Philadelphia, PA: Lippincott Williams & Wilkins; 2015:175, with permission.)

- ▣ **Fluorescein Stain**
  - ✚ Gently touch the fluorescein strip to the lower eyelid conjunctiva and ask the patient to blink two to three times. Wipe away the excess.
  - ✚ Inspect the cornea for abrasions (fluorescein when taken up by the alkaline Bowman membrane, will fluoresce with a cobalt-blue light). Patients with corneal abrasions may have FB sensation in the absence of a retained FB.
- ▣ **Positive Fluorescein Stain** (FIGURE 85.3)
- ▣ **Slit Lamp Inspection**
  - ✚ Examine the fluorescein-stained cornea under the blue light of a slit lamp
  - ✚ Vertical linear lesions on the cornea should raise suspicion for an FB under the eyelids
  - ✚ If you see an FB extending through the full thickness of the cornea, consult an ophthalmologist
  - ✚ Signs of an intraocular FB may be subtle or absent. Look carefully for the following:
    - ✚ Irregular pupil
    - ✚ Shallow anterior chamber
    - ✚ Collapsed iris
    - ✚ Positive Seidel test (extrusion of fluorescent material from the cornea)
    - ✚ Hyphema
    - ✚ Lens opacification
    - ✚ Decreased intraocular pressure

FOREIGN BODY VISIBLE

- ▣ Swab
  - ✚ If easily visualized, remove the particle with a moist sterile cotton-tipped applicator or nasopharyngeal swab
- ▣ Irrigation
  - ✚ FB may be flushed out when the eye is irrigated gently with a stream from an Angiocath connected to a syringe containing saline
  - ✚ If more copious irrigation is required, consider commercial devices such as the Morgan lens
- ▣ Embedded FB
  - ✚ Cornea can be gently scraped with a small 25- or 27-gauge needle, attached to a syringe for stability (under the slit lamp)

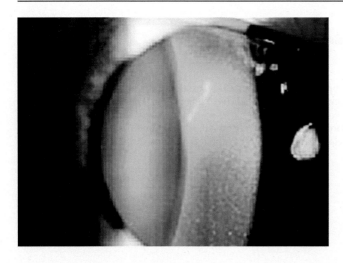

FIGURE 85.3 Corneal abrasion stained with fluorescein under cobalt-blue light. (From Wilson SA, Last A. Management of corneal abrasions. *Am Fam Physician.* 2004;70(1):123–128. http://www.aafp.org/afp/2004/0701/p123.html. Accessed March 30, 2014.)

- Place hand on the patient's cheek bone for increased stability, and hold needle tip *tangential* to the globe surface
- Pick out FB under slit lamp magnification
- Rust rings formed by the oxidation of iron-containing FBs may be removed along with the FB, with repeated picking. Note that rust rings can also be safely removed in 24 to 48 hours in the ophthalmologist's office as well.
- Do not pick or burr in the visual axis. If unsure, consult an ophthalmologist.

AFTERCARE

- May consider topical antibiotics
- Patching not recommended
- Topical anesthetics are not recommended for use at home (corneal toxicity, impairs corneal wound healing)

COMPLICATIONS

- Incomplete removal
- Second FB (patient may not have persistent FB sensation, due to anesthesia)
- Conjunctivitis
- Corneal epithelial injury
- Globe perforation (patch, protect, and call ophthalmology consult service)

SAFETY/QUALITY TIPS

- **Procedural**
  - Everting the upper eyelid is often not done well by emergency physicians. Have the patient look down, place the end of a cotton-tipped applicator across the closed eyelid, then, grasping the lashes, pull the lid inferiorly, then up and over the applicator.
  - If removing an FB using a needle, take special care to stabilize your hand on the patient's face, being mindful that the patient may move his/her head unexpectedly.
- **Cognitive**
  - The most important cognitive error in the management of ocular FBs is failure to find one, or find all of them. Have a low threshold with all eye complaints to perform a slit lamp examination, eyelid eversion, and fluorescein staining.
  - Finding one FB begets the search for the second and third FBs
  - Have special respect for metal-on-metal mechanisms (e.g., metal grinders). Noncontrast computed tomography of the orbits is the right test in these circumstances. Avoid magnetic resonance imaging.

⊕ Acknowledgment

Thank-you to prior author Satchit Balsari.

Suggested Readings

Knoop KJ, Dennis WR. Ophthalmologic procedures. In: Roberts JR, Custalow CB, Thomsen TW, et al. eds. *Roberts and Hedges' Clinical Procedures in Emergency Medicine*. Philadelphia, PA: Elsevier Saunders; 2014:1259–1297.

Weichenthal LA. Corneal abrasion and foreign bodies. In: Wolfson AB, ed. *Harwood-Nuss' Clinical Practice of Emergency Medicine*. 6th ed. Philadelphia, PA: Lippincott William & Wilkins; 2014:344–345.

86

Ear Foreign Body Removal

Diana Kim

INDICATIONS

⊡ Removal of foreign matter lodged within the external auditory canal (FIGURE 86.1)

⊡ **General Basic Steps**
  + **Preparation**
  + **Irrigation**
  + **Removal**

TECHNIQUE

⊡ **Patient Preparation**
  + Place patient in a supine position
    + Restrain patient and immobilize the head
      ▪ Consider sedation for patients unable to cooperate with the procedure
⊡ **Irrigation**
  + Before the procedure, perform pneumatic otoscopy in patients with suspected tympanic membrane (TM) perforation to document an intact TM
    + Pull the pinna superiorly, posteriorly, and laterally in order to straighten the external auditory canal and allow for a more complete visualization of the foreign matter and TM
  + Contraindications for irrigation include patients with suspected or known TM or tympanostomy tubes and organic foreign bodies (FBs) because water may cause the object to swell in the external auditory canal
  + Attach a 20-mL syringe to a 16- or 18-gauge intravenous catheter or a 2-inch section of butterfly needle tubing (cut off the needle assembly)
    + Use water at body temperature to avoid vestibular stimulation

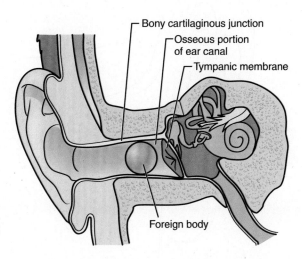

FIGURE 86.1 Foreign body lodged in external auditory canal.

+ Insert the catheter or tubing 1 to 1.5 cm into the canal, aimed superiorly and posteriorly, and irrigate with mild to moderate pressure on the syringe
+ In patients presenting with live insects in the auditory canal, instilling 1 to 2 mL of mineral oil or 2% lidocaine directly into the canal will usually successfully kill the insect within 1 minute. Irrigation with water can then be done to flush out the dead insect **(FIGURE 86.2)**.

INSTRUMENTATION

- Perform only when able to visualize the object
- Various instruments can be used: Alligator forceps, curettes, right-angle hooks, or bayonet forceps
    + Alligator and bayonet forceps are useful to remove insects or other irregular objects, as well as compressible objects (such as paper), which can be "grabbed." Occasionally, separation of the FB may occur, necessitating further attempts.
    + Curettes and right-angle forceps are useful when the hooked end can be passed beyond the FB. At that point, rotate the instrument and allow it to drag the object as you pull **(FIGURE 86.3)**.

SUCTION CATHETER

- May work for round objects that are difficult to grasp
- Inflexible devices such as a Frazier suction device work better than flexible suction catheters. If a flexible catheter is used, choose one with no side holes, or cut the distal portion with the side holes off and be sure to smooth the cut edges.
- Attach a suction catheter device to wall suction and gently advance the catheter tip until it abuts the foreign object. Warn patient about noise, then apply suction and slowly remove the catheter with the FB attached.

CYANOACRYLATE (SUPERGLUE)

- Used for removal of round, dry objects that are difficult to grasp
- Apply a small amount of glue to the wood end of a cotton-tip applicator, place against the object, allow to dry, then slowly remove the applicator with the FB attached
- Avoid/use with caution in uncooperative patients

COMPLICATIONS

- Pain, bleeding, infection due to irritation or manipulation of external auditory canal

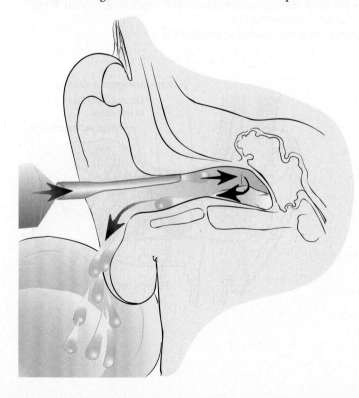

FIGURE 86.2 Syringing cerumen or a foreign body from the auditory canal with an intravenous catheter attached to a 20-mL syringe. The irrigating stream is directed at the posterior, superior wall of the canal. (From Fuerst RS. Removal of cerumen impaction. In: Henretig FM, King C, eds. *Textbook of Pediatric Emergency Procedures.* Philadelphia, PA: Williams & Wilkins; 1997:643, with permission.)

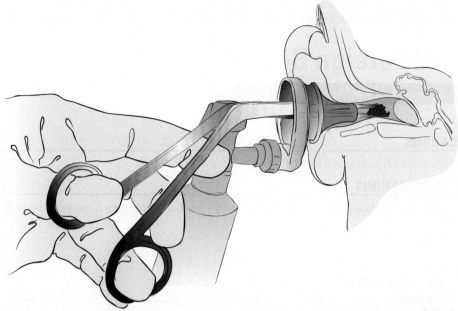

FIGURE 86.3 Cerumen or a foreign body is removed from the auditory canal under direct visualization with an alligator forceps and an operating head otoscope. (From Fuerst RS. Removal of cerumen impaction. In: Henretig FM, King C, eds. *Textbook of Pediatric Emergency Procedures*. Philadelphia, PA: Williams & Wilkins; 1997:644, with permission.)

- ⊡ Nausea, vomiting, vertigo due to irrigation of external canal
- ⊡ Iatrogenic TM perforation
- ⊡ Ossicle disruption

SAFETY/QUALITY TIPS

- ⊡ **Procedural**
  - ✛ A variety of techniques and tools exist to remove ear FBs. After visualization of the FB, consider which of the approaches described is most likely to be successful.
  - ✛ Attempting ear FB removal on an uncooperative/agitated patient, especially a child, is not advised. Removal of an ear FB is usually nonemergent and many of these patients can be managed in the office of an otolaryngologist within 24 to 48 hours.
  - ✛ However, batteries lodged in the external canal should be removed as soon as possible as they can cause corrosion into the middle ear
  - ✛ Always carefully reinspect the canal and TM **after** FB removal
- ⊡ **Cognitive**
  - ✛ Refer all patients to an ENT specialist in cases of:
    - ✛ Inability to adequately sedate an uncooperative patient and failure to removal of FB
    - ✛ FB is abutting the TM
    - ✛ Unable to remove FB after multiple attempts
  - ✛ Local anesthetic drops and/or anti-inflammatory drops can be prescribed (for nonorganic matter) until the follow-up appointment

⊡ **Acknowledgment**

Thank-you to prior authors Elad Bicer and Kathleen G. Reichard.

Suggested Readings

Roberts RR. External auditory canal foreign body removal. In: Reichman EF. *Emergency Medicine Procedures*. 2nd ed. New York, NY: McGraw Hill; 2013.

Riviello RJ. Otolaryngologic procedures. In: Roberts JR, Custalow CB, Thomsen TW, et al. eds. *Roberts and Hedges' Clinical Procedures in Emergency Medicine*. Philadelphia, PA: Elsevier Saunders; 2014:1298–1341.

87

Nasal Foreign Body Removal

Elan S. Levy and Kathleen G. Reichard

INDICATIONS

- Presence of foreign material within the nostril

CONTRAINDICATIONS

- If the foreign body entered the nose traumatically and there is concern it has penetrated the cranial cavity
- If there is danger of obstructing the airway

> **General Basic Steps**
> - **Patient preparation**
> - **Anesthesia**
> - **Choose method of removal**

TECHNIQUE

- **Patient Preparation**
  - An uncooperative child should be properly immobilized or sedated
    - An option is to papoose the child in a blanket in the supine position with the arms at the sides and an assistant holding the head still
  - Using a syringe as a dropper, instill either lidocaine and phenylephrine or lidocaine with epinephrine in the nostril to optimize the visual field and provide anesthesia, decongestion, and hemostasis
  - Dosing for nasal phenylephrine
    - 6 months to 2 years: 1 to 2 drops per nostril of a 0.1255 solution
    - 2 to 6 years: 2 to 4 drops per nostril of a 0.1255 solution
    - Older than 6 years: 2 to 3 drops per nostril of a 0.1255 solution
  - Make sure you have a good light source and suction
  - Consider anxiolysis or sedation in the uncooperative child, especially in those who require more urgent removal of the foreign body, as in the case of button batteries

Methods of removal
Manual removal
Suction catheter
Positive pressure
Foley catheter
Cyanoacrylate glue
Nasal wash

- **Manual Removal**
  - A directly visualized object can be removed with alligator forceps or a curette with or without the assistance of a nasal speculum
  - Alligator forceps are best used for easily grasped, solid or compressible (e.g., paper) objects in the anterior nostril
  - A round and smooth object may be removed with an angled wire loop/curette or right-angle hook. It is inserted along the nasal floor or septum until it is behind the object and rotated so that the angled end is caught behind the object; the object can then be pulled out (**FIGURES 87.1 and 87.2**).

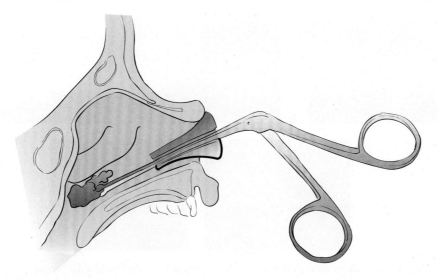

FIGURE 87.1 Removal of an intranasal foreign body using forceps. (From Issacman DJ, Post JC. Nasal foreign body removal. In: Henretig FM, King C, eds. *Textbook of Pediatric Emergency Procedures*. Philadelphia, PA: Williams & Wilkins; 1997:684, with permission.)

+ If no wire loop is available, a makeshift one can be constructed with a paperclip **(FIGURE 87.3)**

✚ **Suction Catheter**
+ Using a small suction catheter connected to wall suction, gently put the suction catheter up to the visible side of the object
  + Be careful not push the object further back
+ When the object becomes attached to the end of the suction catheter, slowly withdraw both the catheter and the foreign body
+ Rigid suction catheters usually work better than flexible catheters
+ The presence of side holes will prevent the vacuum from occurring at the tip. Choose a catheter without side holes, or trim the catheter tip to remove the side holes, leaving only an end opening.
  + Trim any sharp edges from the cut end to prevent trauma

✚ **Positive Pressure**
+ The parent or the physician can do this technique. The parent may assist with this procedure and therefore reduce the child's anxiety.
+ Instruct the parent to gently occlude the nostril without the foreign body with finger pressure
+ Give one quick puff of air into the child's mouth
  + To put the child at ease, the parent can say she/he is going to give the child a big kiss
+ The puff of air should push the foreign body out of the nostril

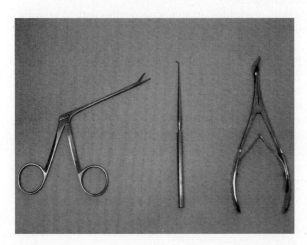

FIGURE 87.2 From left to right—alligator clips, right-angle hook, nasal speculum.

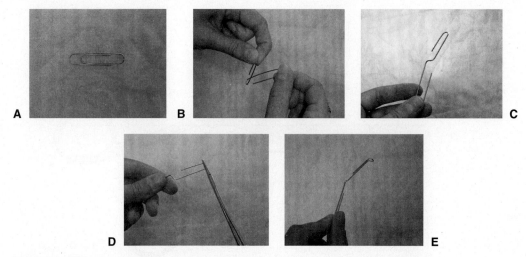

FIGURE 87.3 Pull the paperclip apart as shown and use forceps to bend the end to a right angle.

- Alternatively, the physician can provide positive pressure using an Ambu bag:
  - Place the Ambu bag over the child's mouth leaving the nose free from the mask; gently occlude the unobstructed nostril
  - Give one quick squeeze on the Ambu bag; the resultant positive pressure to the obstructed nostril should push the foreign body out
- This technique is best for large objects that occlude the entire passage and would be difficult to slide an instrument past or grasp onto
- **Foley Catheter**
  - Use a no. 4 to no. 8 Fogarty vascular catheter or a 5- or 6-French balloon Foley catheter
  - Lubricate the balloon end of the catheter with lidocaine jelly or Surgilube and slide the catheter past and behind the object
  - Inflate with 2 to 3 mL of air and pull the Foley catheter forward to force the foreign body out
  - This technique is best used for a visualized, partially obstructing foreign body
- **Cyanoacrylate Glue**
  - On the wooden end of a cotton swab or the cut end of a hollow plastic swab apply a dot of cyanoacrylate glue
    - Use a very small amount so it will not drip
  - Insert the tip into the nostril, making sure not to touch the nasal mucosa
  - Press the tip against the foreign body gently so as not to push the foreign body more posterior, and hold for 30 to 60 seconds to allow for it to dry
  - Withdraw slowly the swab with attached foreign body
  - This technique should be used with caution, or avoided, in an uncooperative patient to avoid the risk of getting glue on the nasal mucosa
- **Nasal Wash**
  - Place the patient in an upright sitting position with the neck in a neutral position
  - Put 7 mL of sterile saline into a bulb syringe, and insert the bulb syringe into the nonobstructed nostril until a good seal is created
  - In one quick squeeze push the sterile saline into the nostril
  - The saline and the foreign body will be expressed out of the opposite nostril
  - This technique should likely be reserved for an older cooperative child because of the risk of saline aspiration **(FIGURE 87.4)**

COMPLICATIONS

- **General**
  - Epistaxis
  - Nasal infection
  - Aspiration of foreign body

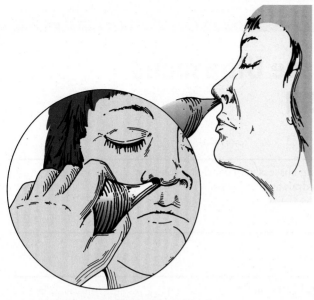

FIGURE 87.4 Nasal wash technique.

+ Partial removal of foreign body
+ Mucosal damage
+ Cribriform plate damage
- Procedure Specific
  + *Nasal wash:* Reflux of saline into the eustachian tubes or aspiration of saline
  + *Positive pressure:* Barotrauma to the tympanic membrane

SAFETY/QUALITY TIPS

- Procedural
  + Sedation is crucial if the patient is uncooperative and cannot be adequately immobilized. Even in a cooperative patient proper immobilization is important because the patient will tend to flinch when instruments are in the nostrils, putting them at risk for trauma.
  + Aspiration of the foreign body is a risk. Take care not to push a foreign body back, so that it falls into the oropharynx, or allow a foreign body to come out of the nose and into the mouth of an upset child.
  + A face-shield mask should be worn during this procedure
- Cognitive
  + If the foreign body is a button battery it should be removed without delay as it can cause ulceration of nasal mucosa and even perforation in a short amount of time
  + Talk with the child through the procedure and involve the parents, if possible, to reduce anxiety
  + An important error is not recognizing that unilateral purulent discharge or epistaxis could be due to a foreign body
  + Patient should be referred to ENT specialist for outpatient treatment in following instances:
    + Unable to adequately sedate an uncooperative patient
    + Unable to remove the object after multiple attempts

- Acknowledgment

Thank-you to prior author Keeli A. Hanzelka.

Suggested Readings

Lichenstein R, Giudice EL. Nasal wash technique for nasal foreign body removal. *Pediatr Emerg Care.* 2000;16(1):59–60.

Reichman EF, Simon RR. *Emergency Medicine Procedures.* New York, NY: McGraw-Hill; 2004:1286–1290.

Simon RR, Brenner BE. *Emergency Procedures and Techniques.* 4th ed. Philadelphia, PA: Lippincott Williams & Wilkins; 2002.

Thomas SH, White BA. Foreign bodies. In: Marx JA, Hockberger RS, Walls RM, et al., eds. *Rosen's Emergency Medicine: Concepts and Clinical Practice.* 8th ed. Philadelphia, PA: Mosby Elsevier; 2013:767–784.

Skin and Soft-Tissue Ultrasound

Daniel Lakoff and Joseph R. Pinero

INDICATIONS

- Identify and differentiate cellulitis from abscess with overlying cellulitis
- Procedural guidance for incision and drainage of abscess
- Assess soft-tissue masses

CONTRAINDICATIONS

- None

RISKS/CONSENT ISSUES

- Contact dermatitis from ultrasound gel (very rare)

TECHNIQUE

- Linear transducer (7.5–10+ MHz)
- Sonographic grip—always have part of the hand, i.e., the little finger, resting upon the body of the patient when possible, as this helps stabilize the probe for fine movements
- Reduce depth
- Adjust gain using a fluid-filled structure as the standard (anechoic fluid or blood should be crisply anechoic)
- Caliper function can be used to measure abscesses in two or three planes
- Assess for vascularity using color Doppler, as the presence of vascularity may result in a contraindication to incision and drainage

NORMAL SKIN AND SOFT TISSUE (FIGURE 88.1)

- Adjust depth to focus only on region of interest, typically 2 to 4 cm
- Scan a wide region, starting away from the region of interest to assess presumably normal skin and soft tissue

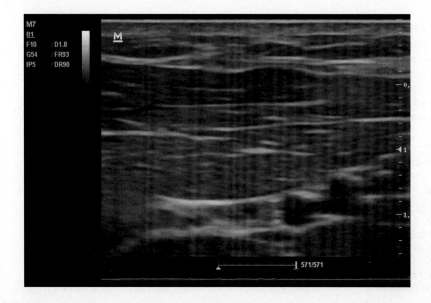

FIGURE 88.1 Normal (vessel, LN, muscle, skin/soft tissue).

◘ Be familiar with the appearance of soft tissue and the structures within it (skin, subcutaneous tissue, blood vessels, lymph node, nerve, muscle fascicles, tendon, bone)

PATHOLOGY

◘ **Cellulitis** (FIGURE 88.2)
+ Diffuse thickened (slightly hyperechoic) subcutaneous layer and fluid (anechoic) dissecting the deeper layers of the skin and fat, creating the pathognomonic cobblestone appearance
+ Can see thin hyperechogenic transverse layers between layers of normal dermis
+ Posterior acoustic enhancement

◘ **Abscess** (FIGURES 88.3–88.5)
+ Variable appearance on ultrasound
+ Typically see well-defined border, but possibly irregular
+ May see anechoic fluid-filled pocket with or without septae supporting loculation (debris)
+ May see posterior acoustic enhancement (shadowing)

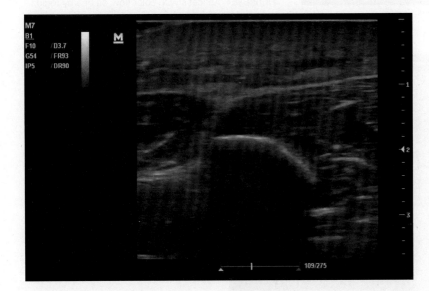

FIGURE 88.2 Cellulitis (cobblestone).

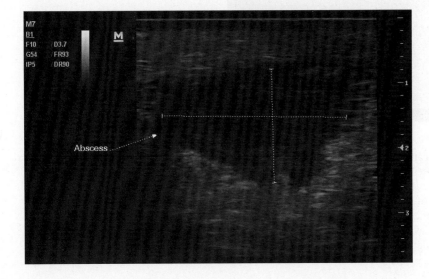

FIGURE 88.3 Abscess.

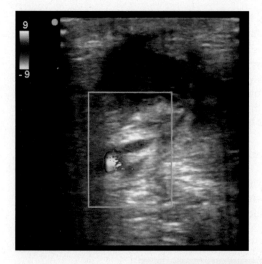

FIGURE 88.4 Abscess with color flow on nearby region.

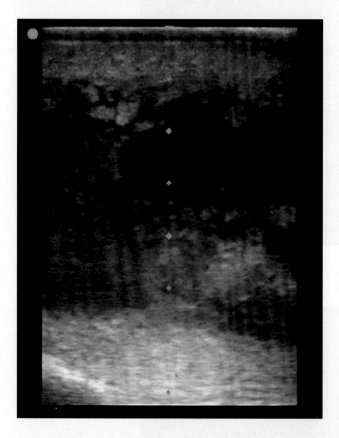

FIGURE 88.5 Abscess with overlying cellulitis.

+ Color Doppler can assess whether or not there is flow in the suspected abscess, indicating it may very well be a pseudoaneurysm, as well as proximity of the abscess from vascular structures
+ Color Doppler can also demonstrate surrounding hyperemia around the abscess to help confirm suspicion of abscess (Figure 88.3)
+ Combination of cellulitis and abscess is quite common (Figure 88.4)
+ Using an endocavitary probe, peritonsillar abscess can also be identified and drained under ultrasound guidance

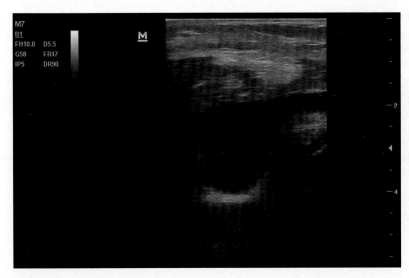

FIGURE 88.6 Baker cyst.

- **Necrotizing Fasciitis**
  + Thickened subcutaneous tissue
  + Layer of fluid >4 mm in depth
  + May see anechoic fluid-filled pocket with or without septae supporting loculation
  + Posterior acoustic enhancement (shadowing) may be seen
  + Air/gas in the subcutaneous tissue
- **Cyst (FIGURE 88.6)**
  + Typically smooth, round, anechoic, hypoechoic or mixed hypoechoic/anechoic, well-defined lesion
  + Should be able to at least minimally compress structure
  + Posterior acoustic enhancement
  + May communicate with a joint (i.e., Baker cyst, popliteal cyst)

SAFETY/QUALITY TIPS

- **Procedural**
  + Use a liberal amount of gel to increase transduction quality or water bath for very superficial structures
  + Scan in multiple planes to best assess the area
  + Do not apply more pressure than required to visualize the image so as not to distort the anatomy of the diseased tissue
  + If uncertain, image the contralateral side to appreciate normal tissue, then view the affected side
- **Cognitive**
  + Vascular lesions like pseudoaneurysms can appear identical to an abscess. Have a very low threshold to "probe before scalpel" suspected abscesses.
  + The cobblestone appearance of cellulitis may be seen in other disease processes, i.e., congestive heart failure, venous stasis, and lymphedema
  + Ultrasound-guided aspiration is the preferred treatment for breast abscesses <3 cm in diameter
  + Be cautious when assessing for abscess in locations with bursa (i.e., knees, elbows), which may appear similar

Suggested Readings

Ahuja AT, Ying M. Sonographic evaluation of cervical lymph nodes. *Am J Roentgenol.* 2005;184(5):1691–1699.

Blaivas M, Adhikari S. Unexpected findings on point-of-care superficial ultrasound imaging before incision and drainage. *J Ultrasound Med.* 2011;30(10):1425–1430.

Carotti M, Ciapetti A, Jousse-Joulin S, et al. Ultrasonography of the salivary glands: the role of grey-scale and colour/power Doppler. *Clin Exp Rheumatol.* 2014;32(1 suppl 80):61–70.

Jaovisidha S, Leerodjanaprapa P, Siriwongpairat P, et al. Emergency ultrasonography in patients with clinically suspected soft tissue infection of the legs. *Singapore Med J.* 2012;53(4):277–282.

Smith S, Salanitri J, Lisle D. Ultrasound evaluation of soft tissue masses and fluid collections. *Semin Musculoskelet Radiol.* 2007;11(2):174–191.

Yen ZS, Wang HP, Ma HM, et al. Ultrasonographic screening of clinically-suspected necrotizing fasciitis. *Acad Emerg Med.* 2002;9(12):1448–1451.

89

Intubation of the Pediatric Patient

Joshua M. Beiner

INDICATIONS

- Inadequate oxygenation or ventilation
- Airway obstruction
- Loss of protective airway reflexes (e.g., depressed cough and gag reflexes)
- Excess work of breathing
- Nonresponsive and apneic

CONTRAINDICATIONS

- **Absolute Contraindications**
  - None for unstable patients (i.e., "crash" airway)
- **Relative Contraindications**
  - *In these circumstances one should consider consultation with anesthesiologist/intensivist, alternative techniques, and/or sedation without paralysis*
    - Infectious: Epiglottitis, croup, retropharyngeal abscess, bacterial tracheitis
    - Noninfectious: Anaphylaxis/angioedema, foreign body, trauma, burns
    - Congenital anomalies (e.g., cleft palate, micrognathia)
    - Unanticipated difficult airway (e.g., multiple failed attempts)

RISKS/CONSENT ISSUES

- Airway trauma
- Arrhythmia (e.g., bradyarrhythmia)
- Aspiration of stomach contents
- Esophageal intubation
- Increase in blood pressure and intracranial pressure (ICP)
- Hypoxemia
- Pain

LANDMARKS

- Anatomical differences in children (FIGURE 89.1):
  - Larger tongue
  - Larger and floppy epiglottis
  - Narrower cricoid ring
  - Larger occiput
  - The glottic opening is more cranial and anterior in children and is located at:
    - C1 in infancy
    - C3–C5 at age 7
    - C4–C6 in the adult (Figure 89.1)
  - Differences are most pronounced under 2 years, transition from 2 to 8 years, then approach small adult anatomy by 8 years

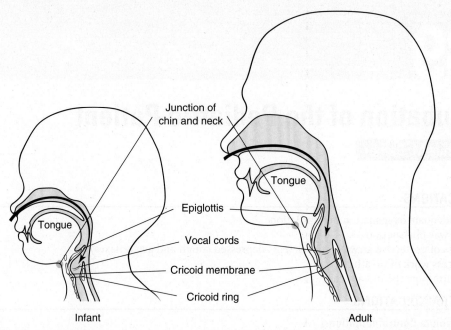

FIGURE 89.1 The anatomic differences particular to children are (a) higher, more anterior position of the glottic opening (note the relationship of the vocal cords to the chin/neck junction); (b) relatively larger tongue in the infant, which lies between the mouth and the glottic opening; (c) relatively larger and more floppy epiglottis in the child; (d) the cricoid ring is the narrowest portion of the pediatric airway versus the vocal cords in the adult; (e) position and size of the cricothyroid membrane in the infant; (f) sharper, more difficult angle for blind nasotracheal intubation; (g) larger relative size of the occiput in the infant.

⊕ General Basic Steps
+ **Preparation**
+ **Preoxygenation**
+ **Pretreatment**
+ **Protection and positioning**
+ **Paralysis and induction**
+ **Placement of tube and proof of tube placement**
+ **Postintubation management**

TECHNIQUE

If crash airway and difficult airway algorithms are not indicated, then rapid sequence intubation (RSI) is the preferred approach. This approach is summarized in seven discrete steps, each beginning with the letter "P."

⊕ **Preparation:** Directed history, physical examination, indications/contraindications for RSI
+ Assemble equipment using the "SOAP ME" mnemonic **(TABLE 89.1)**
+ Size is best estimated using Broselow tape or centimeter measuring tape
  + Oral airway
    ▬ Size using Broselow tape or distance from the angle of the mouth to the ear tragus
  + Nasopharyngeal airway
    ▬ Size using Broselow tape, distance from the tip of the nose to the ear tragus, or largest comfortable size that does not produce skin blanching
  + Laryngoscope blade
    ▬ Straight/Miller blade traditionally has been preferred to the curved blade for infants and young children. However, either blade can be used in any age group depending on availability and operator comfort.
  + Endotracheal tube (ETT) size based on Broselow tape or calculated as follows:
    ▬ Uncuffed: (Age in years/4) + 4 (subtract 0.5−1 for cuffed tube)

TABLE 89.1 EQUIPMENT FOR RSI—"SOAP ME" MNEMONIC		
S	Suction	Yankaur device (children/adolescents) and/or flexible catheters (infants), suction tubing, wall-mounted suction
O	Oxygen	Face mask (preferably nonrebreather), oxygen tubing, high-flow oxygen source, Bag/Valve device (with positive-pressure valve)
A	Airway	Laryngoscope handle with functional light source and blades, endotracheal tubes, airway tape, stylets, oral/nasopharyngeal airways of varying sizes. Rescue equipment (e.g., Bougie, GlideScope, LMA, cricothyrotomy kit, etc.) should be available in case RSI fails.
P	Pharmacology	Weight-based medications should be prepared in advanced. Agent selection will depend on circumstances and may include sedatives, induction agents, neuromuscular-blocking agents, lidocaine, and atropine.
ME	Monitoring equipment	Cardiorespiratory monitoring with pulse oximetry and frequent blood pressure checks through postintubation monitoring phase. Following endotracheal tube placement, secondary confirmation with end-tidal CO_2 calorimeter (qualitative/semiquantitative) and/or capnography (quantitative)

LMA, laryngeal mask airway; RSI, rapid sequence intubation.

- Historically, uncuffed tubes were preferred in infants and young children due to high rates of subglottic stenosis. Currently, either tube may be used in any age group if leak pressures are monitored.
- Prepare extra tubes, both 0.5 size smaller and larger than estimated
  + A stylet can be used to provide rigidity (**TABLE 89.2**)
  + ETT depth by Broselow tape or calculated (if age >1 year)
    - Formula (in cm): (Age in years/2) + 10 or Tube size × 3
  + End-tidal CO_2 monitor
    - If weight <15 kg, use pediatric calorimeter to avoid false negative readings
  + Have airway alternatives available (e.g., GlideScope, Airtraq, laryngeal mask airway [LMA], Bougie, needle cricothyrotomy equipment)

◩ **Preoxygenation**
  + Theoretically, deliver 100% oxygen for 3 minutes. Practically, use nonrebreather facemask (with positive end-expiratory pressure [PEEP] valve) and high-flow nasal cannula once RSI is considered.
  + If child becomes apneic, use bag valve mask (BVM) ventilation prior to intubation
    + Perform neck extension and E-C clamp technique with bag-mask ventilation (BMV) if C-spine injury is not suspected
    + If two providers are available, one person maintains mask seal while the other compresses the bag
    + Use the rhythm "squeeze, release, release" to allow time for exhalation
    + Insert an oral airway in an unconscious patient who is difficult to ventilate

◩ **Pretreatment:** Refers to the administration of medications to attenuate the potential adverse effects of intubation (**TABLE 89.3**)
  + Prior recommendations summarized by "LOAD" (Lidocaine, Opioid, Atropine, Defasciculating agent)
  + No pretreatment agent is recommended routinely for pediatric RSI
  + **Lidocaine:** May limit further rise in ICP in cases of head trauma or elevated ICP
    + No data to suggest or refute use to prevent reflex bronchospasm
  + **Fentanyl:** Analgesic effects may decrease the reflex sympathetic response
    + May cause hypotension or respiratory depression with other sedatives
  + **Atropine:** Used for its anticholinergic effects to prevent or treat bradyarrhythmias
    + Antisialogogue effect is delayed, limiting its use in RSI
    + Interferes with pupillary response of the neurologic examination after paralysis
  + Defasciculating agent: "Defasciculating" and "Priming" doses are no longer recommended

TABLE 89.2

Length (cm)-based pediatric equipment chart

	Pink[a]	Red	Purple	Yellow	White	Blue	Orange	Green
Weight (kg)	6–7	8–9	10–11	12–14	15–18	19–23	23–31	31–41
Length (cm)	60.75–67.75	67.75–75.25	75.25–85	85–98.25	98.25–110.75	110.75–122.5	122.5–137.5	137.5–155
ETT size (mm)	3.5	3.5	4.0	4.5	5.0	5.5	6.0 cuff	6.5 cuff
Lip-to-tip length (mm)	10–10.5	10.5–11	11–12	12.5–13.5	14–15	15.5–16.5	17–18	18.5–19.5
Laryngoscope size+blade	1 straight	1 straight	1 straight	2 straight	2 straight	2 straight or curved	2 straight or curved	3 straight or curved
Suction catheter	8F	8F	8F	8–10F	10F	10F	10F	12F
Stylet	6F	6F	10F	10F	10F	10F	14F	14F
Oral airway (mm)	50	50	60	60	60	70	80	80
Nasopharyngeal airway	14F	14F	18F	20F	22F	24F	26F	30F
Bag/valve device	Infant	Infant	Child	Child	Child	Child	Child/adult	Adult
Oxygen mask	Newborn	Newborn	Pediatric	Pediatric	Pediatric	Pediatric	Adult	Adult
Vascular access	22–24/23–25	22–24/23–25	20–22/23–25	18–22/21–23	18–22/21–23	18–20/21–23	18–20/21–22	16–20/18–21
Catheter/butterfly	Intraosseous	Intraosseous	Intraosseous	Intraosseous	Intraosseous	Intraosseous		
NG tube	5–8F	5–8F	8–10F	10F	10–12F	12–14F	14–18F	18F
Urinary catheter	5–8F	5–8F	8–10F	10F	10–12F	10–12F	12F	12F
Chest tube	10–12F	10–12F	16–20F	20–24F	20–24F	24–32F	24–32F	32–40F
BP cuff	Newborn/infant	Newborn/infant	Infant/child	Child	Child	Child	Child/adult	Adult
LMA[b]	1.5	1.5	2	2	2	2–2.5	2.5	3

Directions for use: (1) measure patient length with centimeter tape or with a Broselow tape; (2) using measured length in centimeters or Broselow tape measurement, access appropriate equipment column; (3) column for ETTs, oral and nasopharyngeal airways, and LMAs; always select one size smaller and one size larger than recommended size.

[a]For infants smaller than the pink zone, but not preterm, use the same equipment as the pink zone.

[b]Based on manufacturer's weight-based guidelines:

Mask size	Patient size (kg)
1	≤5
1.5	5–10
2	10–20
2.5	20–30
3	>30

From Luten RC, Mick NW. Differentiating aspects of the pediatric airway. In: Walls RM, Murphy MF. *Manual of Emergency Airway Management.* 4th ed. Philadelphia, PA: Lippincott Williams & Wilkins; 2012:278.

TABLE 89.3 PHARMACOLOGY FOR RSI

Drug	Dose	Comments
Pretreatment		
Lidocaine	1.5 mg/kg IV	Max dose 100 mg IV Optional for head trauma or elevated ICP
Atropine	0.02 mg/kg IV	Min dose 0.1 mg; Max single dose 0.5 mg child, 1 mg adult Optional in infants >1 y due to disproportionate vagal tone Optional in children <5 y receiving SCh or older children receiving multiple doses of SCh
Induction		
Etomidate	0.3 mg/kg IV	Onset 30–40 sec; Duration 5–8 min Not recommended in septic shock due to transient adrenal suppression No analgesic effect
Ketamine	1–2 mg/kg IV 3–7 mg/kg IM	Onset 30–60 sec IV, 3–4 min IM; Duration 5–10 min IV, 10–25 min IM Provides significant analgesia and amnesia Indicated for RSI with bronchospasm due to bronchodilatory effects Indicated for RSI with septic shock
Propofol	2–3 mg/kg IV	Onset 30–60 sec; Duration 10–15 min Avoid in patients with significant egg/soy allergies No analgesic effect
Midazolam	0.3 mg/kg IV 0.1 mg/kg IV if hypotensive	Max dose 10 mg, administered in 2 mg boluses q2–3 min PRN Onset 2–3 min; Duration 20–40 min No analgesic effect
Paralysis		
Succinylcholine (SCh)	2 mg/kg IV (Infants/children) 1–1.5 mg/kg IV (older children) 3–5 mg/kg IM	Onset 30–40 sec; Duration 3–10 min IV, 10–30 min IM Contraindications: Chronic myopathy; neuromuscular disease; 48–72 h after burn, crush injury, or denervating event; prior malignant hypertension; preexisting hyperkalemia Relative contraindications: Elevated ICP, elevated IOP
Rocuronium	1 mg/kg IV	Onset 30–60 sec; Duration 30–60 min
Vecuronium	0.15–0.2 mg/kg IV	Onset 30–90 sec; Duration 25–120 min Use with caution in difficult airway due to long duration of action

ICP, intracranial pressure; IOP, intraocular pressure; RSI, rapid sequence intubation.

◘ **Protection and Positioning**
+ Perform gentle neck extension to achieve sniffing position and to best align oral, pharyngeal, and laryngeal axes
    + Infants often require a towel behind their shoulders to elevate their torso
    + Children/adolescents often require a towel under their head
+ Maintain C-spine immobilization when concerned about a cervical spine injury

◘ **Paralysis and Induction**
+ Induction agents
    + **Etomidate:** No significant hemodynamic effects and possible neuroprotective effects
    + **Ketamine:** Catecholamine release augments heart rate and blood pressure
        ▪ Previously contraindicated in head trauma due to potential further rise in ICP; however, recent evidence may suggest a neuroprotective effect
        ▪ Anticholinergic premedication (i.e., atropine) is not routinely recommended to counteract the sialogogue effect of ketamine

- + **Propofol:** Usefulness is limited due to hypotension
- + **Midazolam:** May cause respiratory depression and hemodynamic compromise at doses needed for induction of respiratory depression
- + **Thiopental:** Discontinued in US and Canada since 2011
  - – Usefulness limited by effect of hypotension
- ✦ Paralytic agents: Confirm paralysis with absence of spontaneous movements, respiratory effort, blink reflex, and by presence of jaw relaxation
  - + Succinylcholine: May cause elevations in ICP/intraocular pressure (IOP) and/or bradycardia
  - + Rocuronium: Significantly improved intubation conditions at high-dose 1 mg/kg compared to previous ranges, but with prolonged paralysis
  - + Vecuronium: High dose is used for more rapid onset, but with unpredictable duration of paralysis

🔲 **Placement of Tube and Proof of Placement**
- ✦ Blade insertion **(FIGURE 89.2)**
  - + Holding laryngoscope handle in left hand, insert the blade into right side of the mouth
  - + Once the tip of the blade is at the base of the tongue, sweep the tongue to the left side of the mouth with the blade
  - + Using a straight blade, the tip of the blade should lift the epiglottis
  - + Using a curved blade, insert the tip into the vallecula then pull upward in the direction of the long axis of the laryngoscope handle
  - + Use suction as needed to clear the airway
- ✦ Routine cricoid pressure (i.e., Sellick maneuver) is no longer recommended
  - + BURP (Backwards Upwards Rightwards Pressure) of the tracheal cartilage is an optional maneuver to assist with visualization of the glottic opening

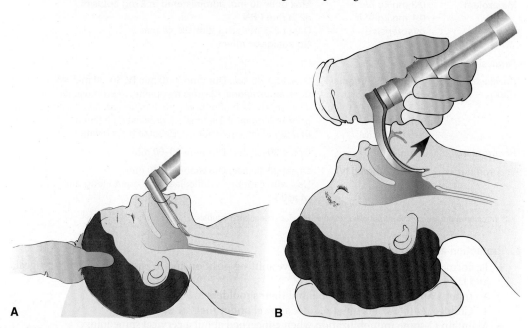

A   **B**

FIGURE 89.2 **A:** Direct laryngoscopy using a straight blade. The tip of the blade is used to directly retract the epiglottis, revealing the vocal cords and glottic opening. (From King C, Stayer SA. Emergent endotracheal intubation. In: King C, Henretig FM, eds. *Textbook of Pediatric Emergency Procedures.* Philadelphia, PA: Williams & Wilkins; 2008:169.) **B:** Direct laryngoscopy using a curved blade. The blade is inserted under direct vision until the tip is positioned in the vallecula. Pulling upward on the laryngoscope handle at 45-degree angle retracts the tongue and at the same time elevates the epiglottis, revealing the vocal cords and glottis. (From King C, Stayer SA. Emergent endotracheal intubation. In: King C, Henretig FM, eds. *Textbook of Pediatric Emergency Procedures.* Philadelphia, PA: Williams & Wilkins; 2008:170.)

- ✛ ETT insertion
  - ✛ Maintain vocal cord visualization at all times and insert the tube through the glottic opening
  - ✛ The black glottic marker should be at the level of the vocal cords
  - ✛ Remove the laryngoscope blade from the mouth and stylet from the tube
  - ✛ Adjust tube depth with calculated number at the level of the lip
  - ✛ Maintain control of the ETT with your hand until properly secured
- ✛ Proof of tube placement
  - ✛ Look for symmetric chest rise and condensation of the tube
  - ✛ Listen for bilateral breath sounds over the lungs apices and axillae, and absence of breath sounds over the stomach
  - ✛ Use end-tidal CO_2 calorimeter (yellow color change indicates proper placement) and continuous capnography monitoring
- ✛ Secure the ETT to the face with tape
- ☐ **Postintubation Management**
  - ✛ Place a nasogastric (NG) or orogastric (OG) tube to decompress the stomach
  - ✛ Obtain a postintubation chest x-ray to assess tube placement
  - ✛ Administer sedation to keep patient comfortable

COMPLICATIONS

- ☐ Incorrect tube placement (e.g., esophageal or mainstem bronchus intubation)
- ☐ Aspiration
- ☐ Broken teeth, bleeding, edema secondary to instrumentation
- ☐ Pneumothorax and pneumomediastinum
- ☐ Cardiac dysrhythmia
- ☐ Adverse effects of pharmacotherapy

SAFETY/QUALITY TIPS

- ☐ **Procedural**
  - ✛ Providers accustomed to intubating adults will generally not encounter difficulty intubating children; the glottis is usually easier to visualize. However, be aware of the important anatomic/physiologic differences: Aligning ear to sternal notch may require chest elevation rather than head elevation and the floppier epiglottis may be easier to control with a straight blade. Perhaps most importantly, when apneic, children desaturate more quickly than adults—have a ventilation plan in mind.
  - ✛ Some centers avoid using succinylcholine in children for concern of undiagnosed muscular dystrophies, which can cause dangerous hyperkalemia if exposed to a depolarizing paralytic
  - ✛ Children's tongues are relatively larger than those of adults. Oral airways are very helpful in overcoming airway obstruction.
  - ✛ If a child could not tolerate a nonrebreather mask, consider blow-by oxygen, high-flow nasal cannula, face tent, or oxygen hood depending on the level of support required
  - ✛ Many pediatric BVM have pop-off valves at size-specific pressures to avoid barotrauma. The valve may need to be closed to deliver sufficient peak pressures in patients with lung disease.
  - ✛ Avoid using the laryngoscope as a lever, which can cause trauma to dentition and gingiva
  - ✛ During passage of the ETT, insert the tube from the right corner of the mouth to avoid obscuring the view of the vocal cords as the tube approaches the glottis
  - ✛ Do not neglect NG or OG tube placement after intubation; BVM ventilation may cause substantial gastric insufflation, which impairs ventilation
  - ✛ Invasive and noninvasive ventilator settings are weight-based
  - ✛ Do not delay bag mask or LMA ventilation after a failed airway attempt. Change patient position, equipment, or provider prior to the next airway attempt.

+ In children who cannot be intubated or ventilated, cricothyrotomy is theoretically contraindicated below the age of eight. In these cases, the recommended approach is cannulation of the trachea with a needle and then a catheter, which can be used for oxygenation.

Cognitive

+ Do not rely on memory or formulas; these will fail under pressure. Use a reference or a Broselow tape to determine proper equipment size—the best technique cannot overcome incorrectly sized equipment.
+ Consider alternatives to RSI when appropriate (cardiac or respiratory arrest, concerning difficult airway features or airway lesions like epiglottitis)
+ Infants are obligate nose breathers until at least 2 to 3 months of age
+ Crying dramatically increases a child's work of breathing due to dynamic obstruction. Keep a conscious child with an airway lesion (e.g., croup) in a position of comfort with the family for as long as feasible.
+ Even in severe upper airway obstruction, the positive pressure of BMV may stent open the malleable trachea while preparing for definitive airway management

Acknowledgment

Thank-you to prior authors Joshua S. Easter and Kevin M. Ban.

Suggested Readings

King C, Rappaport LD. Emergent endotracheal intubation. In: King C, Henretig FM, eds. *Textbook of Pediatric Emergency Procedures*. 2nd ed. Philadelphia, PA: Lippincott Williams & Wilkins; 2008:147–190.

Walls RM, Murphy MF, eds. *Manual of Emergency Airway Management*. 4th ed. Philadelphia, PA: Lippincott Williams & Wilkins; 2012:276–314.

Yamamoto LG. Emergency airway management-rapid sequence intubation. In: Fleisher GR, Ludwig S. *Textbook of Pediatric Emergency Medicine*. 6th ed. Philadelphia, PA: Lippincott Williams & Wilkins; 2010:74–84.

90

Sedation and Analgesia for the Pediatric Patient

Michelle N. Vazquez

INDICATIONS

- ⊡ To provide anxiolysis, analgesia, sedation, and motor control during unpleasant diagnostic or therapeutic procedures. Decisions regarding appropriate sedation practices depend on:
  - ✚ Type of procedure or treatment
  - ✚ Age and medical condition of the patient
  - ✚ Skill and experience of practitioner
  - ✚ Available staff
  - ✚ Policies and procedures of the institution

CONTRAINDICATIONS

- ⊡ No absolute contraindications to analgesia other than significant allergies
  - ✚ Pain control is an essential component of good emergency care
  - ✚ Choice of agent depends on level of pain, speed of action, medical condition, and age of patient
- ⊡ **Relative Contraindications**
  - ✚ Presence of acute or chronic conditions which make the patient American Society of Anesthesiologists (ASA) class III or higher (anesthesiology should be involved in the care of these patients; general anesthesia in the operating room [OR] may be indicated)
  - ✚ Inadequate personnel available
    - ✚ Except for mild anxiolysis (oral benzodiazepines) or analgesia without sedation, person administering sedation cannot be the same person performing the procedure
    - ✚ The Centers for Medicare and Medicaid Services (CMS) recommends two physicians (one to manage sedation, one to perform procedure) and a nurse be present for the duration of the sedation. The American College of Emergency Physicians (ACEP) Clinical Policy on Procedural Sedation and Analgesia in the Emergency Department recommends one physician (performing the procedure) and one nurse be present for the sedation.

RISK/CONSENT ISSUES

- ⊡ Inadvertent deep sedation or general anesthesia
- ⊡ Hypoxia/hypoventilation
- ⊡ Nausea and vomiting
- ⊡ Medication reactions
  - ✚ Fentanyl: Respiratory depression, rigid chest (more likely with rapid delivery)
  - ✚ Morphine: Histamine release *and hypotension*
  - ✚ Benzodiazepines, barbiturates: Paradoxical reaction of restlessness or agitation
  - ✚ Ketamine: Laryngospasm, emergence reactions, *and hypertension*
  - ✚ Propofol: Hypotension

CLASSIFICATION

- ⊡ Often, moderate sedation is the goal for emergency department procedural sedation; however, the depth of sedation should be determined by the procedure being performed and the patient characteristics. One must be aware of the possibility of the patient passing into a state of deep sedation and be able to manage this occurrence. Advanced airway management skills are required for anyone performing procedural sedation.
  - ✚ **Minimal/mild sedation:** Impaired cognitive function and coordination but unaffected ventilatory and cardiovascular functions; able to respond to verbal commands

+ **Moderate sedation:** Blunted anxiety/pain responses but intact airway reflex; normal cardiovascular function; patient should respond to verbal commands (possibly with addition of light tactile stimulation).
+ **Dissociative sedation:** Profound analgesia and amnesia with retention of airway reflexes, spontaneous respirations, and cardiovascular function
  + State induced by ketamine
+ **Deep sedation:** Difficult to arouse; can respond purposefully to repeated or painful stimulation; partial or complete loss of airway reflexes is possible; cardiovascular function usually intact

PRESEDATION CONSIDERATIONS

All patients should have a presedation assessment, which includes the following:

☐ Consider type and severity of underlying medical conditions; consult anesthesiology for patients of ASA class III and higher **(TABLE 90.1)**

☐ Consider current medications and allergies especially regarding previous adverse experiences with analgesia/anesthesia

☐ Inspect airway for abnormalities or limited neck mobility that may impair rescue airway intervention (short neck, obesity, large tonsils/tongue, small mandible)

☐ Determine time and nature of last meal: Fasting recommendations for elective procedures are 2 to 3 hours for liquids and 4 to 8 hours for solids; in an emergency situation, these guidelines are often not realistic; document the time of last intake and the need for emergent treatment.

☐ Perform a general physical examination, concentrating on cardiac and lung auscultation, presence of active upper respiratory infection (URI) or asthma exacerbation, and baseline neurologic state

☐ Assemble all equipment you may need for sedation and potential complications:
  + Suction
  + Oxygen delivery system (face mask or nasal cannula of appropriate size)
  + Airway equipment
  + Monitors (pulse oximeter, electrocardiography, blood pressure, capnography)
  + Medications, including reversal agents

☐ **General Basic Steps**
  + **Presedation evaluation**
  + **Choosing appropriate agent**
  + **Induction of sedation**
  + **Monitoring**
  + **Recovery**

TABLE 90.1 AMERICAN SOCIETY OF ANESTHESIOLOGISTS PHYSICAL STATUS CLASSIFICATION

ASA class	Examples
I: Healthy patient	Unremarkable past medical history
II: Mild systemic disease—no functional limitation	Mild asthma without active wheezing, well-controlled diabetes, VSD without failure
III: Severe systemic disease with functional limitation	Active wheezing, poorly controlled diabetes or seizure disorder, history of CHF
IV: Severe systemic disease that is a constant threat to life	Advanced degree of cardiac, pulmonary, renal, or endocrine insufficiency
V: Moribund patient who is not expected to survive without procedure	Septic shock, severe trauma

ASA, American Society of Anesthesiologists; CHF, congestive heart failure; VSD, ventricular septal defect.

TECHNIQUE

- Choice of agent depends on the following:
  + Age of patient
  + Goal of your intervention **(TABLE 90.2)**
  + Type of procedure **(TABLE 90.3)**
  + Duration of procedure
- Titrate dose to desired effect or to predetermined maximum **(TABLE 90.4)**
- Continue monitoring through recovery period
- See **TABLE 90.5** for information on selected agents

TABLE 90.2 GOAL OF INTERVENTION

Goal	Recommended medication or intervention
Motion control	Sedative or dissociative
Anxiolysis	Guided imagery/distraction, nitrous, sedative or dissociative
Sedation	Sedative or dissociative
Analgesia alone	Acetaminophen, ibuprofen, opioid
Amnesia	Opioids, dissociative, sedative

TABLE 90.3 TYPE OF PROCEDURE

Type of procedure	Specific examples	Recommended medication or intervention
Nonpainful	Diagnostic imaging	Pentobarbital (PO, PR, IM, IV)
		Midazolam (PO, PR, IV)
		Propofol (IV)
		Etomidate (IV)
Minimally painful	Minor trauma	Nitrous oxide
	Instrumentation	Topical/local anesthesia (LET/EMLA)
	Peripheral access	Midazolam (PO, PR, IV)
		Sucrose (PO—infants only)
Painful	Fracture reduction	Ketamine (IM, IV)
	Central access	Fentanyl + midazolam (IV)
		Propofol ± fentanyl (IV)
		Regional anesthesia/hematoma block

EMLA, eutectic mixture of local anesthetic; LET, lidocaine epinephrine tetracaine.

TABLE 90.4 DOSES OF SELECTED ANALGESICS

Medication	Dose	Comments
Sucrose	0.5–1 mL PO, then dip pacifier in solution	Newborn to 3–6 months
Acetaminophen (PO, PR)	10–15 mg/kg	
Ibuprofen (PO)	5–10 mg/kg	Do not use if <6 months of age
Ketorolac	0.5–1 mg/kg, (maximum 30 mg)	
Morphine	0.1 mg/kg/dose; repeat q5–10 min until desired effect	Monitor respiratory status

TABLE 90.5 LIST OF SELECTED AGENTS

Sedative hypnotic	Dose	Onset	Duration	Comments
Midazolam	IV: Initially 0.1 mg/kg; titrate to maximum 0.5 mg/kg	2–3 min	20–60 min	1.5–5 times stronger than diazepam Dose in small increments Wait 2 min in between doses
	IM: 0.1–0.15 mg/kg	10–20 min	60–120 min	
	PO: 0.5–1 mg/kg; maximum 20 mg	15–30 min	60–90 min	Use IV formulation added to flavored syrup
	IN, PR: 0.3 mg/kg	IN: 60 min PR: 10–30 min	IN: 60 min PR: 60–90 min	Intranasal route is uncomfortable
Pentobarbital	IV: 1–6 mg/kg, adjust increments of 2 mg/kg	1 min		
	IM: 2–6 mg/kg to a maximum of 100 mg			
	PO or PR age <4 y: 6 mg/kg to maximum: 100 mg	10–15 min	60–120 min	
	PO or PR age >4 y: 3 mg/kg to maximum: 100 mg	15–60 min	60–240 min	
Etomidate	IV: 0.1–0.3 mg/kg/dose	30–60 sec	3–5 min	May cause emesis, myoclonus
Methohexital	PR: 25 mg/kg; maximum 500 mg	10–15 min	60 min	
Thiopental	PR: 10–25 mg/kg	10–15 min	60–120 min	
Analgesic	**Dose**	**Onset**	**Duration**	**Comments**
Fentanyl	IV: 1 µg/kg/dose; may repeat every 2–3 min; titrate to desired effect	2–3 min	30–60 min	Exhibits little hypnosis Rare histamine release May cause respiratory depression May cause chest wall rigidity (more likely with higher doses, rapid rate)
Dissociative agent	**Dose**	**Onset**	**Duration**	**Comments**
Ketamine	IV: 1–2 mg/kg; repeat dose 0.5 mg/kg; maximum 500 mg or 5 mg/kg, whichever is less	1–5 min	10–150 min	Administer IV: over 1–2 min. Note: Prior to ketamine, may give atropine 0.01 mg/kg or glycopyrrolate, 0.005 mg/kg
	IM: 4 mg/kg of ketamine mixed with atropine in the same syringe	5–15 min		May cause hallucinations up to 48 hr Patients may not perform skilled or hazardous tasks for 48 hr

TABLE 90.5   LIST OF SELECTED AGENTS *(continued)*

Sedative hypnotic	Dose	Onset	Duration	Comments
				Contraindicated in patients with URI with significant nasal discharge or for procedures which stimulate posterior pharynx May cause increased intracranial or intraocular pressure

Inhalation agent	Dose	Onset	Duration	Comments
Nitrous oxide	30%–70% concentration; continuous flow or demand valve	<5 min	<5 min after discontinuation	Up to 80% nonresponders Do not use in combination with other drugs

Reversal agents	Dose	Onset	Duration	Comments
Naloxone	IV, IM, SQ: 0.1 mg/kg to maximum of 2 mg; may repeat every 2 min	IV: 2 min IM, SQ: 10–15 min	IV: 20–40 min IM, SQ: 60–90 min	*Do not* use routinely May cause hypertension and pulmonary edema Use cautiously in opiate dependence
Flumazenil	IV: 0.01–0.03 mg/kg; maximum 0.2 mg	1–2 min	30–60 min	Contraindicated in patients on benzodiazepine for seizures Administer IV over 15 sec

URI, upper respiratory infection.

SAFETY/QUALITY TIPS

⬚ **Procedural**

+ Prepare for Procedural Sedation and Analgesia (PSA) using a full intubation setup, so that you are able to manage all airway and breathing insults that may occur during PSA
+ Assiduously monitor the patient for hypoventilation. If hypoventilation occurs, respond to it using a stepwise approach that starts with discontinuing the PSA agents, repositioning the patient, and performing a jaw thrust. Bag-mask (or laryngeal mask airway [LMA]) ventilation should generally be performed after these less risky maneuvers have failed to restore ventilation.
+ If bag-mask ventilation is required, bag very slowly and gently, using two hands on the mask (an assistant compresses the bag)
+ If a reversal agent is given, the patient must be monitored well beyond the duration of action of the PSA agent, noting that the duration of the reversal agent may be shorter than the PSA agent
+ Chloral hydrate and the "lytic cocktail" or "DPT" (combination of meperidine, promethazine, and chlorpromazine) are no longer recommended due to unpredictable depth of sedation, long duration of action, and associated adverse events
+ The highest risk time of the procedural sedation is often after the procedure is completed, the painful stimuli end, and the providers walk away. Generally, an airway-capable provider should remain at bedside until the patient responds to a verbal stimulus.

Cognitive

+ The notion that neonates/infants cannot feel or remember pain is inaccurate. If you are uncomfortable providing PSA to a very small child, consider referring to anesthesiology.
+ Use of the age-appropriate nonpharmacologic techniques such as dimmed lighting, stereo headphones, movies, video games, toys, storytelling, guided imagery, and singing can decrease the dose of medication needed, or eliminate it entirely
+ Encourage the parents to calm the child as they greatly reduce the child's stress
+ Warn the parents about the nystagmus and trancelike cataleptic state resulting from ketamine
+ Be prepared for the possibility of disinhibitory effects of benzodiazepines and postprocedure nausea and vomiting

Acknowledgment

Thank-you to prior authors Veda Maany, Oscar Rago, and Angela M. Tangredi.

Suggested Readings

Asadi P, Ghafouri HB, Yasinzadeh M, et al. Ketamine and atropine for pediatric sedation: a prospective double-blind randomized controlled trial. *Pediatr Emerg Care*. 2013;29(2):136–139.

Chong JH, Chew SP, Ang AS. Is prophylactic atropine necessary during ketamine sedation in children? *J Pediatr Child Health*. 2013;49(4):309–312.

Filho EM, de Carvalho WB. Dealing with ketamine sedation adverse events: are co-administered anticholinergics necessary? *Pediatr Emerg Care*. 2013;29(8):955–956.

Kye YC, Rhee JE, Kim K, et al. Clinical effects of adjunctive atropine during ketamine sedation in pediatric emergency patients. *Am J Emerg Med*. 2012;30(9):1981–1985.

Lee JH, Jung HK, Lee GG, et al. Effect of behavioral intervention using smartphone application for preoperative anxiety in pediatric patients. *Korean J Anesthesiol*. 2013;65(6):508–518.

Pacheco GS, Ferayorni A. Pediatric procedural sedation and analgesia. *Emerg Med Clin North Am*. 2013;31(3):831–852.

91

Umbilical Vein Catheterization

Jennifer E. Sanders

INDICATIONS

- To provide rapid vascular access in neonates up to 2 weeks of age for resuscitation in which all other access attempts have failed
- To provide rapid administration of intravenous fluids, medications, and blood

CONTRAINDICATIONS

- None for the unstable newborn with respiratory failure or cardiovascular compromise
- **Relative Contraindications**
  + Successful peripheral or central venous access
  + Umbilical vein catheter (UVC) placement in newborns with omphalocele, gastroschisis, omphalitis, peritonitis, or necrotizing enterocolitis
  + Cellulitis or impetigo of the abdominal skin

LANDMARKS

- The umbilicus consists of one large, thin-walled vein and two smaller, thick-walled arteries
- Picture the vessels as a face in which the arteries form the eyes, and the vein forms the mouth (FIGURE 91.1)

EQUIPMENT

- Personal protective equipment (face mask, eye protection, gown, sterile gloves)
- Cardiac monitor with pulse oximetry
- Antiseptic prep solution, sterile drapes, gauze pads, antibiotic ointment
- External heat source (i.e., radiant warmer or heat lamps)
- Umbilical catheter tray (if not available, then equipment listed below)
  + Scalpel (No. 11 or 15)
  + Small hemostat
  + Needle holder
  + Umbilical tape or silk suture (3-0 or 4-0) on straight or curved needle
  + Size 5-French umbilical catheter
- A 10-mL saline-filled syringe
- Three-way stopcock
- Bag of saline solution
- Adhesive tape

- **General Basic Steps**
  + **Prepare catheter**
  + **Tie umbilicus**
  + **Cut cord**
  + **Identify vessels**
  + **Pass catheter**
  + **Confirm placement**
  + **Secure catheter**

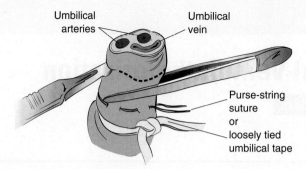

FIGURE 91.1 Introduction of the umbilical vein catheter. (From Lipton JD, Schafermeyer RW. Umbilical vessel catheterization. In: Henretig FM, King C, eds. *Textbook of Pediatric Emergency Procedures*. Philadelphia, PA: Williams & Wilkins; 1997:519, with permission.)

TECHNIQUE

▣ **Preparation**
+ Place newborn in the supine and frog-leg position (Place soft limb restraints only if necessary.)
+ Continuously monitor vital signs and oxygen saturation
+ Use universal precautions
+ Sterilize the umbilicus and entire abdomen with antiseptic solution
+ Drape the area with sterile towels, leaving the prepped umbilicus exposed
+ Consider placement of nasogastric tube (NGT) to prevent aspiration of gastric contents **(FIGURE 91.2)**

▣ **Equipment Preparation**
+ Connect umbilical catheter to one port of three-way stopcock, syringe to second port, and tubing to bag of saline solution to third port
+ Flush catheter with saline solution

▣ **Tie Umbilicus**
+ Using umbilical tape or silk suture, loosely tie a purse string at the base of the umbilicus

▣ **Cut Cord**
+ Cut the umbilical cord transversely with a scalpel 1 to 2 cm from abdominal wall, being careful to cut only cord and not infant skin

▣ **Identify Vessels**
+ Expose the umbilical vessels by attaching two clamps/hemostats to the stump, thereby everting the edges
+ Identify the larger, thin-walled vein and dilate its lumen with forceps
+ Remove any visible clot with forceps

▣ **Pass Catheter**
+ Holding the umbilical catheter near its distal end, advance the catheter tip until blood returns freely
+ If the goal is to perform central venous pressure monitoring, pass the catheter approximately two-thirds the length of the shoulder to umbilicus distance

▣ **Confirm Placement**
+ Blood return confirms placement for a low lying catheter
+ Radiograph of the thorax and abdomen is required to confirm placement of a central venous umbilical catheter

▣ **Secure Catheter**
+ Tightening the purse-string suture or the umbilical tape
+ Tape or suture the catheter in place

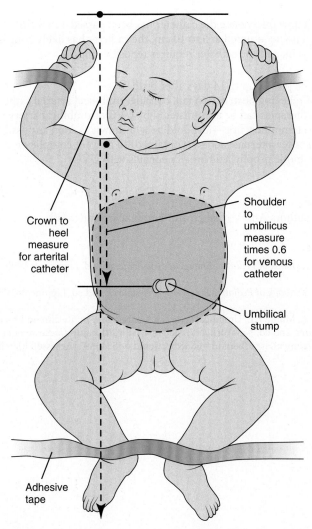

FIGURE 91.2 Positioning of infant, measurement of for central venous catheter. The red area represents the area that should be sterilized prior to catheter insertion. (From King C, Henretig FM. *Textbook of Pediatric Emergency Procedures*. 2nd ed. Lippincott Williams & Wilkins; 2008:483–491.)

COMPLICATIONS

- Infection
- Thrombosis or embolism
- Perforation
- Portal vein thrombosis
- Hemorrhage

SAFETY/QUALITY TIPS

- **Procedural**
  - If the catheter does not pass freely during the first few centimeters of catheter advancement, consider loosening the purse string/umbilical tape
  - If the catheter still does not advance, apply gentle continuous pressure, and put caudal or cephalad traction on the cord, while performing a gentle twisting motion

+ Blood should flow freely once the catheter has been passed 4 to 5 cm
+ If obstruction is encountered at 5 to 10 cm, the catheter has likely gone into a branch of the portal vein, and the catheter requires repositioning

⊡ **Cognitive**

+ A UVC may be placed up to 14 days after birth
+ If attempts at relieving obstruction fail, consider umbilical arterial catheterization as an alternative—therapies can be administered by UVC or umbilical artery catheter
+ The UVC is a temporary line—it should be withdrawn as soon as possible after resuscitation (after alternate access is obtained) to prevent complications
+ Consider antibiotic prophylaxis for all neonates with UVCs

⊡ **Acknowledgment**

Thank-you to prior authors Ann Vorhaben and Ramona S. Sunderwith.

Suggested Readings

Fleisher G, Ludwig S. *Textbook of Pediatric Emergency Medicine*. 6th ed. Lippincott Williams & Wilkins; 2010:1759.

King C, Henretig FM. *Textbook of Pediatric Emergency Procedures*. 2nd ed. Lippincott Williams & Wilkins; 2008:483–491.

Reichman EF, Noland A, Muniz AE. Umbilical vessel catheterization. In: Reichman EF. ed. *Emergency Medicine Procedures*. 2nd ed. New York, NY: McGraw-Hill; 2013. http://accessemergencymedicine.mhmedical.com/content.aspx?bookid=683&Sectionid=45343695. Accessed March 08, 2014.

92

Reduction of Nursemaid's Elbow (Radial Head Subluxation)

Kimberly Kahne

DEFINITION

- Radial head subluxation is frequently referred to as "nursemaid's elbow"
- The annular ligament of the radius displaces into the radiocapitellar articulation (FIGURE 92.1A)
- A common injury in children between the ages of 2 and 5 years, after which the annular ligament strengthens and the injury becomes uncommon

INDICATIONS

- Clinical suspicion of a nursemaid's elbow based on:
  + Refusal to use affected arm
  + Typical posture: Affected arm adducted or held at the side, with the elbow slightly flexed and forearm pronated. The child is usually in no distress unless the arm is moved.
  + Suggestive mechanism of injury

CONTRAINDICATIONS

- Gross deformity, swelling, or significant point tenderness suggesting fracture

- **General Basic Steps**
  + **Analgesia (if indicated)**
  + **Patient preparation**
  + **Reduction**
  + **Reevaluation**

TECHNIQUE

- **Patient Preparation**
  + Caretaker/parent holds child in her/his lap, restraining the unaffected arm
- **Hyperpronation Method** (FIGURE 92.1B)
  + With one hand, encircle the elbow with the thumb over the region of the radial head, keeping the elbow flexed at 90 degrees
  + With the other hand, grasp the wrist, and firmly pronate at the wrist
- **Supination/Flexion Method** (FIGURE 92.1C and D)
  + With one hand, encircle the elbow with the thumb over the region of the radial head, keeping the elbow position in some flexion
  + With the other hand, grasp the wrist and apply gentle traction before supination
  + In one motion, supinate the forearm fully and flex the elbow to the ipsilateral shoulder
- **Postprocedure**
  + Reevaluate child in 10 to 15 minutes to note use of arm. The child will generally regain use of the arm quickly.
  + If the child has not regained use of the arm within 10 to 15 minutes of attempted reduction and no click was detected during procedure, the procedure should be repeated
  + Radiography should be performed if the child has not regained use of arm after a reasonable time and no click was detected

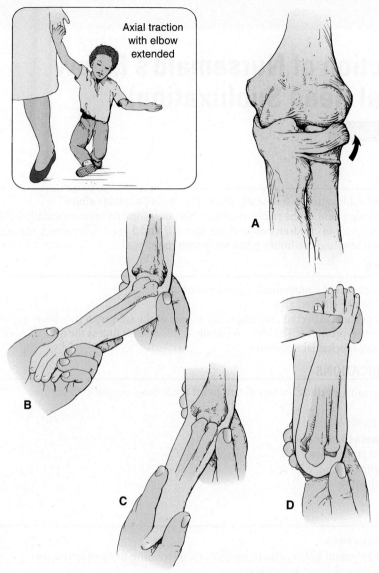

Figure 92.1 A–D: Nursemaid's elbow. (From Cimpello LB, Deutsch RJ, Dixon C, et al. Illustrated techniques of pediatric emergency procedures. In: Fleisher GR, Ludwig S. *Textbook of Pediatric Emergency Medicine.* 6th ed. Philadelphia, PA: Lippincott Williams & Wilkins; 2010:1832.)

COMPLICATIONS

✚ Pain
✚ Unsuccessful reduction
✚ Vascular or musculoskeletal damage can occur if performed on a child with a fracture

SAFETY/QUALITY TIPS

⊡ Procedural

+ Reduction is generally performed without premedication. If subluxation has been present for hours, oral anxiolysis can be used to overcome the child's anxiety.
+ Explain to caretaker that reduction causes transient discomfort
+ A palpable click signifies reduction but may not always be present
+ The hyperpronation technique has been shown to be at least as successful as the supination/flexion technique, and is less painful. A good approach is to start with hyperpronation, if unsuccessful, attempt supination/flexion.
+ If successful, patients do not require any studies or immobilization

⊡ Cognitive

+ The most important error is to attempt a nursemaid's reduction on a fractured arm. Children with radial head subluxation have minimal pain if undisturbed, and are nontender. If concerned, image before attempting reduction.
+ Fractured clavicle can present similarly
+ If reduction has been achieved clinically and maintained, analgesics and follow-up visits are unnecessary
+ Caution parents of the risk of repeat subluxation, try to avoid the precipitating mechanism of tugging on the arms

⊡ Acknowledgment

Thank-you to prior authors Adrian Martinez and Emilola Ogunbameru.

Suggested Readings

Fleisher GR, Ludwig S. *Textbook of Pediatric Emergency Medicine.* 6th ed. Philadelphia, PA: Lippincott Williams & Wilkins; 2010:1832–1833.

Gunaydi YK, Katirci Y, Duyma H, et al. Comparison of success and pain levels of supination-flexion and hyperpronation maneuvers in childhood nursemaid's elbow cases. *Am J Emerg Med.* 2013;31(7):1078–1081.

King C, Henretig FM. *Textbook of Pediatric Emergency Procedures.* Philadelphia, PA: Lippincott Williams & Wilkins; 2008:964.

Tintinalli JE, Stpczynski JS, Ma OJ, et al. *Tintinalli's Emergency Medicine: A Comprehensive Study Guide.* 7th ed. New York, NY: McGraw-Hill; 2011.

INDEX